CANCER ETIOLOGY, DIAGNOSIS AND TREATMENTS

# LUNG CANCER

# A COMPREHENSIVE OVERVIEW

# CANCER ETIOLOGY, DIAGNOSIS AND TREATMENTS

Additional books in this series can be found on Nova's website
under the Series tab.

Additional e-books in this series can be found on Nova's website
under the e-book tab.

CANCER ETIOLOGY, DIAGNOSIS AND TREATMENTS

# LUNG CANCER

## A COMPREHENSIVE OVERVIEW

KATHY GATELY
EDITOR

New York

For permission to use material from this book please contact us:
Telephone 631-231-7269; Fax 631-231-8175
Web Site: http://www.novapublishers.com



**Library of Congress Cataloging-in-Publication Data**

ISBN: 978-1-62618-447-3

Library of Congress Control Number: 2013935077

*Published by Nova Science Publishers, Inc. † New York*

# Contents

# Preface

Lung cancer is the leading cause of cancer death among both men and women. Each year, more people die of lung cancer than of colon, breast, and prostate cancers combined. Lung tumours are heterogeneous with diverse molecular profiles between patients, making them difficult to treat. We now understand that we must exploit these differences by characterising each patient's distinct molecular signature and design treatment protocols that target specific tumours more effectively with reduced toxicities. Recent advances in both molecular diagnostics and targeted therapeutic agents for cancer patients, have changed the way we manage lung cancer treatment.

Although our understanding of the molecular biology of lung carcinogenesis and the mechanisms involved in acquired resistance to treatment is constantly evolving we still have much to learn in order to significantly reduce the burden caused by this devastating disease. Therefore, I am delighted to present here a comprehensive overview of lung cancer in the 21$^{st}$ century. This book was written by international experts in the field of lung cancer and we are grateful to them for their thorough review and detailed analysis provided in each chapter.

This book provides a valuable resource for anyone who wants up-to-date information on the pathology, epidemiology, biology and treatment options for lung cancer. I anticipate that the material in this textbook which applies to clinical practice will provide an excellent reference guide for medical students, graduate students, epidemiologists, oncologists, pathologists and researchers. We hope that an increased understanding of the complexities of this disease will ultimately provide patients with improved treatment options and a better prognosis.

**Kathy Gately BSc; PhD**
Institute of Molecular Medicine
Trinity College Dublin
St. James's Hospital
Dublin, Ireland

In: Lung Cancer: A Comprehensive Overview
Editor: Kathy Gately
ISBN: 978-1-62618-447-3


*Chapter I*

# The Pathology of Lung Cancer

***Niamh Leonard***
Consultant Histopathologist, St James's Hospital, Dublin, Ireland

## Abstract

Lung cancer is the most common cause of cancer-related death. There have been significant recent advances in oncology and molecular pathology which have led to improved response rates and survival times. Both cytological and histopathological specimens are used to make a diagnosis of lung cancer so that the appropriate treatment can be planned.

Most lung cancers are carcinomas. Adenocarcinoma is now the most common type of carcinoma followed by squamous cell carcinoma and small cell carcinoma. Adenocarcinomas are carcinomas which show glandular differentiation. A new classification has been recommended for adenocarcinomas. A major change is that the term bronchioloalveolar is no longer to be used, the terms lepidic pattern, adenocarcinoma in situ and minimally invasive carcinoma are preferred. Squamous cell carcinomas tend to be central tumours, although there has been an increase in peripheral tumours. It used to be sufficient for treatment to make a distinction on biopsy of small cell carcinoma versus non-small cell carcinoma but recent advances in oncology mean that further categorisation of non-small carcinomas into adenocarcinomas and squamous cell carcinomas is very important. There are specific treatments and contraindications for both entities so that the distinction of each on biopsy has, for the first time, been specifically addressed by a classification system. This determines whether molecular screening of the biopsy is required to detect mutations in the epidermal growth factor receptor (EGFR), KRAS genes or anaplastic lymphoma kinase (ALK) gene.

Other lung cancers include small cell carcinoma which has a distinctive appearance on hematoxylin and eosin (HandE) staining as well as large cell carcinomas and the group of neuroendocrine carcinomas. The lung is also a common site for metastases which may occasionally be difficult to distinguish from primary lung tumours.

The staging of lung cancer is important and cases should be discussed at multidisciplinary team meetings so that correlation can be made between the clinical, pathological and radiological features.

# Introduction

Lung cancer is the most common cause of cancer-related death with a 5 year survival of 15%. This poor survival rate had changed little for years, however, recent advances in oncology and molecular pathology have led to improvements in patient response and survival times. One result of recent advances is that radical changes have been suggested to the classification of adenocarcinomas, which now represent the largest group of lung cancer.

Lung cancer patients often present with respiratory symptoms such as persistent infection or cough. Alternatively, routine imaging may show up an asymptomatic lesion which is suspicious for malignancy. A tissue diagnosis needs to be made before treatment options can be considered.

Both cytological and histopathological specimens can be used to make a diagnosis of lung cancer and correlation of findings from both techniques produces the most accurate results. Cytological specimens available for analysis include sputum, bronchial brushings, bronchial lavage and endobronchial ultrasound biopsy (EBUS). Sputum cytology was the most common cytology specimen as it is easy to obtain but bronchial brushings and lavage specimens are now more commonly used. At flexible bronchoscopy a brush is applied to the surface of a lesion to sample cells for a bronchial brushing sample or saline can be flushed onto the surface and aspirated for a bronchial lavage specimen. Bronchial lavage is used for tumours just beyond the reach of the bronchoscope. Tumours that lie underneath the bronchial surface or mediastinal lymph nodes can be sampled using EBUS. EBUS sampling of lymph nodes is used to stage patients and is less invasive than an open operation to sample nodes.

Histopathology specimens include bronchial biopsy performed at flexible bronchoscopy. Tumours which are more peripheral and thus harder to reach may require core biopsy performed in radiology or, very infrequently, a wedge resection performed at surgery.

Once a tissue diagnosis has been made, treatment can be considered. Patients with more advanced disease may not be suitable for surgery so that radiotherapy and/or chemotherapy will be considered. Patients with earlier stage disease will be offered surgery and the resected tumour will be analysed to confirm the diagnosis and stage disease.

# Common Lung Cancers

The vast majority of lung cancers are carcinomas. Squamous cell carcinoma used to be the most common type in the 1980s but the incidence of adenocarcinoma has continued to rise so that it is now the most frequent form in men in the USA with an increasing incidence in women [1]. Small cell carcinomas are less common and account for 14% of all lung cancers [2].

Squamous cell carcinomas were more likely to arise centrally (Figure 1) whereas many adenocarcinomas arose peripherally from lung parenchyma (Figure 2). However, peripheral squamous cell carcinomas became more common than central tumours around 2001. It has been suggested that the introduction of filters in cigarettes in the late '60s and early '70s led to deeper inhalation of carcinogenic fumes and hence the development of peripheral tumours (Nicholson AG, personal communication). Small cell carcinomas behave and are treated very differently from other types of carcinoma so that, for practical purposes, primary lung carcinomas were divided into small cell and non small cell carcinomas. Cases without specific morphologic features of adenocarcinoma or squamous cell carcinoma were diagnosed as 'non-small cell carcinoma, not otherwise specified'. Recent advances in molecular pathology and oncology have meant that further subclassification of non small cell carcinomas is important. Specific chemotherapy is available which is effective for specific types of non-small cell carcinoma but which may have significant adverse side effects in other tumour types. For example, a chemotherapeutic agent called pemetrexed works best on adenocarcinomas rather than squamous cell carcinomas and bevacizumab, an angiogenesis inhibitor, has increased toxicity with squamous cell carcinomas so that distinction of adenocarcinoma from squamous cell carcinoma is extremely important [3].

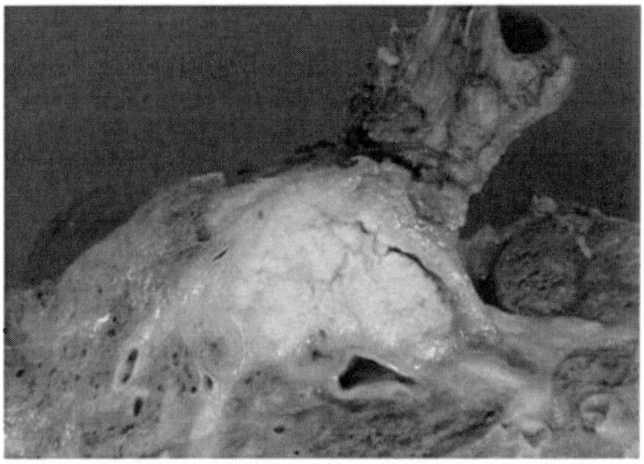

**(A)**

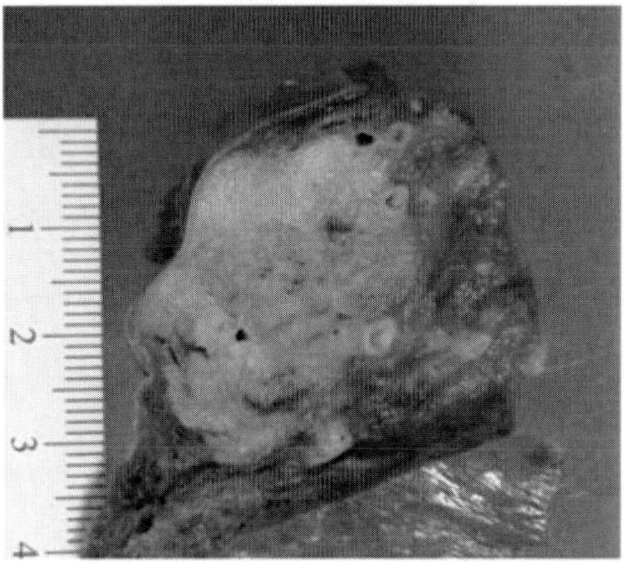


**(B)**

Figure 1. A) Squamous cell carcinoma near hilum of lung. Tumour can be seen growing into the lumen of a main bronchus. B) Adenocarcinoma of lung arising in the periphery and reaching the pleura.

# Adenocarcinoma

Adenocarcinomas are carcinomas which show glandular differentiation and/or mucin production. They are most likely to present as nodules in the periphery of the lung. A significant proportion of adenocarcinomas do not present clinically and are detected as an incidental finding on radiological examination. In contrast to squamous cell carcinoma and small cell carcinoma which show a strong association with cigarette smoking, adenocarcinoma is the most common tumour type seen in non-smokers.

The major morphological types defined in the WHO Classification of Tumours [4] are acinar, papillary, bronchioloalveolar and solid. Most tumours have a mixture of these subtypes and therefore were classified as mixed. The diagnosis of an adenocarcinoma as mixed type did little to distinguish entities with possibly different prognoses and treatment responses. Recent advances in the molecular pathology and oncology of lung adenocarcinoma led to a new classification which was sponsored by the International Association for the Study of Lung Cancer, the American Thoracic Society and the European Respiratory Society and published in February 2011 [5].

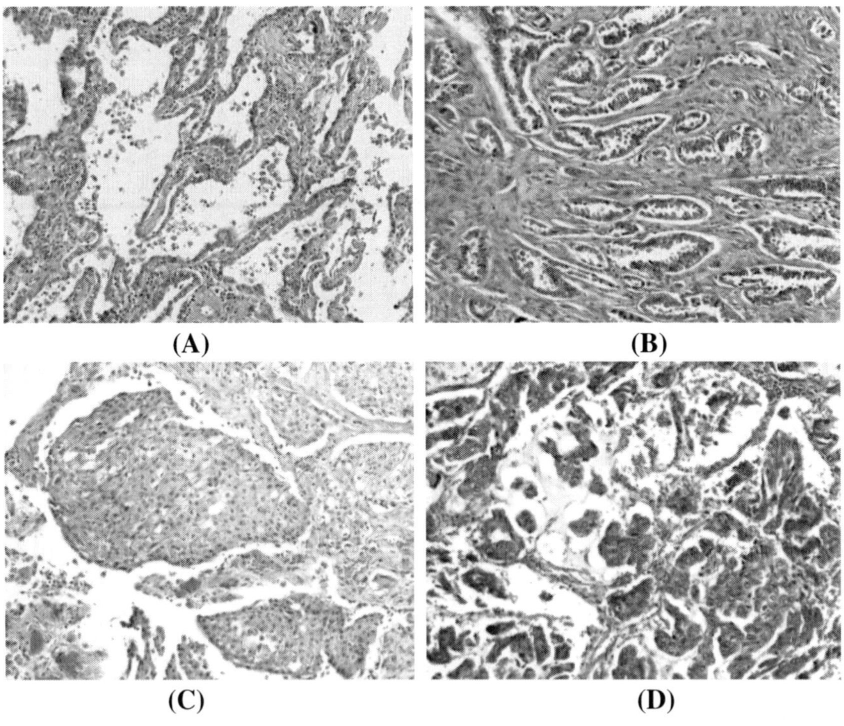


Figure 2. A) Adenocarcinoma, lepidic type. Tumour cells grow along alveolar walls but do not invade the stroma. B) Adenocarcinoma, acinar type. The tumour forms well defined acini with surrounding desmoplastic stroma. C) Adenocarcinoma, solid type. The tumour forms solid groups of cells with poorly defined glandular spaces. Immunohistochemistry is often required to confirm that this tumour type is an adenocarcinoma. D) Adenocarcinoma, micropapillary type. The tumour forms papillae which lack a fibrovascular core and are termed micropapillary rather than papillary (which have a fibrovascular core).

The new classification defines major histological types of adenocarcinoma as lepidic pattern, acinar, papillary, micropapillary and solid (Figure 2a-2d). Tumours with a lepidic pattern belong to a favourable prognosis group, the moderate prognosis group includes papillary and acinar patterns and poor prognosis is associated with solid and micropapillary patterns [6].

The term bronchioloalveolar carcinoma has been in use for a long time. However, it was felt to be a poorly defined entity which could include good prognosis tumours with a purely in situ component and also advanced tumours with invasion. The terms adenocarcinoma in situ and minimally invasive carcinoma are now recommended instead [5]. The use of the term lepidic indicates a tumour with an in situ pattern. This represents a major change to the current classification schemes although it only applies to very early, usually small, lesions which are not especially common.

It has also been recommended that the term mixed be abandoned and that pathologists should report the predominant adenocarcinoma type and list other patterns in 5% increments. For the first time, very specific guidelines have been suggested for use in the reporting of biopsies (see below) [5].

Premalignant lesions have been identified in lung resections for adenocarcinoma and these are called atypical adenomatous hyperplasia (AAH). One study found that 23% of resections for adenocarcinoma had solitary AAH lesions as well [7]. They are asymptomatic but may be detected as ground glass lesions using high resolution CT scanning.

## Squamous Cell Carcinoma

The majority of squamous cell carcinomas occur in smokers and ex-smokers. Most squamous cell carcinomas arose in central parts of the lung, although peripheral tumours have increased in incidence to become more common [8]. The tumours are white or grey and when they become large, may show central cavitation caused by tumour necrosis [4].

Microscopically the tumour cells show keratinisation and/ or intercellular bridges (Figure 3). The tumour may be well, moderately or poorly differentiated. There are recognized variants which include papillary, clear cell, small cell and basaloid squamous cell carcinoma. Basaloid squamous cell carcinoma has a poorer prognosis than other types of squamous cell carcinoma.

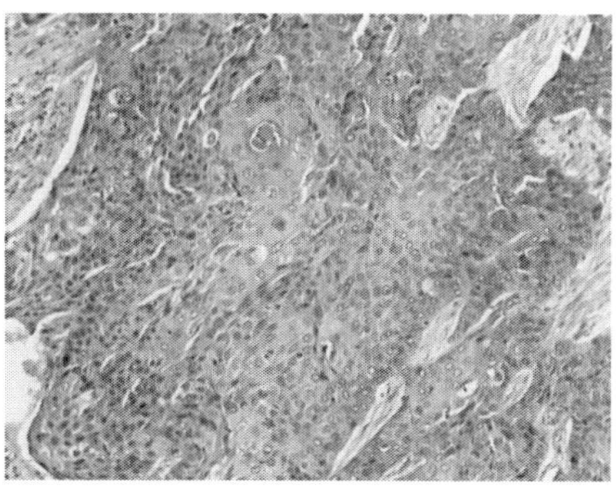

Figure 3. Squamous cell carcinoma. The tumour cells are large with eosinophilic cytoplasm and focal keratin production.

A precursor lesion of squamous cell carcinoma is well recognised. Normal bronchial mucosa consists of cuboidal cells with cilia. In smokers, damage to the mucosa from inhaled carcinogens leads to squamous metaplasia of the mucosa which may then become dysplastic and progress to squamous cell carcinoma in situ.

## Distinction of Adenocarcinoma from Squamous Cell Carcinoma on Biopsy Specimens

The distinction of small cell carcinoma from non small cell carcinoma has historically been critical in the pathological diagnosis of lung cancer as the treatment for each is very different. Several recent clinical observations have made the further categorisation of non small cell carcinomas into squamous cell carcinomas and adenocarcinomas important. First, lung cancer patients treated with bevacizumab have an increased risk of potentially fatal haemorrhage if their tumours are squamous cell so that the treatment is contraindicated in such patients [9], second, patients with adenocarcinoma or large cell carcinoma do better if treated with pemetrexed than squamous cell cancer patients and third, EGFR mutation is associated with adenocarcinoma morphology and can be treated with EGFR tyrosine kinase inhibitors. Additionally, adenocarcinomas may have a mutation leading to fusion of the genes EML4 and ALK [10] which can be targeted by the drug crizotinib. Pathologists have therefore been advised to reduce the use of the term 'non-small cell carcinoma' as a biopsy diagnosis [3].

There are many cases with well differentiated features that can be easily distinguished on HandE. However, a significant proportion will need further investigation using immunohistochemistry. A panel of stains should be used which leaves tissue available for molecular analysis. This is usually done from histopathological material although cell blocks can sometimes be made from cytological specimens if enough material is available.

Thyroid transcription factor-1 (TTF1) is the most reliable marker for adenocarcinoma and p63 is a reliable squamous marker [5] (Figure 4). Tumours tend not to stain with both markers, however, if they do, a tumour which expresses TTF1 and p63 in the same cells should be reported as 'favour adenocarcinoma'.

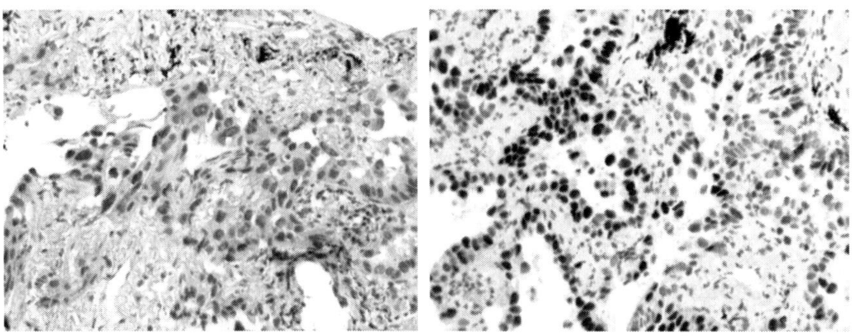

(A) (B)

Figure 4. A) Bronchial biopsy which contains a non small cell tumour with few distinguishing characteristics. B) There is positive nuclear staining with TTF1 and negative staining with p63 (not shown) indicating that this is an adenocarcinoma.

A tumour in which the markers are expressed by different populations of cells may be an adenosquamous carcinoma, but it is not possible to confirm this diagnosis on a small biopsy as the whole tumour needs to be seen. It is recommended that biopsies which are negative with TTF1 and only weakly or focally positive with a squamous marker are reported as 'non small cell carcinoma, not otherwise specified' rather than 'non small cell carcinoma, favour squamous cell carcinoma' [5]. This is so that cases with adenocarcinomatous differentiation which may respond to EGFR inhibitor therapies are not missed. Many new markers are emerging which indictates that recommended antibody panels for tumour evaluation are evolving over time.

## Small Cell Carcinoma

Small cell carcinoma accounts for up to one fifth of all lung cancers and is almost invariably associated with smoking (11). It is an aggressive tumour with a poor prognosis and only 10% are confined to the lung at presentation.

It has a characteristic appearance on HandE and is made up of small cells with large nuclei and very little cytoplasm. The nuclei have finely granular chromatin with few or no nucleoli. Nuclear moulding is seen with necrosis and numerous mitoses [2] (Figure 5).

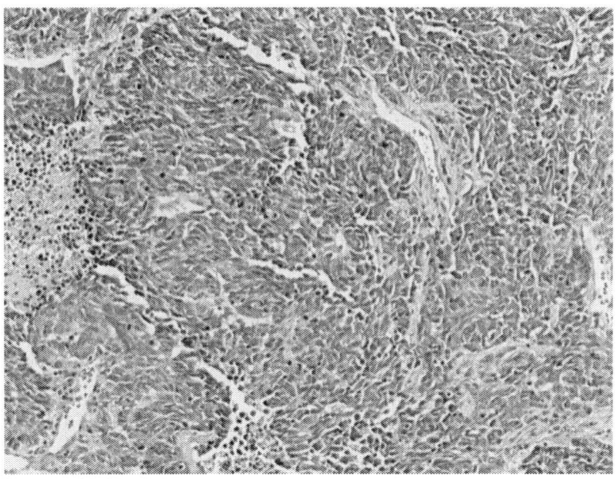

Figure 5. Small cell carcinoma. The cells have very little cytoplasm and so the tumour looks more blue than other tumour types. There is often crush artefact as well as a high mitotic and apoptotic rate.

Although the features are usually distinctive enough to make a diagnosis, crush artefact may distort the tissue and make the diagnosis difficult. Malignant lymphomas can look similar and immunohistochemical stains may be needed. Small cell carcinomas stain with CD56, Synaptophysin and Chromogranin with TTF1 staining in 70-90% in contrast to lymphomas which will stain with CD45.

Small cell carcinomas are part of a group of neuroendocrine tumours which also include large cell neuroendocrine carcinoma, carcinoid tumours and atypical carcinoid tumours.

Some small cell carcinomas contain larger cells so that the differential includes large cell neuroendocrine carcinoma. Large cell neuroendocrine carcinomas have cells that are more than 3 times the size of a resting lymphocyte, in contrast to small cell carcinomas. They also have prominent nucleoli. In rare cases, it may be difficult to distinguish between small cell carcinoma and large cell neuroendocrine carcinoma. It should also be appreciated that small cell carcinomas may be seen in combination with a non-small cell carcinoma.

## Large Cell Carcinoma

Large cell carcinoma is a carcinoma which lacks features of small cell carcinoma, squamous cell carcinoma and adenocarcinoma and accounts for about 9% of all lung cancers (4). They present as large peripheral lung masses. Variants include large cell neuroendocrine carcinoma (see below), basaloid carcinoma, lymphoepithelioma-like carcinoma, clear cell carcinoma and large cell carcinoma with rhabdoid phenotype, all of which have a worse prognosis than large cell carcinoma of usual type.

## Neuroendocrine Tumours

Carcinoid tumours are the most common entity in this group and have an excellent prognosis. They are firm well defined tumours and often grow into bronchi.

They are made up of uniform cells with eosinophilic cytoplasm often growing in packets or nests (Figure 6). Typical carcinoids have no evidence of necrosis and less than 2 mitoses per 10 high power fields in contrast to atypical carcinoids which can have one or both features. Atypical carcinoids have lower 5- and 10-year survivals than typical carcinoids. Other tumours within the neuroendocrine group include large cell neuroendocrine carcinomas and small cell carcinomas, already discussed above.

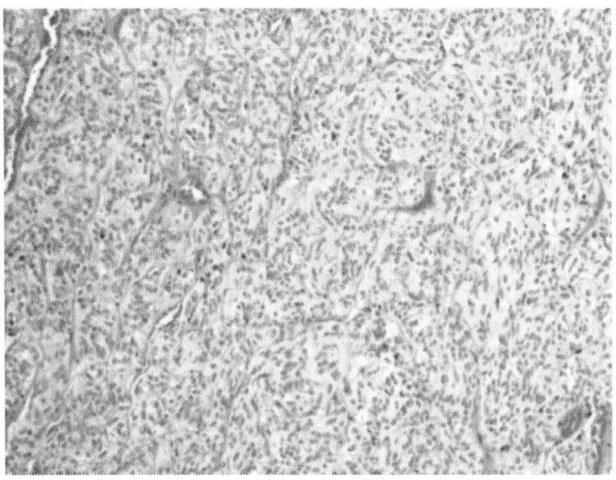

Figure 6. Carcinoid tumour formed of packets of uniform cells with regular nuclei.

## Metastases

The lungs are the commonest site for metastases in the body. Breast cancer is the most common malignancy to spread to lung, following in descending order by colon, stomach, pancreas, kidney, melanoma, prostate, liver, thyroid, adrenal, male genital tract and female genital tract [4].

Lung metastases are more likely to be multiple than single and, combined with the relevant clinical history, are not usually a diagnostic problem. Single lesions may be more difficult to diagnose and may require biopsy. Some may have characteristic morphological features although immunohistochemistry will usually be used as well to characterise the tumour.

Primary adenocarcinomas of lung are Cytokeratin 7 positive, TTF1 positive and Cytokeratin 20 negative. In contrast, metastatic breast carcinomas will show oesotrogen receptor positivity and metastastic colon cancers will be Cytokeratin 7 negative, TTF1 negative and Cytokeratin 20 positive as well as being CDX-2 positive (Figure 7). There is a primary adenocarcinoma of lung of so-called enteric type which can have a similar immunoprofile to metastatic colonic carcinoma so that distinction of these two entities may be difficult.

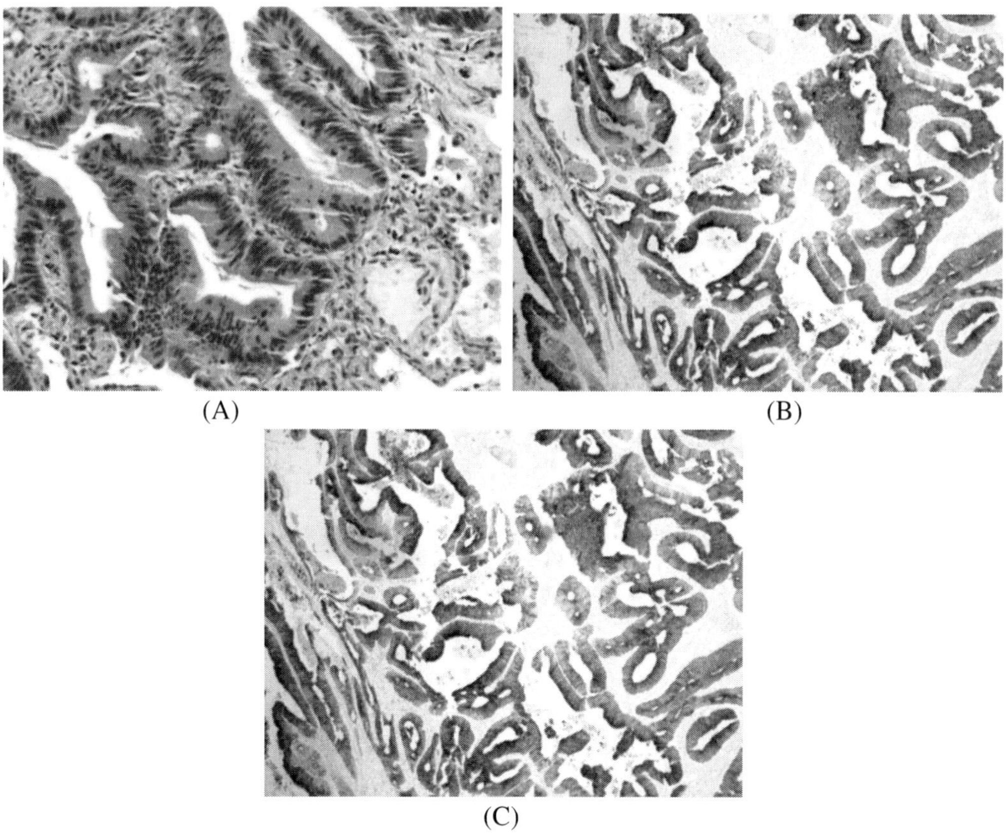


Figure 7. A) Solitary lesion in lung which is an adenocarcinoma which showed positive staining with Cytokeratin 20 (B) and CDX-20 (C) with negative staining for Cytokeratin 7. This is a metastasis from a colorectal primary.

Surgical resection is now undertaken as a curative treatment for selected patients with lung metastases [12]. Confirmation of the diagnosis as well as the size of the metastasis and status of resection margins is required from the pathology report.

## Other Tumours

There are many uncommon tumours which can affect the lung. For example, salivary gland tumours such as mucoepidermoid carcinoma, adenoid cystic carcinoma and epithelial-myoepithelial carcinomas may arise from bronchial glands. Lymphomas can arise from the lung's lymphocytes and mesenchymal lesions from blood vessels, cartilage and other connective tissue.

## Staging

The staging of any tumour is critical as it determines the treatment that the patient receives and their prognosis. The TNM system maintained by the American Joint Committee on Cancer (AJCC) and the Union for International Cancer Control (UICC) is widely used. TNM stands for tumour, nodes and metastasis. The most recent edition is the $7^{th}$ and has been in use since Jan $1^{st}$ 2010. It involved analysis of a database of more than 100,000 patients (13) along with their clinical outcomes so that features having an effect on prognosis could be identified.

The T stage is defined by tumour size and also involvement of pleura and structures beside the lung. The stages are as follows:

T0 No evidence of primary tumour

T1 Tumour 2cm or less in maximum dimension (1a) or between 2 and 3cm (1b)

T2 Tumour more than 3cm but 5cm or less in maximum dimension (2a) or between 5 and 7cm (2b). Also any tumour which invades visceral pleura.

T3 Tumour more than 7cm or one that directly invades any of the following: parietal pleura, chest wall, diaphragm, phrenic nerve, mediastinal pleura, parietal pericardium or tumour in main bronchus or separate tumour nodule(s) in same lobe.

T4 Tumour of any size invading any of the following: mediastinum, heart, great vessels, trachea, recurrent laryngeal nerve, oesophagus, vertebral body, carina, separate tumour nodule in a different ipsilateral lobe.

The N stage is defined by regional lymph node involvement.

NX Regional lymph nodes cannot be assessed

N0 No regional lymph node metastases

N1 Metastasis in ipsilateral peribronchial and/or ipsilateral hilar lymph nodes

N2 Metastasis in ipsilateral mediastinal and/or subcarinal lymph nodes

N3 Metastasis in contralateral mediastinal, contralateral hilar, ipsilateral or contralateral scalene or supraclavicular lymph nodes.

The M stage is defined as follows:

M0 No distant metastases
M1a Separate tumour nodule(s) in a contralateral lobe, tumour with pleural nodules or malignant pleural effusions
M1b Distant metastasis in extrathoracic organs

The resected tumour is examined both macroscopically and microscopically for classification and staging of the tumour. For the purposes of staging, the most advanced feature is the most important. For instance, a 2cm tumour which would usually be T1a becomes T2a if there is invasion of visceral pleura and T3 if it invades the diaphragm.

The pathological stages then get grouped into clinical prognostic groups (occult, 0, IA, IB, IIA, IIB, IIIA, IIIB, IV).

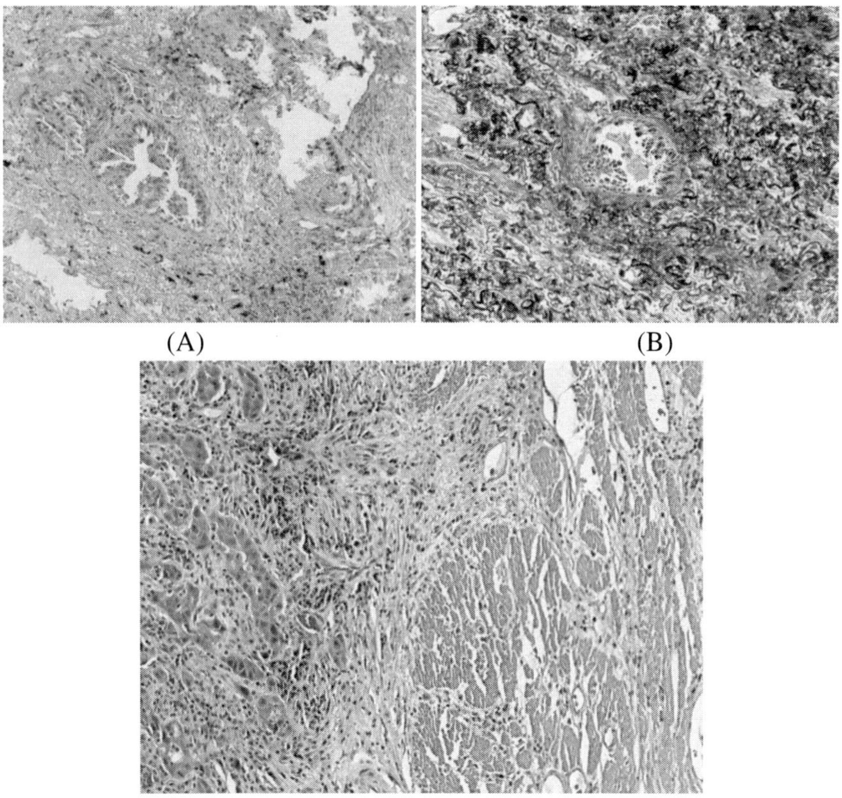

(A) (B) (C)

Figure 8. A) Islands of tumour are present near the pleural surface of the lung. B) An elastin stain of the same area which stains elastin fibres black. This shows that the tumour has invaded into the pleura which has elastin fibres. The tumour is therefore staged as T2 on the basis of this finding. C) Tumour invading into muscle of the oesophagus and this will be staged as T4.

Although the staging process is fairly well defined, some areas may be difficult to assess. Pleural involvement may be difficult to assess on routine HandE staining and an Elastic Van Gieson (EVG) stain to highlight elastin fibres may be useful (Figure 8a-c). The prognostic significance of pleural involvement is uncertain at present but may become more obvious once more data is collected [14]. The staging system is constantly updated as new information becomes available. Another area of difficulty occurs when a patient presents with two lung tumours. The pathologist must distinguish between synchronous primary tumours which could be staged as early as T1 each and a satellite tumour nodule which would be staged as T3 if in the same lobe, T4 if in a different ipsilateral lobe and M1a if in a contralateral lobe. The recent recommendation that adenocarcinomas are described in terms of their different types in 5% increments has been shown to be of use in determining whether or not tumours are synchronous primaries or one secondary to the other [15].

Multidisciplinary team working has become standard practice in pathology. All patients with a clinical suspicion of cancer should have their cases discussed at a multidisciplinary meeting where all the relevant findings can be discussed and correlated. The patient can be staged correctly and optimum treatment planned.

## Molecular Analysis

The identification of specific mutations in lung cancers has now become routine. Mutations in EGFR (epidermal growth factor receptor), KRAS and ALK (anaplastic lymphoma kinase) genes are important and may determine the types of treatments offered to patients.

In 2004 reports appeared that adenocarcinoma patients with mutations in EGFR had a better response to the treatments gefitinib and erlotinib, which are EGFR tyrosine kinase inhibitors, than patients without mutations [16-18]. EGFR mutations are more likely to occur in adenocarcinomas from female, never smokers with an East Asian background. In the USA 15% of patients with primary lung adenocarcinoma are estimated to have EGFR mutations [19].

ALK mutations occur in about 4% of patients and in general, EML4–ALK and EGFR and KRAS mutations are mutually exclusive, however, counterexamples have also been reported [20]. The patients tend to be younger, lighter smokers with adenocarcinomas with a solid pattern and signet ring cells (21). The drug crizotinib has been approved to treat ALK positive tumours and has shown improved response rates [22].

KRAS mutations are found in 15-30% of lung adenocarcinomas. They are more common in smokers or former smokers than non-smokers and also in Caucasian patients rather than East Asian patients [10].

It would be useful if specific histopathological patterns were associated with specific mutations and the lepidic pattern is associated with EGFR mutations, the presence of a signet ring component with ALK and of a mucinous pattern with KRAS. However, this is not universal and the fact that patients without a specific mutation do better with conventional therapy means that molecular assessment is necessary.

## Conclusion

Lung cancer is the number one cause of cancer death. Long associated with a poor prognosis, recent advances have lead to a small but significant improvement in response rates and survival times. The proposed changes in pathological classification of tumours is a response to these new developments. Correlations between the disciplines involved in the diagnosis and treatment of lung cancer should make it easier to investigate and progress new discoveries and treatments.

# References

[1] Travis WD, Lubin J, Ries L, Devesa S. United States lung carcinoma incidence trends: declining for most histologic types among males, increasing among females. *Cancer* 1996; 77:2464-2470.

[2] Travis WD. Update on small cell carcinoma and its differentiation from squamous and other non-small cell carcinomas. *Modern Pathology* 2012;25: S18-S30.

[3] Travis WD, Rekhtman N, Riley GJ, et al. Pathologic diagnosis of advanced lung cancer based on small biopsies and cytology, a paradigm shift. *J Thorac Oncol* 2010; 5(4):411-414.

[4] Travis WD, Brambilla E, Muller-Hermelink HK and Harris CC. World Health Organization Classification of Tumours. *Pathology and Genetics, Tumours of the lung, pleura, thymus and heart.* IARC Press Lyon 2004.

[5] Travis WD, Brambilla E, Noguchi M, et al, International Association for the Study of Lung Cancer/American Thoracic Society/European Respiratory Society International Multidisciplinary Classifcation of Lung Adenocarcinoma. *J Thorac Oncol* 2011;6:244-285.

[6] Warth A, Muley T, Meister M, et al. The novel histologic International Association for the Study of Lung Cancer/American Thoracic Society/European Respiratory Society classification system of lung adenocarcinoma is a stage-independent predictor of survival. *J Clin Oncol* 2012; 30:1438-1446.

[7] Nakahara R, Yokose T, Nagai K, et al. Atypical adenomatous hyperplasia of the lung: a clinicopathological study of 118 cases including cases with multiple atypical adenomatous hyperplasia. *Thorax* 2001; 56:302-305.

[8] Funai K, Yokose T, Ishii G, et al. Clinicopathological characteristics of peripheral squamous cell carcinoma of the lung. *Am J Surg Pathol* 2003; 27:978-984.

[9] Johnson DH, Fehrenbacher L, Novotny WF, et al. Randomized phase II trial comparing bevacizumab plus carboplatin and paclitaxel with carboplatin and paclitaxel alone in previously untreated locally advanced or metastatic non-small-cell lung cancer. *J Clin Oncol* 2004; 22:2184-91.

[10] Brandao GDA, Brega EF and Spatz A. The role of molecular pathology in non-small cell lung carcinoma- now and in the future. Curr Oncol 2012;19: S24-S32.

[11] Krug LM, Pietanza MC, Kris MG, et al. Small cell and other neuroendocrine tumours of the lung. In: DeVita VT, Lawrence TS, Rosenberg SA. (eds). DeVita, Hellman and Rosenberg's Cancer, Principle and Practice of Oncology, 9th edn. Wolters Kluwer; Lippincott Williams and Wilkins: Philadephia 2011, pp 848-870.

[12] Onaitis MW, Petersen RP, Haney JC ,et al. Prognostic factors for recurrence after pulmonary resection of colorectal cancer metastases. *Ann Thorac Surg* 2009; 87:1684-9

[13] AJCC Staging Manual, Seventh Edition, Springer 2010.

[14] Detterbeck FC, Boffa DJ, Tanoue LT, Wilson LD. Details and difficulties regarding the new lung cancer staging system. *Chest* 2010; 137(5):1172-1180.

[15] Girard N, Deshpande C, Lau C, et al. Comprehensive histologic assessment helps to differentiate multiple lung primary nonsmall cell carcinomas from metastases. *Am J Surg Pathol* 2009;33(12): 1752-1764. 2009.

[16] Paez JG, Janne PA, Lee JC, et al. EGFR mutations in lung cancer:correlation with clinical response to gefitinib therapy. *Science* 2004;304:1497-1500.

[17] Lynch TJ, Bell DW, Sordella, et al. Activating mutations in the epidermal growth factor receptor underlying responsiveness of non-small-cell lung cancer to gefitinib. *N Engl J Med* 2004; 350:2129-2139.

[18] Pao W, Miller V, Zakowski M, et al. EGF receptor gene mutations are common in lung cancers from 'never smokers' and are associated with sensitivity of tumors to gefitinib and erlotinib. *Proc Natl Acad Sci USA* 2004;101:13306-13311.

[19] Keedy VL, Temin S, Somerfield MR, et al. American Society of Clinical Oncology provisional clinical opinion: epidermal growth factor receptor (EGFR) testing for patients with advanced non-small-cell lung cancer considering first-line EGFR tyrosine kinase inhibitor therapy. *J Clin Oncol* 2011;29:2121-7.

[20] Tiseo M, Gelsomino F, Boggiani D, et al. EGFR + EML4-ALK mutations in NSCLC: a case report of erlotinib-resistant patient with both concomitant mutations. *Lung Cancer* 2011;71:241-3.

[21] Rodig SJ, Mino-Kenudson M, Dacic S, et al. Unique clinicopathologic features characterize ALK-rearranged lung adenocarcinoma in the Western population. *Clin Cancer Res* 2009;15:5216-23.

[22] Kwak EL, Bang YJ, Camidge DR, et al. Anaplastic lymphoma kinase inhibition in non-small-cell lung cancer. *N Engl J Med* 2010;363:1693-703.

In: Lung Cancer: A Comprehensive Overview
Editor: Kathy Gately
ISBN: 978-1-62618-447-3


*Chapter II*

# Introduction to Lung Cancer, its Epidemiology and Diagnosis

***Stephen A. Deppen***[1,2,3] **and Eric L. Grogan**[1,3,4]*
[1]Department of Thoracic Surgery, Vanderbilt University Medical Center, Nashville, TN, US
[2]Department of Epidemiology, Vanderbilt University, Nashville, TN, US
[3]Veterans Affairs, Tennessee Valley Healthcare System, Nashville, TN, US
[4]Institute for Medicine and Public Health, Vanderbilt University, Nashville, TN, US

## Abstract

Lung cancer is the leading cause of death among those with cancer. As the smoking epidemic spreads to the developing world, so too will lung cancer. This chapter examines the epidemiology of lung cancer and describes the major risk factors for lung cancer from the literature. Recent developments on screening for lung cancer using low dose computed tomography scans are introduced. The current guidelines and algorithms for diagnosis of lung cancer in a screening population as well as those who present to the clinician with symptomatic disease or incidentally discovered lung nodules are described in detail. Accessing the lung to obtain a pathological diagnosis can be difficult and the patient and clinician must develop an individualized treatment plan that takes into consideration the status of the patient and likelihood of cancer.

## Introduction

Lung cancer is the most common cause of cancer related death in the United States (US) and kills more people than breast, prostate, kidney, colon, liver and skin cancers combined.

* Email: steve.deppen@Vanderbilt.Edu.

More than 220,000 new cases and nearly 160,000 deaths from lung cancer occurred in the US in 2010, accounting for approximately 17% of annual incident cancers and 28% of all cancer deaths [1, 2]. The overall 5-year survival for lung cancer is a dismal 15.6%, largely resulting from advanced stage at the time of diagnosis. Localized, pathological stage IA lung cancer, has a 73% 5-year survival rate while metastatic, stage IV disease has a 7% survival rate [3]. Lung cancer diagnosis and treatment exerts a significant economic burden as well. The US spends an estimated $10.3 billion on direct lung cancer care which comprises 10% of all cancer related healthcare expenditures [4]. These direct costs are dwarfed by the estimated $83 billion lost in productivity from caregiving and lost wages due to early mortality from the disease. Lung cancer contributes 27% of all cancer such productivity related losses [5].

Lung cancer, like most cancers, is a complex and diverse disease. It is caused primarily by environmental factors. Known risk factors for lung cancer include tobacco smoking, radon exposure, air pollutants, second hand smoke, occupational exposures and individual genetics. The most significant exposure risk for both small cell (SCLC), which comprises 14% of all lung cancers, and non-small cell lung cancer (NSCLC), which comprises the remaining 86%, is tobacco smoking. Approximately 85% of the population attributable risk for lung cancer is due to tobacco smoking [6, 7]. Among non-smokers lung cancer is a relatively rare disease, <15 per 100,000, in those under age 70.

The age-adjusted incidence rates for lung cancer in the US, according to SEER data, peaked in 1992 at 69.4 cases per 100,000. The trend in incidence is down 0.6 cases per 100,000 per year since 1992 and was 58.8 per 100,000 in 2009, the most recently available data [8]. Among women, age-adjusted incidence has decreased to 51.2 per 100,000 since reaching its peak of 53.5 in 2005 (Figure 1). The incidence rate of lung cancer in men has steadily declined from its peak of 102.1 per 100,000 in 1984 to 69.2 in 2009. Age-adjusted mortality rates in the US have seen slight declines in recent years for women (38.6 per 100,000) from their peak in 2002 of 41.6 per 100,000.

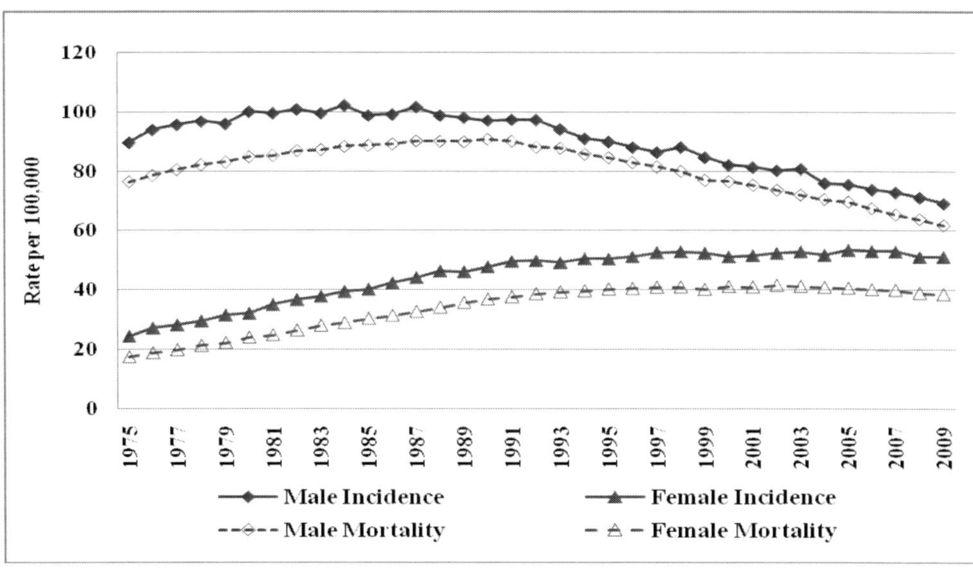


Figure 1. Age Adjusted U.S. Lung and Bronchus Cancer Incidence and Mortality Rates by Sex, 1975-2009. Source: SEER 2012.

A more dramatic decline in mortality among men has been observed from an age-adjusted high in 1990 of 90.6 to 62 per 100,000 in 2009 [9].

There is a 4 fold geographic variation in lung cancer incidence across the US. Kentucky has the highest rate among both men (125.1 per 100,000) and women (80.3 per 100,000), and Utah has the lowest rates (29.2 for men and 19.0 per 100,000 for women) [9]. Incidence rate differences match the historical smoking prevalence in those states and have remained fairly consistent over time. The variation in lung cancer rates follows smoking rates across the country. Geographic variation has been observed in other countries as well.

## International Variation in Lung Cancer Prevalence

World-wide lung cancer incidence generally follows the smoking epidemic with developed countries having the highest but declining incidence rates. The latency period for smoking caused lung cancer is approximately 30 years. Thus, current cancer rates can be easily estimated using historical cigarette smoking prevalence as other causes have minimal impact on population incidence rates compared to that from smoking [10].

Incidence rates are increasing among developing countries with the greatest increases occurring in Asia and Eastern Europe, while the African continent has the lowest incidence rates (Figure 2) [11].

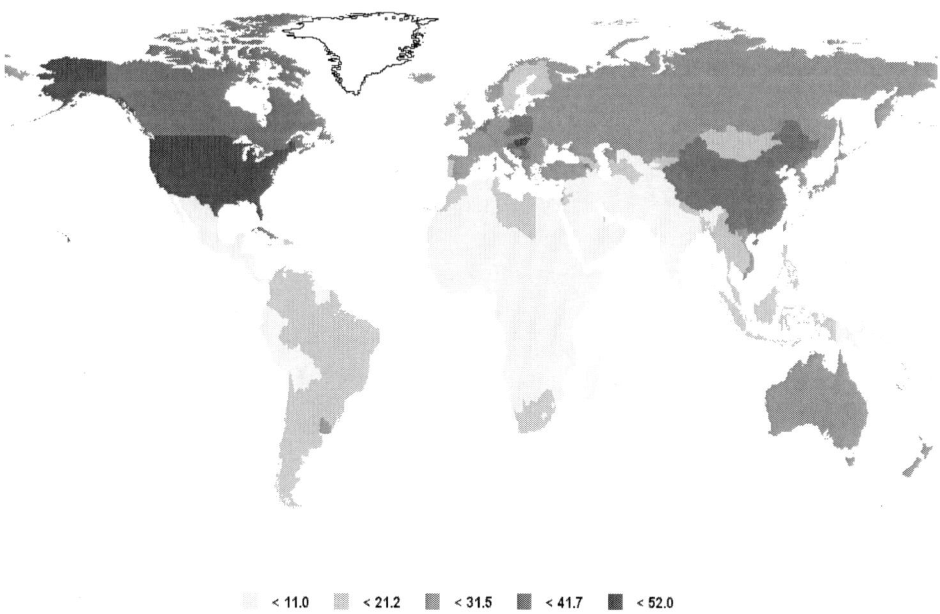


Figure 2. Lung cancer estimated age-standardized incidence rate per 100,000: both sexes, all ages. SOURCE: GLOBOCAN 2008(IARC) – 7/30/2012.

For men, the highest incidence rates occur in Eastern Europe and in North America. Among women, the highest incidence rates occur in North American and Northern Europe [12]. Some of the greatest geographic variability in lung cancer rates within a country have been observed in China. A 20 fold difference in lung cancer mortality between women in northwest China compared to those in southern China was observed [13]. A higher proportion of lung cancer, especially among women, is attributable to non-smoking causes in less developed countries. Survival is similar in developing countries to that in developed countries with 14% of men and 18% of women diagnosed with lung cancer surviving at least five years [14].

## Age and Lung Cancer

Lung cancer is generally a disease of the elderly. Less than 1 in 100,000 individuals under age 30 develop lung cancer [7]. Lung cancer risk increases with age for both smokers and non-smokers. The increased risk appears to be similar among never smokers irrespective of race, except for Hispanics and African-American men of which there is too little data [15]. Nearly two-thirds of incident lung cancers occur in those over age 65. The median age at initial diagnosis is 71[16]. After age 70 lung cancer incidence increases even among non-smokers to a rate similar that of kidney or liver cancer.

## Host Factors and Lung Cancer Risk from Smoking

Smoking has been a known cause of lung cancer for nearly six decades [17, 18]. Doll and Hill's seminal findings from their prospective cohort confirmed previous retrospective studies that tobacco smoking causes lung cancer [17]. Approximately 80% of women and 90% of men diagnosed with lung cancer were smokers. In the US smoking prevalence peaked among males in the 1940s and 50s at around 67%. Smoking prevalence peaked for US females in the late 1960s at approximately 44%. Active tobacco smoking remains the greatest risk factor for lung cancer, although passive tobacco smoke exposure is a contributing risk factor especially among non-smokers. Tobacco smoke and the carcinogenic chemicals in the smoke act on the lung to generate cancer through a number of biological processes.

Polycyclic aromatic hydrocarbons (PAH) and N-nitrosamines are both presentin tobacco smoke and exert their effects on the lung and carcinogenesis through both gene mutationsand the formation of DNA adducts (Figure 3).

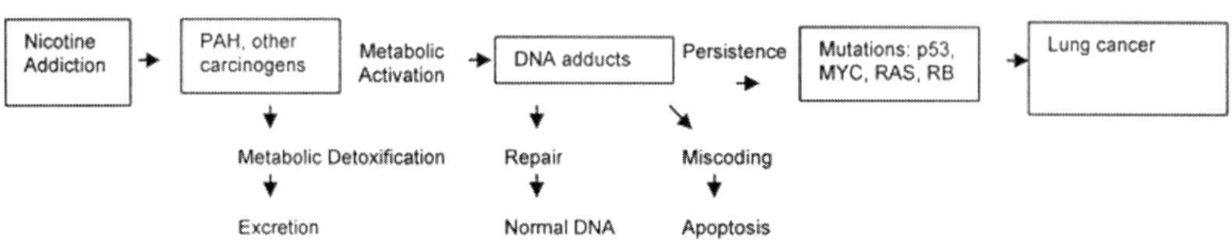


Figure 3. Schema depicting individual differences in response to carcinogens (from Hecht JNCI 1999).

The subsequent cellular changes and mutation proliferation result in lung cancer [19, 20]. There is an observed dose-response between smoking and lung cancer risk [1, 21, 22]. The relative risk per year of contracting lung cancer increases between 8 and 17% per 10 cigarettes per day additionally smoked [23, 24]. The change in risk due to smoking is generally monotonic [25, 26]. The age at which smoking began, the number of cigarettes smoked per day, and the duration of smoking all influence the likelihood of developing lung cancer [27, 28]. Current smokers have a 20-fold increase in lung cancer risk compared to never-smokers [6]. The cumulative risk of dying from lung cancer before age 85 was 22.1% for a male smoker and 11.9% for a female smoker of European descent, in the absence of competing causes of death. This compares to a 1.1% probability for a man and 0.8% probability for a woman non-smoker dying from lung cancer before age 85[15].

## Gender Differences in Lung Cancer Incidence

Gender differences in lung cancer risk from smoking in the US have been observed in the past, and women were considered more susceptible to developing lung cancer [29-31]. More men are diagnosed with lung cancer than women but smoking prevalence among men has historically been higher compared to women. The gap in smoking rates between men and women has greatly narrowed and in 2009 23.5% of men and 17.9% of women smoked [32]. As the rates of smoking among both men and women have become more similar since the 1960s, their lung cancer incidences and age adjusted lung cancer death rates have converged (Figure 1) [33, 34]. After controlling for smoking duration, time of initiation and intensity, no gender specific differences in lung cancer risk have been found [25, 28, 34, 35]. However, the adjusted risk for lung cancer death is lower in women when compared to men, and this result has been consistent over time [36, 37].

Separating gender specific risk for lung cancer from that associated with smoking habits has been difficult. Some researchers investigating incident lung cancers found women smokers had higher risks for lung cancer when compared to male smokers, especially after age 70 [30]. Women have been found to have different distributions of cancer histology. Specifically, non-smoking women of all races are two to four times more likely to have bronchioloalveolar cancer compared to men [38-40]. Among non-smokers, age and temporal biases within the cohorts studied may have influenced the relationship given that women live longer than men [41].

A recent study examined gender specific risk for lung cancer by pooling non-smokers from 13 cohorts and 22 cancer registries from around the world [15]. Thun and colleagues found no differences in lung cancer age-standardized incidence rates between men and women age 40 and higher [15]. Some differences were found after further stratification by race. Incidence among Asian and Pacific Islander women was 71% which was twice that found in Hispanic women and 31% more than the incidence observed in non-Hispanic whites [15]. In non-smokers the lung cancer death rate is slightly higher in men, 17.1 per 100,000, when compared to women, 14.7 per 100,000 [42]. This increased risk of lung cancer related mortality in men compared to women is seen among smokers who develop lung cancer as well.

## Race

A number of population studies have found that racial differences in response to smoking and lung cancer risk may occur due to intensity, what types of cigarettes are smoked or other environmental factors like access to care or socio-economic status. Incidence rates of lung cancer among smokers are higher among African American men compared to Caucasian men [1].

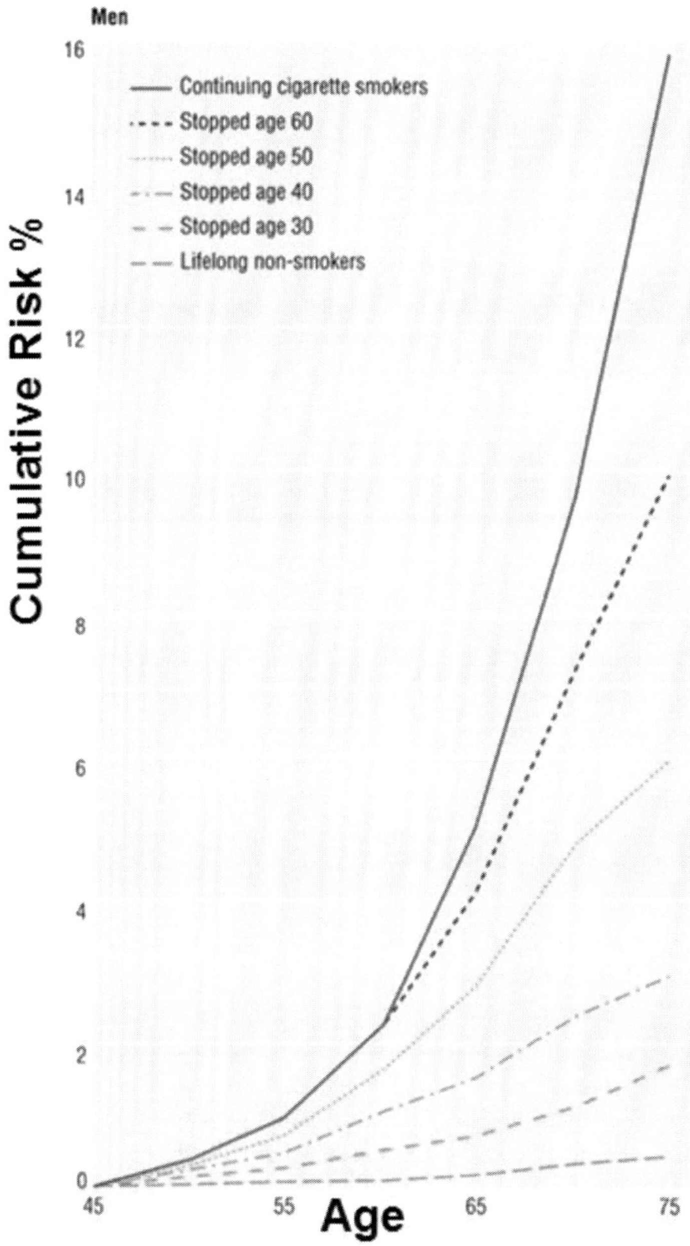


Figure 4. Age adjusted cumulative risk after smoking cessation (from Peto et al, 2000).

Smoking prevalence among black men is slightly higher than that observed among white men. However, the literature remains mixed as to whether race is an independent host factor for smoking related risk for lung cancer incidence. African Americans and Native Hawaiians appear to have higher risk of lung cancer at lower smoking concentrations (<31 cigarettes a day). Lung cancer risks were similar among heavy smokers across races and sexes in one large multi-racial cohort [43], and only African American heavy smokers had higher lung cancer risks in a case-control study [44].

One conjectured cause of the observed higher lung cancer risks among African Americans was their higher prevalence of mentholated cigarette smoking, 62% among African Americans compared to 23% among Caucasian smokers [45]. Menthol cigarettes were thought to be more difficult to quit compared to non-flavored cigarettes and to contribute to the lung cancer burden from smoking [45, 46].

A recent study in the Southern Community Cohort examined menthol cigarettes and compared incidence and rates of smoking cessation between African American smokers and Caucasian smokers. This study found lower incidence of lung cancer among menthol smokers irrespective of race and similar odds of quitting [47]. Other prospective studies similarly found no increased risk from mentholated cigarettes [48].

Smoking cessation decreases all cause and lung cancer related mortality irrespective of age at which one stops smoking [49, 50]. The benefits of quitting for reducing lung cancer risk are also well documented (Figure 4) [51, 52]. The benefits of smoking cessation on lung cancer risk reduction stops at around two times the risk for former smokers when compared to never smokers [53, 54]. Decreased risk of lung cancer changes little after 15 years post cessation and remains elevated up to 30 years after cessation [24]. Prevention of smoking initiation followed by smoking cessation remains the best, least costly methods of lung cancer risk reduction. Smoking cessation can benefit anyone, irrespective of age or smoking duration [6, 55].

## Second-Hand Tobacco Smoke

Exposure to second-hand or environmental tobacco smoke as a cause of cancer was first reported in 1981 in a study of non-smoking Asian women married to smokers [56, 57]. More recent studies and meta-analyses found a dose-response relationship between lung cancer and environmental tobacco smoke exposure which strengthened the causal relationship found in earlier studies and by review groups [58-60]. The excess risk for lung cancer of a non-smoking spouse married to a smoker is between 25% and 30% [61, 62]. Workplace exposure to environmental tobacco smoke was associated with a 16% increase in risk in a large European study [63] and 17% in the meta-analysis by Boffetta [(61]. Population exposure to second hand smoke is estimated to be around 40%. An estimated one fourth of lung cancer cases among non-smokers or 3,000 deaths per year are attributable to environmental tobacco smoke in the United States (US) [59]. Non-smokers exposed to environmental tobacco smoke also have increased likelihood of mortality from cardiovascular and cerebrovascular diseases as well as other respiratory diseases [64]. "Misclassification of exposure to second hand smoke is inevitable," according to one review of the environmental tobacco smoking literature [65]. However, misclassification does not explain the extent of observed risk. Also assuming that any misclassification is non-differential with respect to case and control status, then it will likely dilute the estimate and attenuate the estimated risk. If the estimates of risk for lung cancer from involuntary smoking are smaller than estimated, it remains a significant carcinogen given the large historical prevalence of exposure to second hand smoke. Reduction of this exposure through workplace and public area restrictions of tobacco smoking has resulted in cotinine serum levels dropping 2 to 3 fold [66]. These reductions in environmental tobacco smoke exposure may reduce lung cancer from this source by 60%.

## Non-Smoking Related Exposures for Lung Cancer

Other environmental exposures associated with increased lung cancer risk include: naturally occurring radon (10-15% population attributable risk), asbestos and metal dusts and other occupational exposures (9-15%), second-hand tobacco smoke exposure (5-10%) and outdoor air pollutants (1-2%).

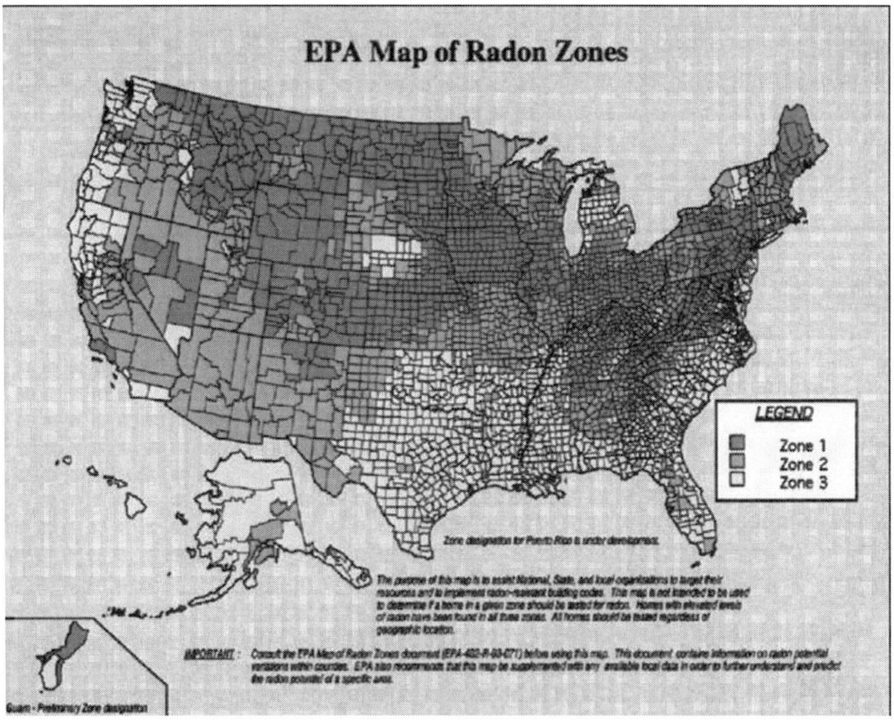


Figure 5 U.S. map of radon (from USEPA, 2003).

## Radon

Radon gas and its polonium decay products are naturally occurring in rocks and soils across the US (Figure 5). In 1988 the International Agency for Research on Cancer (IACR) found that radon was a cause for human lung cancer, and the Environmental Protection Agency (EPA) has given guidance on residential abatement of radon [67, 68].

Residential and occupational radon exposure may be responsible for 10% to 15% of all lung cancer deaths per year in the US, thus making radon the second leading cause of lung cancer behind cigarettes [69]. Radon is the primary cause of lung cancer among lifetime non-smokers and those without other significant occupational exposure, like asbestos, small particulates or other known carcinogenic chemicals. An estimated half of the average individuals annual radiation dose is from radon and its decay products[70]. An assessment by the EPA found that approximately 12% of lung cancer deaths among smokers were radon related, and among non-smokers 26% of the lung cancer deaths were radon related [68]. Similar results have been found in European case-control studies, and an increased relative risk from radon appears to be linear in exposure for both smokers and non-smokers. Multiplicative effect modification wasnot found in the combined European studies. However, in other studies, radon exposure synergistically increased lifetime lung cancer risk among smokers 9 to 10 times compared to the risk among non-smokers [68]. In a case-control study of American miners, the interaction of radon and smoking was greater than additive and less than multiplicative [71]. Turner and colleagues used the large Cancer Prevention Study-II cohort and over 310,000 residential radon measurements across 1601 counties in the US to estimate the association between radon and lung cancer mortality while controlling for smoking, ambient air quality, occupational exposures and socio-economic factors. A positive, linear trend was observed between ambient radon and lung cancer. For each 100Bq/m$^3$ increase in radon related dose, a 15% increase in the risk of lung cancer mortality was observed.

## Occupational Exposures

Asbestos, arsenic, chromium, nickel, beryllium and silica have been shown to increase risk for developing lung cancer among exposed, non-smoking workers. Other chemicals, including organic solvents, pesticides and non-ferrous metal dust or fumes have not consistently been shown to cause cancer in non-smokers [72-74]. A large European prospective study of individual industry exposures found that asbestos (HR 1.5; 95%CI: 1.2-1.9), heavy metals (HR 1.4: 95%CI: 1.1-1.8) and polycyclic aromatic hydrocarbon (HR 1.6; 95%CI: 1.2-2.1) (PAH) related exposures had the highest hazard ratios for lung cancer related mortality. The population attributable risk for employment within at least one at risk industry was 16% for men. Most occupational lung cancer studies are nested case-control studies which suffer from possible residual confounding from smoking and lack of lung cancer among non-smokers exposed to the carcinogen being studied within the cohort [55]. However, individual industry specific cohort studies have consistently found that occupational exposures to known lung carcinogens increase the risk for lung cancer among those employed in those industries after controlling for other risk factors [75].

In a comprehensive survey of occupational exposures across Britain using International Agency for Reaseach on Cancer (IARC)designated causative or possibly causative carcinogens, Brown and colleagues estimated over 5400 lung cancers attributable to occupational exposure [75]. Occupational exposures are estimated to cause 13% of the expected lung cancer in 2012 in Britain [76]. This estimated attributable fraction is higher than that previously estimated by Doll and Peto due to the higher rates of smoking related lung cancer among men in the earlier study [77]. Brown found that asbestos alone comprised 41% of the lung cancer cases estimated to arise from occupational exposures. Boffetta and colleagues found lower cancer rates among men and higher rates among women in a French study of occupational exposures and lung cancer [78] and rates half that of Brown for both sexes in a survey of Central and Northern Europe [79]. The discrepancy between the studies arise from the definition of carcinogen exposure, where the British study included possible carcinogens (IARC class 2A), the Olsson and Boffetta studies included only those known human carcinogens (IARC class 1) and prevalence of asbestos exposure differed greatly based on locally specific industries. Even given the wide variance in estimated occupational exposures observed in the literature, occupational exposure remains a significant burden for lung cancer in the US and across much of the developed world.

## Air Pollutants

Controversy best characterizes the literature regarding air pollutants and lung cancer risk. A recent review of European studies examining lung cancer risk from air pollution found no clear association, but questions remain around measurement error and latency of outcome [80]. A large cohort study in the US found strong evidence for an association between elevated fine particulate air pollution exposures and significant increases in lung cancer mortality [67, 81]. Another systematic review not limited to studies performed in Europe found weak evidence of a causal relationship between air pollution and lung cancer. The heterogeneity across studies limited conclusions to be drawn. However, the strongest associations were observed in populations near point sources of known carcinogens, primarily benzene and arsenic. Environmental exposures and their risks were small relative to risks from smoking and occupational exposure. Withrow and colleagues found that tobacco smoking and occupational carcinogen exposures were often incompletely controlled in the assessment of risk and inadequate latency periods for lung cancer to develop were also cited, thus limiting reported results [82]. In developing countries, indoor air contamination from cooking and heating are significant contributors to lung cancer risk among non-smokers [83-85]. Fortunately, simple improvements in ventilation or fuel substitution have been shown to reduce the risk for lung cancer and other respiratory diseases in these populations [86].

## Body Mass Index as a Risk Factor for Lung Cancer

The evidence for body mass index (BMI) as a risk factor for lung cancer independent from smoking is generally weak and conflicting. A small case control study in non-smokers found those with a BMI over 30 had twice the odds of developing cancer when compared to those with a BMI below 21[87]. In a more recent study of the Women's Health Initiative, BMI was found to be inversely related to lung cancer risk in smokers. No association was found among non-smokers between BMI and lung cancer after adjusting for other lung cancer risk factors. BMI has been found to be inversely related to cancer incidence in populations with a history of tobacco use in a number of studies [47, 88, 89]. BMI independent of smoking has not been found to be associated with lung cancer in a prospective cohort to date. Studies examining the relationship between BMI and lung cancer may suffer from residual confounding from smoking, or some other unknown biological mechanism occurs or is associated with higher BMI being protective for lung cancer. Additional studies are needed to determine whether BMI is a lung cancer risk factor independent of smoking.

## Non-Cancer Lung Disease

Recent studies have shown a strong association between lung disease and lung cancer. An estimated 25% of heavy smokers develop chronic obstructive pulmonary disease (COPD) [90] and 12 to 17% of heavy smokers develop lung cancer yet 40 to 70% of those with lung cancer have COPD as well [91]. Of those with COPD, 85% have tobacco smoke exposure. COPD has been found to be an independent risk factor for lung cancer in a number of studies [91-93]. Patients with lung cancer and COPD are more likely to have squamous cell histology and a 2 fold higher risk for lung cancer compared to those without COPD. Exploration of the biological and genetic factors that cause differences in bronchus epithelial cells through the inflammatory process and DNA repair of the two diseases are thought to possibly predict high risk individuals for lung cancer [94, 95]. Asthma was associated with decreased risk of lung cancer in males in one study [93]. Pulmonary fibrosis and interstitial lung disease exhibit a similar inflammatory response and have been found to be a risk factor for lung cancer in some studies [96, 97]. Non-cancer lung disease is an inclusion criteria proposed for lung cancer screening and is an important risk factor for early detection [98].

## Genetic Factors in Lung Cancer Risk

A minority of individuals exposed to tobacco smoke contract lung cancer which leads to the hypothesis that significant heritable risk factors exist. Studies showing an association between family history of lung cancer and increased risk support this hypothesis [6, 99]. Aggregation of lung cancer within families has been shown in both case-control and cohort studies. One study examining the genetic evidence among twins and a second in non-smokers and their first degree relatives found higher risks for lung cancer within families. Furthermore, association results were stronger in those cancers occurring at a younger ages [100, 101]. Genetic factors of risk should be grouped into two distinct categories: germline mutations which are inherited that make one more susceptible to the carcinogens in tobacco smoke or increase cancer risk independent of tobacco smoke exposure and somatic mutations that are caused by tobacco smoke or other injuries to the lung or from other environmental exposures. To understand possible mutations and their effects, three biological pathways that regulate cells and detoxify tobacco smoke must be understood.

First, the compounds in tobacco smoke are metabolized primarily under the control of two pathways. The initial pathway metabolizes non-reactive compounds in tobacco smoke, primarily polycyclic aromatic hydrocarbons for example, into highly reactive intermediates. This metabolism occurs, for the most part, through the cytochrome-p450 pathway. These reactive compounds may bind to DNA and cause genetic injury (Figure 3). Furthermore, these intermediates are transformed into complexes that are more easily excreted. Glutathione s-transferase dominates this second pathway. Germline mutations to genes which regulate either pathway may influence lung cancer risk. CPY1A1 and other p450 related enzymes with polymorphisms to their underlying gene promoter regions have been associated with lung cancer risk [102, 103]. Similarly, mutations that influence enzymes from this pathway have been shown to increase lung cancer risk [104, 105].

A second area of genetic interest is the tumor suppressor gene, p53. This gene influences multiple cellular response pathways relevant to the carcinogenesis of various cancers and is not unique to lung cancer. The types of mutations in this gene in populations with lung cancer appear to be different between smokers and non-smokers. As such, some mutations in p53 gene are likely somatic rather than germline.

A third pathway for lung cancer susceptibility involves DNA repair and DNA repair capacity. Both germline and somatic mutations occur in the capacity of DNA repair enzymes to overcome miscoding or promote apoptosis.

For example, DNA methylation, both hyper-methylation and hypo-methylation depending upon gene regions, increases risk [106]. Comprehensive review of genetic variations in the cause of lung cancer is beyond the scope of this chapter and other sources better serve this purpose [107-110].

Research in risk factors independent of tobacco smoking requires investigation of non-smokers. Such research is problematic as very few people with lung cancer have not had some exposure to primary or environmental tobacco smoke. The best studies actively measure cotinine blood levels but rarely do so 20 to 30 years prior to the development of lung cancer or over the normal latency period of lung cancer development. Therefore, misclassification in studies examining genetic mutations in non-smokers is likely [55]. Even a pooled analysis of non-smokers was unable to determine incident cancer associations by race for African American or Asian men, and little data exists for non-smoking or environmental tobacco smoke free incidence in Hispanics [55]. In some Asian countries 70% of the lung cancer among non-smokers occurs in women. However, tobacco smoke exposure misclassification in Asian women may be a factor, and Asian women are exposed to high levels of indoor pollution and other environmental risk factors for lung cancer compared to their European and North American counterparts [83]. The initial studies linking environmental tobacco smoke and lung cancer were conducted in populations of Asian women married to spouses who smoked [56, 111].

The wide variation of lung cancer incidence between and within Asian countries confounds estimates of association between gender and lung cancer. Whether Asian women are more susceptible to lung cancer due to gender or race specific genetic factors and not greater environmental exposures is not known at this time. One suggested argument for a genetic difference in lung cancer risk arises from the higher prevalence of epidermal growth factor receptor positive (EGFR) tumors in certain populations. Somatic mutations in EGFR are found with greater frequency among non-smokers and Asian women. Presence of this tumor mutation greatly influences treatment when present [112]. Currently, no serum biomarker or other genetic tests are recommended to assess risk for screening or diagnostic purposes [113].

# Diagnosis of Lung Cancer

An individual can present to a clinician for evaluation and diagnosis from three sources: symptomatic, incidentally discovered pulmonary nodule and periodic screening. Irrespective of source, the diagnosis of lung cancer begins with radiographic imaging of the chest and detailed history and physical of the individual. Previously, most lung cancer was diagnosed symptomatically (estimated 75%), but with the proliferation of imaging modalities, more lung anomalies are being discovered incidentally [114]. Diagnosis of lung cancer depends on presentation, the type (non-small cell lung cancer or small cell lung cancer) location and size of the lesion, the presence of metastasis and status of the patient.

# Symptomatic Lung Cancer Detection

Currently, lung cancers are detected after the patient develops symptoms. Clinically present symptoms for NSCLC are varied and categorized simply as either pulmonary, extrapulmonary thoracic and extrathoracic symptoms. Pulmonary symptoms include persistent cough, dyspnea, wheezing, hemoptysis or pneumonic symptoms. Cough is common among cigarette smokers and nonspecific. Dyspnea occurs in 50-60% of patients with NSCLC. Dyspnea is also common in smokers with chronic obstructive pulmonary disease which is often comorbid with their lung cancer. Hemoptysis presents more frequently in those with centrally located tumors or SCLC and occurs in 25-40% of patients [115]. Compression of the bronchus by the tumor or enlarged lymph nodes may cause dyspnea or wheezing. Finally, many of the symptoms of NSCLC mimic those from postobstructive pneumonitis or atelectasis and are nonspecific, delaying diagnosis.

Extrapulmonary thoracic symptoms arise from invasion of the chest wall or mediastinal structures by tumor or enlarged lymph nodes. Peripheral tumors can invade through the visceral pleura causing somatic pain of ribs, muscle and shoulder pain, or radicular pain due to neurovascular bundle invasion. Symptoms from mediastinal involvement directly relate to the structure invaded. Phrenic nerve involvement may result in chronic hiccups or diaphragmatic paralysis. Voice alteration may signal laryngeal node invasion or recurrent aspiration due to nerve paralysis. Vena caval obstruction may result in superior vena cava syndrome or distention of venous drainage or edema of the upper body and is caused by extensive right mediastinal lymph node involvement. These symptoms arise more often from SCLC. Pericardial invasion can occur, leading to symptomatic effusion or tamponade. Vertebral body invasion can also occur with concomitant back pain [115].

Finally, extrathoracic symptoms include paraneoplastic syndromes and metastatic symptoms. Pananeoplastic syndromes include those symptoms related to the primary tumor or its metastases by hormonal intermediates. Manifestations include skeletal syndromes or endocrine manifestation such as cachexia, hypercalcemia, and hypertrophic pulmonary osteoarthropathy. Among skeletal syndromes, clubbing from hypertrophic pulmonary osteoarthropathy occurs in an estimated 5% of NSCLC patients and is the most common such syndrome [116]. Inappropriate antidiuretic hormone secretion is an endocrine manifestation that occurs in up to 46% of SCLC patients. Symptoms include anorexia, nausea, vomiting, confusion, lethargy and seizures. Hypercalcemia develops in 10% of lung cancer patients and is associated with squamous cell cancer.

Lung cancer most frequently metastasizes to the brain, spinal cord, bone, liver, lung, adrenal glands and soft tissues. Approximately 25% of lung cancer patients develop bony metastases. An estimated 10% of patients present with and another 10 to 15% eventually develop central nervous system related metastases, most of which are asymptomatic. Anorexia, unplanned weight loss and fatigue are common symptoms nonspecific to possible metastases and should be discussed with patients by clinicians as their presence should initiate a search for metastatic disease [115].

## Asymptomatic Disease: Incidental and Screening Detection

Individuals presenting for diagnosis of nodules or anomalies found on screening low dose computed tomography (LDCT) represent a novel population for clinicians. Only since May and June of 2012 have a number of societies proposed interim guidelines for screening of lung cancer. Cancers which present with symptoms commonly are later stage disease (stage IV, 40% and stage III, 30%-40%) and subsequently have poor prognosis for survival [117, 118]. Given the poor survival of late stage lung cancer and cost of treatment, early detection of lung cancer through screening of high risk populations may be a clinically viable and cost-effective intervention.

The recently concluded National Lung Screening Trial (NLST) screened individuals at high risk for lung cancer with LDCT or chest x-ray. The study found a 20% decrease in lung cancer related mortality in the LDCT arm compared to those randomized to the chest x-ray arm. All-cause mortality was 7% less in the LDCT arm as well. The success of low dose computed tomography in reducing mortality compared to chest radiograph in the NLST has caused the leading physician and patient advocate groups to propose screening guidelines for lung cancer.

The American College of Chest Physicians (ACCP), American Society of Clinical Oncology, National Comprehensive Cancer Network (NCCN), American Association of Thoracic Surgery, American Cancer Society, American Lung Association and American Thoracic Society all endorse using the NLST study criteria as the basis for lung cancer screening, see Table 1 [117].

In addition, the NCCN also expanded the possible pool of those to be screened to persons age 50 to 74 with more than 20 pack year history of smoking who also have a secondary risk factor including any, family history of lung cancer in first degree relative, previous cancer, asbestos or radon exposure, chronic obstructive pulmonary disease, or occupational exposure to a known lung carcinogen [119]. Cost effectiveness of LDCT screening has been estimated as low as $19,000[120] to over $110,000 per quality adjusted life year using the NLST based risk criteria [121] for screening inclusion and accepted screening guidelines described above. More accurate estimates of cost-effectiveness within the NLST are expected to be published shortly [122].

**Table 1. Screening Criteria Risk Status – National Comprehensive Cancer Network**

| High Risk | Moderate Risk | Low Risk |
|---|---|---|
| Age 55 -74 | Age ≥ 50 | Age < 50 |
| ≥ 30 pack year history | ≥ 20 pack year history OR second-hand smoke exposure | < 20 pack year history of smoking |
| Current smoker OR Smoking cessation ≤ 15 years | No additional risk factors | |
| *OR*[a] Age ≥ 50 | | |
| ≥ 20 pack year history OR second-hand smoke exposure | | |
| One additional risk factor (other than second-hand smoke)[b] | | |

[a] NCCN criteria category 2B level of evidence.

[b] Risks include - Radon exposure, asbestos exposure, occupational exposure, cancer history, family history, other lung disease (COPD or pulmonary fibrosis).

# Diagnosis of Suspected Lung Cancer

The diagnosis of suspected lung cancer is as much art as science. The clinician must individualize care by weighing the risks of increasingly invasive procedures, the patient's physiological status, with the need to timely treat the most deadly of cancers. The diagnosis of lung cancer, as described hereafter, relies upon NCCN, ACCP as well as Fleischner Society guidelines which both the NCCN and ACCP guidelines incorporate into their clinical guidelines [113, 114, 119, 123-125]. Additional guidance for lung cancer screening and diagnosis are included as well since the experience and clinical issues arising from screening CT scans are addressed in most recent guidance [119]. Readers should refer to the primary literature referenced and individual societies' websites for updates to clinical guidelines discussed here.

Suspected lung cancer can present in three ways: symptomatically, incidentally from imaging for another diagnostic purpose or an anomaly from periodic screening. Anomalies or lesions of the lung are generally classified according to size at maximum average diameter and morphological characteristics that are observable on radiograph. Lung nodules are larger than 3mm in maximum diameter and less than 30mm (Figure 6A). Lung masses are 30mm and larger in size. Nodules and masses appear as generally solid collections of tissue on CT scan (Figure 6B). Ground glass opacities and ground glass nodules can vary widely in size and are characterized by their non-solid appearance or consistency on imaging (Figure 6C).

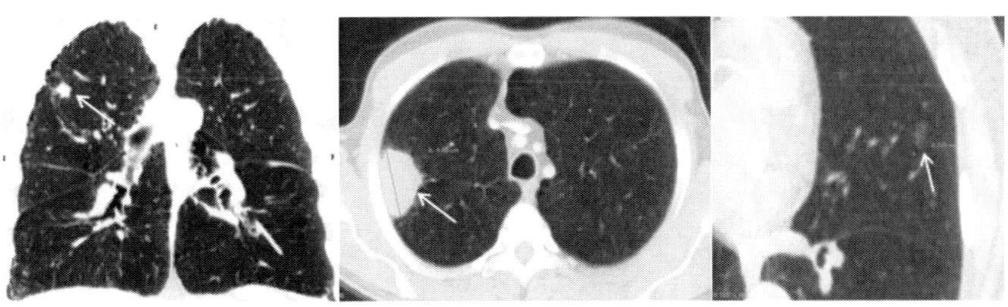

A B C

Figure 6(A). Spiculated Nodule; (B). Spiculated Lung Mass; (C). Ground Glass Opacity.

## Diagnosis Based on Imaging Characteristics

Other important physical characteristics of a lung lesion are calcification and edge shape. Partial or complete calcification is an indication of benign etiology. Smooth edges of a lesion are an indication of likely calcification or another benign disease process. Irregular edge characteristics including lobulated and especially coronal or spiculated edge (Figures 6A and 6B) are more likely to be cancer [126]. The location of the lesion within the lung often determines the applicable method of biopsy and may influence whether the individual is a candidate for surgical treatment. Peripheral lesions occur in the outer third of the lung and are more amenable to transthoracic CT guided fine needle aspiration. Central lesions occur in the interior two thirds and may be more accessible by bronchoscopic techniques [123].

Lung nodule diagnosis is different when the nodule is solid or partially solid compared to nodules with ground glass consistency or non-solid. The diagnostic regimen for solid or partially solid nodule without patterns of calcification or other characteristics of benign disease depends upon the lesions maximum size. For lesions 4mm or smaller in size, monitoring with annual LDCT is recommended for at least 2 years. Lesions 4 to 6mm in maximum diameter should receive a follow-up LDCT in 6 months while lesions 6-8mm in diameter should receive a follow-up LDCT in 3 months. If on any follow-up LDCT growth occurs, then the individual should be evaluated for biopsy or surgical excision. Growth on serial radiographs is defined as an increase in mean diameter of 2mm for nodules initially less than 15mm in size and an increase of at least 15% compared to baseline scan for nodules more than 15mm in size at baseline [119]. However, a rapid increase in size should raise the suspicion of an inflammatory process or the possibility of cancer other than NSCLC. If inflammation or infection is suspected, then a round of antibiotics which also includes anaerobic spectrum should be considered.

Nodules greater than 8mm are candidates for evaluation by combined 18-fluorodeoxyglucose positron emission tomographic and computed tomographic scan (FDG-PET). A negative FDG-PET scan indicates low likelihood of cancer and continued monitoring in 3 months with a LDCT is sufficient. A scan with hypermetabolism above the background of surrounding parenchyma, regardless of absolute or maximum uptake value is indicative of possible cancer. Biopsy or surgical excision should then be pursued to obtain pathological tissue diagnosis. Endobronchial nodules should be evaluated by LDCT within a month of discovery and if the lesion is symptomatic or doesnot resolve, then bronchoscopy and tissue diagnosis pursued. For any nodule that is stable or decreases in size on subsequent LDCT, continued surveillance with decreasingly frequent LDCT with a maximum annual interval is warranted for an additional two years. Continued annual LDCT should be considered for those patients who are eligible for lung cancer screening until the individual is no longer eligible for definitive treatment of a lung cancer that could occur.

Nodules with ground glass or nonsolid characteristics are also evaluated based upon size at baseline. Those nodules that are less than 5mm in diameter on baseline radiograph should be re-evaluated by annual LDCT. Similar nodules whose diameter is between 5 and 10mm should receive a follow-up LDCT in 6 months and nodules larger than 10mm should get a LDCT in 3 to 6 months. If growth is observed or if the nodule becomes increasingly solid on subsequent LDCT irrespective of size on baseline radiograph, then biopsy or surgical excision should be explored. For those lesions under 5mm on baseline radiograph, the clinician may also consider an additional LDCT scan in 3-6 months rather than biopsy. For ground glass lesions larger than 10mm on initial scan, the clinician may consider biopsy or excision over waiting 3-6 months for another scan as these nodules are more likely cancerous. If the nodule is stable on subsequent LDCT and its size is not greater than 10mm, then continued surveillance with annual LDCT is warranted for an additional two years or until the individual is no longer eligible for definitive treatment.

# Diagnostic Strategies

Clinicians evaluating a patient with a symptomatic or asymptomatic nodule should estimate the probability of cancer. This estimate should be based upon either clinical judgment or by a validated prediction model using all information available including previous radiographs and biopsies at the time of evaluation [114, 123].

Currently, a number of predictive models have been validated for lung cancer. The most widely used in the US are the Mayo [126, 127] and the Bach models [28, 128]. Other models including those by Spitz and Cassidy have been validated and published in the literature [129-132]. A single institution model developed in a chinese populationhas not been validated in separate populations but may be more accurate in the population it was developed or in the case of the Solitary Pulmonary Nodule model developed by Gurney and colleagues and validated by Isbell et. al. (2011), the model includes a wider variety of information available to the surgeon or pulmonologist [21, 133, 134]. Clinician estimation of lung cancer risk was found to be similarly accurate to the Mayo model in a study comparing predictive accuracy [135].

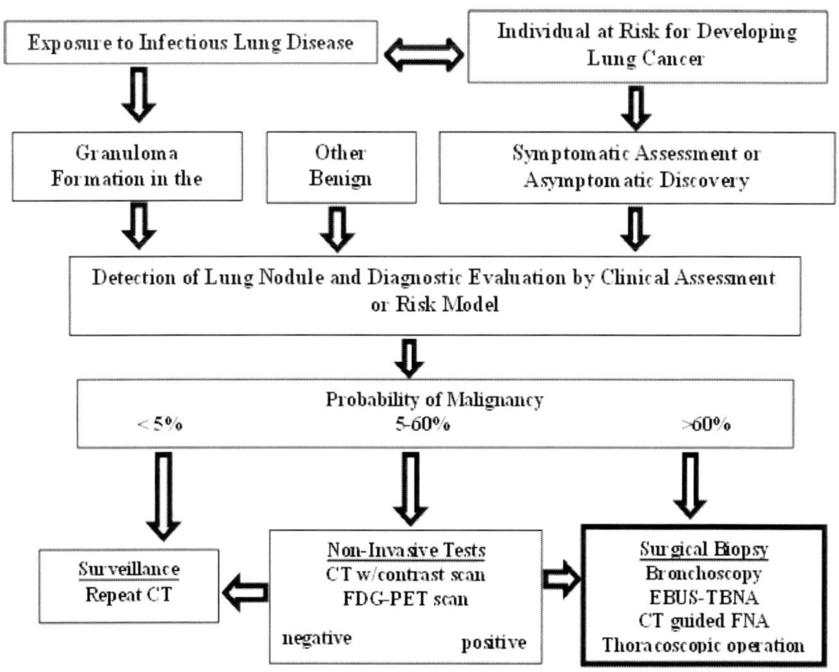


Figure 7. Diagnostic Guidelines of Nodules, Suspicious for Lung Cancer (from Wahidi, 2007).

Model accuracy for predicting lung cancer measured by area under the receiver operator curve (ROC) ranges from 75 to 90%. Predictive accuracy is generally lower in the validation population with ROC of 70-85%.

When the estimated probability of cancer is below 5% then continued surveillance is warranted with additional LDCT imaging based upon lesion size as described above or high dose thin slice CT with contrast media followed by annual LDCT. If after 2 years of surveillance no change is observed or indications of benign disease occur, e.g. calcification, smooth edges or shrinkage of lesion diameter, then active surveillance should be stopped. In surgical candidates with an indeterminate nodule that measures at least 8mm in diameter a tissue diagnosis is preferred when the probability is greater than 60% or moderate to high (Figure 7).

In patients with an intermediate probability of cancer (5 to 60%) additional evaluation is warranted including FDG-PET scan or thin slice CT with contrast if contrast will be tolerated by the patient. Whenever growth or hypermetabolic activity are observed, then definitive tissue diagnosis should be obtained by the most appropriate means including surgical resection, transthoracic needle biopsy, endobronchial ultrasound and biopsy, CT guided needle biopsy or bronchoscopy. Three studies have found that FDG-PET scans are less accurate due to granulomatous lung disease in their geographic regions [136-138]. Granulomatous disease most frequently arises from fungal lung diseases in the US and from tuberculosis in regions where it is prevalent. The three major mycotic infections in order of North American prevalence are histoplasmosis, coccidioidomycosis and blastomycosis. Granuloma formation in the lung is one possible result for all three of the most common fungal infections found in the US. Granulomatous disease of the lung can look identical to cancerous tissue on CT or PET scan and can have all the hallmarks of a cancerous lesion including symptomatic hemoptysis, growth on repeated CT scans, spiculated edge characteristics and lack of calcification [139]. In those instances FDG-PET scans are plagued by false positive results and previous CT scans or a CT scan with contrast for diagnosis may provide similar information [136, 137].

Because the lung is difficult to access, obtaining a tissue diagnosis is not without significant risk. Fine needle aspiration and transthoracic needle lung biopsy are frequently complicated by pneumothorax (15-25%) and other complications [140-143]. The accuracy of bronchoscopy is highly dependent on the location and size of the tumor relative to the airway and has a lower complication rate for bleeding or pneumothorax than needle biopsy. Non-diagnostic results can occur in up to 30% of case series, greatly limiting its utility especially for peripheral lesions [144]. Thoracoscopic surgery in the NLST had a 24% benign disease result rate at final pathology [122]. These individuals also experienced a 1% mortality rate from their lung operation and others have found the mortality rate for thoracoscopic surgery to be even higher between 1 and 5%, depending upon the population and specialization of the surgeon [145, 146].

## Conclusion

Lung cancer remains the most deadly of cancers. However, the advent of LDCT screening may reduce the mortality from the disease and increase the number of survivors. A debate regarding screening, its efficacy, overdiagnosis and cost effectiveness began well before the results of the National Lung Screening Trial were released and continues [117, 146-150]. Implementation of a national screening program for lung cancer will result in an enormous increased volume of pulmonary nodules in need of a diagnosis. A personalized diagnostic plan developed for patients with suspected lung cancer depends upon the patient's risk factors for developing cancer and the accuracy of the diagnostic imaging that is specific to the patient's geographic location. The clinician must weigh the risks and discuss those risks candidly with their patients and their options of care.

# References


[1] Siegel R, Ward E, Brawley O, Jemal A. Cancer statistics, 2011. *CA: A Cancer Journal for Clinicians.* 2011;61(4):212-36.

[2] Kohler BA, Ward E, McCarthy BJ, Schymura MJ, Ries LAG, Eheman C, et al. Annual Report to the Nation on the Status of Cancer, 1975–2007, Featuring Tumors of the Brain and Other Nervous System. *Journal of the National Cancer Institute.* 2011 May 4, 2011;103(9):714-36.

[3] Vallieres EMDF, Shepherd FAMDF, Crowley JP, Van Houtte PMD, Postmus PEMDP, Carney DMDP, et al. The IASLC Lung Cancer Staging Project: Proposals Regarding the Relevance of TNM in the Pathologic Staging of Small Cell Lung Cancer in the Forthcoming (Seventh) Edition of the TNM Classification for Lung Cancer. *Journal of Thoracic Oncology.* 2009;4(9):1049-59.

[4] National CI. *Cancer Trends Progress Report - 2009-2010* Update. National Cancer Institute; 2010 [updated 4/15/2010; cited 2012 01/20/2012].

[5] Bradley CJ, Yabroff KR, Dahman B, Feuer EJ, Mariotto A, Brown ML. Productivity Costs of Cancer Mortality in the United States: 2000–2020. *Journal of the National Cancer Institute.* 2008 December 17, 2008;100(24):1763-70.

[6] Alberg A, Ford J, Samet J. Epidemiology of lung cancer: ACCP evidence-based clinical practice guidelines (2nd edition). *Chest.* 2007;132:29S - 55S.

[7] Howlader N, Noone A, Krapcho M, Neyman N, Aminou R, Altekruse S, et al. SEER Cancer Statistics Review, 1975-2009. Bethesda, MD: National Cancer Institute; 2012 [updated April, 2012; cited 2012 6/8/2012]; Available from: *http://seer.cancer.gov/csr/1975_2009_pops09/index.html.*

[8] National Cancer Institute. *Fast Stats.* National Cancer Institute; 2012 [updated 4/11/2011; cited 2012 01/23/2012].

[9] National Cancer Institute. State cancer profiles. 2011 [updated 11/18/2011; cited 2011 12/01/2011]; Available from: *http://statecancerprofiles.cancer. gov/.*

[10] Shibuya K, Inoue M, Lopez AD. Statistical modeling and projections of lung cancer mortality in 4 industrialized countries. *International Journal of Cancer.* 2005;117(3):476-85.

[11] Jemal A, Center MM, DeSantis C, Ward EM. Global patterns of cancer incidence and mortality rates and trends. *Cancer Epidemiol Biomarkers Prev.* 2010 Aug;19(8):1893-907.

[12] WHO. GLOBOCAN 2008: World Cancer statistics. 2008 [cited 2011 04-11-2012]; Available from: *http://globocan.iarc.fr/factsheets/populations/ factsheet.asp?uno=900.*
[13] Liu B-Q, Peto R, Chen Z-M, Boreham J, Wu Y-P, Li J-Y, et al. Emerging tobacco hazards in China: 1. Retrospective proportional mortality study of one million deaths. *BMJ*. 1998 November 21, 1998;317(7170):1411-22.
[14] Youlden DR, Cramb SM, Baade PD. The International Epidemiology of Lung Cancer: Geographical Distribution and Secular Trends. *Journal of Thoracic Oncology*. 2008;3(8):819-31 10.1097/JTO.0b013e31818020eb.
[15] Thun MJ, Hannan LM, Adams-Campbell LL, Boffetta P, Buring JE, Feskanich D, et al. Lung Cancer Occurrence in Never-Smokers: An Analysis of 13 Cohorts and 22 Cancer Registry Studies. *PLoS Med*. 2008;5(9):e185.
[16] National Cancer Institute. Table I-11 Median Age of Patients at Diagnosis, 2004-2008. National Cancer Institute; 2011 [cited 2012 01/23/2012]; Available from: *http://seer.cancer.gov/csr/1975_2008/results_single/sect _01_table.11_2pgs.pdf.*
[17] Doll R, Hill A. The mortaltiy of doctors in relation to theri smoking habits; a preliminary report. *British Medical Journal*. 1954;1(4877):1451-5.
[18] US Department of Health and Welfare. Smoking and health: a report of the Advisory Committee to the Surgeon General. In: *US Department of Health and Welfare*, editor. Washington DC: US Printing Office; 1964.
[19] Hecht SS. Tobacco smoke carcinogens and lung cancer. *J Natl Cancer Inst*. 1999;91(14):1194-210.
[20] Paz-Elizur T, Krupsky M, Blumenstein S, Elinger D, Schechtman E, Livneh Z. DNA repair activity for oxidative damage and risk of lung cancer. *J Natl Cancer Inst*. 2003 Sep 3;95(17):1312-9.
[21] Gurney JW, Lyddon DM, McKay JA. Determining the likelihood of malignancy in solitary pulmonary nodules with Bayesian analysis. Part II. Application. *Radiology*. 1993 February 1993;186(2):415-22.
[22] Tammemagi MCP, Freedman MTMD, Pinsky PFP, et al. Prediction of True Positive Lung Cancers in Individuals with Abnormal Suspicious Chest Radiographs-A Prostate, Lung, Colorectal, and Ovarian Cancer Screening Trial Study. *Journal of Thoracic Oncology*. 2009;4(6):710-21.
[23] Song Y-M, Sung J, Cho H-J. Reduction and Cessation of Cigarette Smoking and Risk of Cancer: A Cohort Study of Korean Men. *Journal of Clinical Oncology*. 2008 November 1, 2008;26(31):5101-6.
[24] Ebbert JO, Yang P, Vachon CM, et al. Lung Cancer Risk Reduction After Smoking Cessation: Observations From a Prospective Cohort of Women. *Journal of Clinical Oncology*. 2003 March 1, 2003;21(5):921-6.
[25] Alberg AJ, Nonemaker J. Who Is at High Risk for Lung Cancer? Population-Level and Individual-Level Perspectives. *Semin Respir Crit Care Med*. 2008 02.06.2008;29(03):223,32.
[26] Lubin JH, Caporaso N, Wichmann HE, et al. Cigarette Smoking and Lung Cancer: Modeling Effect Modification of Total Exposure and Intensity. *Epidemiology*. 2007;18(5):639-48.
[27] Burns D, Anderson C, Gray N. Has the lung cancer risk from smoking increased over the last fifty years? *Cancer Causes and Control*. 2011;22(3):389-97.

[28] Bach PB, Kattan MW, Thornquist MD, et al. Variations in lung cancer risk among smokers. *J Natl Cancer Inst.* 2003 Mar 19;95(6):470-8.
[29] Henschke CI, Miettinen OS. Women's susceptibility to tobacco carcinogens. *Lung Cancer.* 2004;43(1):1-5.
[30] Henschke CI, Yip R, Miettinen OS. Women's susceptibility to tobacco carcinogens and survival after diagnosis of lung cancer. *JAMA*. 2006 Jul 12;296(2):180-4.
[31] Risch HA, Howe GR, Jain M, et al. Are Female Smokers at Higher Risk for Lung Cancer than Male Smokers? *American Journal of Epidemiology.* 1993 September 1, 1993;138(5):281-93.
[32] American Lung Association. *Trends in tobacco use*, 2011.
[33] Jemal A, Travis WD, Tarone RE, Travis L, Devesa SS. Lung cancer rates convergence in young men and women in the United States: Analysis by birth cohort and histologic type. *International Journal of Cancer.* 2003;105(1):101-7.
[34] Bain C, Feskanich D, Speizer FE, et al. Lung Cancer Rates in Men and Women With Comparable Histories of Smoking. *Journal of the National Cancer Institute.* 2004 June 2, 2004;96(11):826-34.
[35] Freedman N, Leitzmann M, Hollenbeck A, et al. Cigarette smoking and subsequent risk of lung cancer in men and women: analysis of a prospective cohort study. *Lancet Oncol.* 2008;9:649 - 56.
[36] Thun MJ, Jemal A. How much of the decrease in cancer death rates in the United States is attributable to reductions in tobacco smoking? *Tob Control.* 2006 Oct;15(5):345-7.
[37] Jemal A, Ward E, Thun M. Declining death rates reflect progress against cancer. *PLoS One.* 2010;5(3):e9584.
[38] Wong MP, Fung L-F, Wang E, et al. Chromosomal aberrations of primary lung adenocarcinomas in nonsmokers. *Cancer.* 2003;97(5):1263-70.
[39] Patel JD. Lung Cancer in Women. *Journal of Clinical Oncology.* 2005 May 10, 2005;23(14):3212-8.
[40] Kligerman S, White C. Epidemiology of Lung Cancer in Women: Risk Factors, Survival, and Screening. *American Journal of Roentgenology.* 2011 February 1, 2011;196(2):287-95.
[41] Davis DL. Trends in Nonsmoking Lung Cancer. *Epidemiology.* 1993;4(6):489-91.
[42] Thun MJ, Henley SJ, Burns D, et al. Lung Cancer Death Rates in Lifelong Nonsmokers. *Journal of the National Cancer Institute.* 2006 17 May 2006;98(10):691-9.
[43] Haiman CA, Stram DO, Wilkens LR, et al. Ethnic and Racial Differences in the Smoking-Related Risk of Lung Cancer. *New England Journal of Medicine.* 2006;354(4):333-42.
[44] Stellman SD, Chen Y, Muscat JE, et al. Lung cancer risk in white and black Americans. *Ann Epidemiol.* 2003 Apr;13(4):294-302.
[45] Kabat GC, Shivappa N, Hébert JR. Mentholated cigarettes and smoking-related cancers revisited: An ecologic examination. *Regulatory Toxicology and Pharmacology.* 2012;63(1):132-9.
[46] Okuyemi KS, Faseru B, Sanderson Cox L, et al. Relationship between menthol cigarettes and smoking cessation among African American light smokers. *Addiction.* 2007;102(12):1979-86.

[47] Blot WJ, Cohen SS, Aldrich M, et al. Lung cancer risk among smokers of menthol cigarettes. *J Natl Cancer Inst.* 2011 May 18;103(10):810-6.

[48] Murray RP, Connett JE, Skeans MA, Tashkin DP. Menthol Cigarettes and Health Risks in Lung Health Study Data. *Nicotine and Tobacco Research.* 2007 January 1, 2007;9(1):101-7.

[49] Westmaas J, Brandon T. Reducing Risk in Smokers. *Current Opinion in Pulmonary Medicine.* 2004;10(4):284-8.

[50] Halpern MT, Gillespie BW, Warner KE. Patterns of Absolute Risk of Lung Cancer Mortality in Former Smokers. *Journal of the National Cancer Institute.* 1993 March 17, 1993;85(6):457-64.

[51] Peto R, Darby S, Deo H, et al. Smoking, smoking cessation, and lung cancer in the UK since 1950: combination of national statistics with two case-control studies. *Bmj.* 2000;321(7257):323-9.

[52] US Department of Health and Human Services. The Health Consequences of Smoking: A Report of the Surgeon General. In: *U.S. Department of Health and Human Services PHS*, editor. Rockville, MD: Centers for Disease Control 2004.

[53] Ando M, Wakai K, Seki N, et al. Attributable and absolute risk of lung cancer death by smoking status: Findings from the Japan collaborative cohort study. *International Journal of Cancer.* 2003;105(2):249-54.

[54] Burns DM. Primary prevention, smoking, and smoking cessation: implications for future trends in lung cancer prevention. *Cancer.* 2000;89(11 Suppl):2506-9.

[55] Samet JM, Avila-Tang E, Boffetta P, et al. Lung Cancer in Never Smokers: Clinical Epidemiology and Environmental Risk Factors. *Clinical Cancer Research.* 2009 September 15, 2009;15(18):5626-45.

[56] Hirayama T. Non-smoking wives of heavy smokers have a higher risk of lung cancer: a study from Japan. *BMJ.* 1981 1981-01-17 00:00:00;282(6259):183-5.

[57] Trichopoulos D, Kalandidi A, Sparros L, MacMahon B. Lung cancer and passive smoking. *Int J Cancer.* 1981;27(1):1-4.

[58] Fontham Eh CPRP, et al. Environmental tobacco smoke and lung cancer in nonsmoking women: A multicenter study. *JAMA: The Journal of the American Medical Association.* 1994;271(22):1752-9.

[59] US Environmental Protection Agency. Respiratory health effects of passive smoking: lung cancer and other disorders. In: *EPA*, editor. Washington, DC: US Government Printing Office; 1992.

[60] Hackshaw AK, Law MR, Wald NJ. The accumulated evidence on lung cancer and environmental tobacco smoke. *BMJ.* 1997 October 18, 1997;315(7114):980-8.

[61] Boffetta P. Involuntary smoking and lung cancer. *Scand J Work Environ Health.* 2002;28(suppl 2):30-40.

[62] Taylor R, Gumming R, Woodward A, Black M. Passive smoking and lung cancer: a cumulative meta-analysis. *Australian and New Zealand Journal of Public Health.* 2001;25(3):203-11.

[63] Brennan P, Buffler PA, Reynolds P, Wu AH, Wichmann HE, Agudo A, et al. Secondhand smoke exposure in adulthood and risk of lung cancer among never smokers: A pooled analysis of two large studies. *International Journal of Cancer.* 2004;109(1):125-31.

[64] Hill SE, Blakely T, Kawachi I, Woodward A. Mortality among Lifelong Nonsmokers Exposed to Secondhand Smoke at Home: Cohort Data and Sensitivity Analyses. *American Journal of Epidemiology*. 2007 March 1, 2007;165(5):530-40.
[65] US Department of Health and Human Services. The Health Consequences of Involuntary Exposure to Tobacco Smoke: A Report of the Surgeon General. In: *U.S. Department of Health and Human Services CfDCaP,* Coordinating Center for Health Promotion, National Center for Chronic Disease Prevention and Health Promotion, Office on Smoking and Health, editor. Atlanta, GA:: U.S. Government Printing Office; 2006.
[66] Pirkle JL, Bernert JT, Caudill SP, et al. Trends in the Exposure of Nonsmokers in the U.S. Population to Secondhand Smoke: 1988–2002. *Environ Health Perspect.* 2006;114(6).
[67] Turner MC, Krewski D, Pope CA, et al. Long-term Ambient Fine Particulate Matter Air Pollution and Lung Cancer in a Large Cohort of Never-Smokers. *American Journal of Respiratory and Critical Care Medicine*. 2011 December 15, 2011;184(12):1374-81.
[68] EPA. *EPA Assessment of Risks from Radon in Homes*. EPA, editor. Washington DC: Office of Radiation and Indoor Air; 2003. p. 98.
[69] Committee on Health Risks of Exposure to Radon BV. *Health Effects of Exposure to Radon*. Council NR, editor: National Academies Press; 1999.
[70] Krewski D, Lubin JH, Zielinski JM, et al. A Combined Analysis of North American Case-Control Studies of Residential Radon and Lung Cancer. *Journal of Toxicology and Environmental Health, Part A*. 2006 2006/05/01;69(7-8):533-97.
[71] Schubauer-Berigan MK, Daniels RD, Pinkerton LE. Radon Exposure and Mortality Among White and American Indian Uranium Miners: An Update of the Colorado Plateau Cohort. *American Journal of Epidemiology*. 2009 March 15, 2009;169(6):718-30.
[72] Zeka A, Mannetje At, Zaridze D, et al. Lung Cancer and Occupation in Nonsmokers: A Multicenter Case-Control Study in Europe. *Epidemiology*. 2006;17(6):615-23.
[73] Veglia F, Vineis P, Overvad K, et al. Occupational Exposures, Environmental Tobacco Smoke, and Lung Cancer. *Epidemiology*. 2007;18(6):769-75.
[74] De Matteis S, Consonni D, Lubin JH, et al. Impact of occupational carcinogens on lung cancer risk in a general population. *Int J Epidemiol.* 2012 March 31, 2012.
[75] Brown T, Darnton A, Fortunato L, Rushton L. Occupational cancer in Britain. *Br J Cancer*. 2012;107(S1):S56-S70.
[76] *UK CR. UK Cancer Incidence (2009) and Mortality (2010) Summary*, May 2012.
[77] Doll R, Peto R. The causes of cancer: quantitative estimates of avoidable risks of cancer in the United States today. *J Natl Cancer Inst.* 1981;66(6):1191-308.
[78] Boffetta P, Autier P, Boniol M, et al. An Estimate of Cancers Attributable to Occupational Exposures in France. *Journal of Occupational and Environmental Medicine*. 2010;52(4):399-406.
[79] Olsson AC, Gustavsson P, Zaridze D, et al. Lung Cancer Risk Attributable to Occupational Exposures in a Multicenter Case-Control Study in Central and Eastern Europe. *Journal of Occupational and Environmental Medicine*. 2011;53(11):1262-7.
[80] Gallus S, Negri E, Boffetta P, et al. European studies on long-term exposure to ambient particulate matter and lung cancer. *European Journal of Cancer Prevention*. 2008;17(3):191-4.

[81] Pope CA, Burnett RT, Thun MJ, et al. Lung cancer, cardiopulmonary mortality, and long-term exposure to fine particulate air pollution. JAMA: *The Journal of the American Medical Association*. 2002;287(9):1132-1141.

[82] Whitrow MJ, Smith BJ, Pilotto LS, et al. Environmental exposure to carcinogens causing lung cancer: Epidemiological evidence from the medical literature. *Respirology*. 2003;8(4):513-21.

[83] Lan Q, He X, Shen M, et al. Variation in lung cancer risk by smoky coal subtype in Xuanwei, *China. International Journal of Cancer*. 2008;123(9):2164-9.

[84] Kodgule R, Salvi S. Exposure to biomass smoke as a cause for airway disease in women and children. *Current Opinion in Allergy and Clinical Immunology*. 2012;12(1):82-90.

[85] Hosgood HD, Wei H, Sapkota A, et al. Household coal use and lung cancer: systematic review and meta-analysis of case–control studies, with an emphasis on geographic variation. *Int J Epidemiol*. 2011 June 1, 2011;40(3):719-28.

[86] Lan Q, Chapman RS, Schreinemachers DM, et al. Household Stove Improvement and Risk of Lung Cancer in Xuanwei, China. *Journal of the National Cancer Institute*. 2002 June 5, 2002;94(11):826-35.

[87] Rauscher GH, Mayne ST, Janerich DT. Relation between Body Mass Index and Lung Cancer Risk in Men and Women Never and Former Smokers. *American Journal of Epidemiology*. 2000 September 15, 2000;152(6):506-13.

[88] Smith L, Brinton LA, Spitz MR, et al. Body Mass Index and Risk of Lung Cancer Among Never, Former, and Current Smokers. *Journal of the National Cancer Institute*. 2012 March 27, 2012.

[89] Tarnaud C, Guida F, Papadopoulos A, et al. Body mass index and lung cancer risk: results from the ICARE study, a large, population-based case–control study. *Cancer Causes and Control*. 2012;23(7):1113-26.

[90] Crapo JD. Preclinical vascular disease identifies smokers at risk for COPD. *Proceedings of the National Academy of Sciences*. 2010 May 11, 2010;107(19):8503-4.

[91] Young RP, Hopkins RJ, Christmas T, et al. COPD prevalence is increased in lung cancer, independent of age, sex and smoking history. *European Respiratory Journal*. 2009 August 1, 2009;34(2):380-6.

[92] de Torres JP, Marín JM, Casanova C, et al. Lung Cancer in Patients with Chronic Obstructive Pulmonary Disease. *American Journal of Respiratory and Critical Care Medicine*. 2011 October 15, 2011;184(8):913-9.

[93] Koshiol J, Rotunno M, Consonni D, et al. Chronic Obstructive Pulmonary Disease and Altered Risk of Lung Cancer in a Population-Based Case-Control Study. *PLoS One*. 2009;4(10):e7380.

[94] Beane J, Sebastiani P, Liu G, et al. Reversible and permanent effects of tobacco smoke exposure on airway epithelial gene expression. *Genome Biol*. 2007;8(9):R201.

[95] Brody JS, Spira A. State of the art. Chronic obstructive pulmonary disease, inflammation, and lung cancer. *Proc Am Thorac Soc*. 2006 Aug;3(6):535-7.

[96] Usui K, Tanai C, Tanaka Y, et al. The prevalence of pulmonary fibrosis combined with emphysema in patients with lung cancer. *Respirology*. 2011;16(2):326-31.

[97] Mizuno S, Takiguchi Y, Fujikawa A, Motoori K, Tada Y, Kurosu K, et al. Chronic obstructive pulmonary disease and interstitial lung disease in patients with lung cancer. *Respirology*. 2009;14(3):377-83.

[98] Sekine Y, Katsura H, Koh E, et al. Early detection of COPD is important for lung cancer surveillance. *European Respiratory Journal. 2011* November 16, 2011.
[99] Matakidou A, Eisen T, Houlston RS. Systematic review of the relationship between family history and lung cancer risk. *Br J Cancer*. 2005;93(7):825-33.
[100] Braun MM, Caporaso NE, Hoover RN, Page WF. Genetic component of lung cancer: cohort study of twins. *The Lancet*. 1994;344(8920):440-3.
[101] Bailey-Wilson JE, Amos CI, Pinney SM, Petersen GM, de Andrade M, Wiest JS, et al. A major lung cancer susceptibility locus maps to chromosome 6q23-25. *Am J Hum Genet*. 2004 Sep;75(3):460-74.
[102] Ji Y-n, Wang Q, Lin X-q, Suo L-j. CYP1A1 MspI polymorphisms and lung cancer risk: An updated meta-analysis involving 20,209 subjects. *Cytokine*. 2012;59(2):324-34.
[103] Pavanello S, Fedeli U, Mastrangelo G, et al. Role of CYP1A2 polymorphisms on lung cancer risk in a prospective study. *Cancer Genetics*. 2012;205(6):278-84.
[104] McWilliams JE, Sanderson BJ, Harris EL, et al. Glutathione S-transferase M1 (GSTM1) deficiency and lung cancer risk. *Cancer Epidemiol Biomarkers Prev*. 1995;4(6):589-94.
[105] Ye Z, Song H, Higgins JP, et al. Five glutathione s-transferase gene variants in 23,452 cases of lung cancer and 30,397 controls: meta-analysis of 130 studies. *PLoS Med*. 2006 Apr;3(4):e91.
[106] Tsou JA, Hagen JA, Carpenter CL, Laird-Offringa IA. DNA methylation analysis: a powerful new tool for lung cancer diagnosis. *Oncogene*. 2002 Aug 12;21(35):5450-61.
[107] Schwartz AG, Prysak GM, Bock CH, Cote ML. The molecular epidemiology of lung cancer. *Carcinogenesis*. 2007 Mar;28(3):507-18.
[108] Chen L-S, Saccone NL, Culverhouse RC, et al. Smoking and Genetic Risk Variation Across Populations of European, Asian, and African American Ancestry—A Meta-Analysis of Chromosome 15q25. *Genetic Epidemiology*. 2012;36(4):340-51.
[109] Truong T, Hung RJ, Amos CI, et al. Replication of Lung Cancer Susceptibility Loci at Chromosomes 15q25, 5p15, and 6p21: A Pooled Analysis From the International Lung Cancer Consortium. *Journal of the National Cancer Institute*. 2010 July 7, 2010;102(13):959-71.
[110] Hung RJ, Christiani DC, Risch A, et al. International Lung Cancer Consortium: Pooled Analysis of Sequence Variants in DNA Repair and Cell Cycle Pathways. *Cancer Epidemiology Biomarkers and Prevention*. 2008 November 1, 2008;17(11):3081-9.
[111] Gao Y, Blot WJ, Zheng W, et al. Lung cancer among Chinese women. *Int J Cancer*. 1987;40(5):604-9.
[112] Ladanyi M, Pao W. Lung adenocarcinoma: guiding EGFR-targeted therapy and beyond. *Mod Pathol*. 2008;21(S2):S16-S22.
[113] Alberts WM. Epidemiology of Lung Cancer ACCP Evidence-Based Clinical Practice Guidelines (2nd Edition). *Chest*. 2007;132:29S-55S.
[114] Gould MK, Fletcher J, Iannettoni MD, et al. Evaluation of patients with pulmonary nodules: when is it lung cancer?: ACCP evidence-based clinical practice guidelines (2nd edition). *Chest*. 2007 Sep;132(3 Suppl):108S-30S.
[115] Patterson GA, editor. *Pearson's Thoracic and Esophageal Surgery 3ed:* Elsevier; 2008.
[116] Izumi M, Takayama K, Yabuuchi H, et al. Incidence of hypertrophic pulmonary osteoarthropathy associated with primary lung cancer. *Respirology*. 2010;15(5):809-12.

[117] Bach PB, Mirkin JN, Oliver TK, et al. Benefits and harms of ct screening for lung cancer: A systematic review. *JAMA: The Journal of the American Medical Association*. 2012;307(22):2418-29.

[118] Corner J, Hopkinson J, Fitzsimmons D, et al. Is late diagnosis of lung cancer inevitable? Interview study of patients' recollections of symptoms before diagnosis. *Thorax*. 2005 April 1, 2005;60(4):314-9.

[119] National Comprehensive Cancer Network. Lung Cancer Screening v1.2012. NCCN Clinical Practice Guidelines in Oncology (NCCN Guidelines) [serial on the Internet]. 2011 [cited 2011 10-26-2011]: Available from: *http://www.nccn.org/professionals/physician_gls/recently_updated.asp*.

[120] Pyenson BS, Sander MS, Jiang Y, Kahn H, Mulshine JL. An Actuarial Analysis Shows That Offering Lung Cancer Screening As An Insurance Benefit Would Save Lives At Relatively Low Cost. *Health Affairs*. 2012 April 1, 2012;31(4):770-9.

[121] McMahon PM, Kong CY, Bouzan C, et al. Cost-Effectiveness of Computed Tomography Screening for Lung Cancer in the United States. *Journal of Thoracic Oncology*. 2011;6(11):1841-8.

[122] National Lung Screening Trial Research Team, Aberle DR, Adams AM, Berg C, Black WC, Clapp JD, et al. Reduced Lung-Cancer Mortality with Low-Dose Computed Tomographic Screening. New England Journal of Medicine. 2011;365(5):395-409.

[123] Rivera MP, Mehta AC. Initial diagnosis of lung cancer: ACCP evidence-based clinical practice guidelines (2nd edition). *Chest*. 2007 Sep;132(3 Suppl):131S-48S.

[124] Wahidi MM, Govert JA, Goudar RK, et al. Evidence for the treatment of patients with pulmonary nodules: when is it lung cancer?: ACCP evidence-based clinical practice guidelines (2nd edition). *Chest*. 2007 Sep;132(3 Suppl):94S-107S.

[125] MacMahon H, Austin J, Gamsu G, et al. Guidelines for management of small pulmonary nodules detected on CT scans: a statement from the Fleischner Society. *Radiology*. 2005;237:395 - 400.

[126] Swensen SJ, Silverstein MD, Ilstrup DM, et al. The Probability of Malignancy in Solitary Pulmonary Nodules: Application to Small Radiologically Indeterminate Nodules. *Arch Intern Med*. 1997 April 28, 1997;157(8):849-55.

[127] Herder GJ, van Tinteren H, Golding RP, et al. Clinical Prediction Model To Characterize Pulmonary Nodules*. *Chest*. 2005 October 2005;128(4):2490-6.

[128] Cronin KA, Gail MH, Zou Z, et al. Validation of a model of lung cancer risk prediction among smokers. *J Natl Cancer Inst*. 2006 May 3;98(9):637-40.

[129] Gould MK, Ananth L, Barnett PG. A clinical model to estimate the pretest probability of lung cancer in patients with solitary pulmonary nodules. *Chest*. 2007 Feb;131(2):383-8.

[130] Schultz EM, Sanders GD, Trotter PR, et al. Validation of two models to estimate the probability of malignancy in patients with solitary pulmonary nodules. *Thorax*. 2008 Apr;63(4):335-41.

[131] Cassidy A, Duffy SW, Myles JP, et al. Lung cancer risk prediction: A tool for early detection. *International Journal of Cancer*. 2007;120(1):1-6.

[132] Spitz MR, Etzel CJ, Dong Q, et al. An Expanded Risk Prediction Model for Lung Cancer. *Cancer Prev Res*. 2008 September 1, 2008;1(4):250-4.

[133] Li Y, Chen K-Z, Wang J. Development and Validation of a Clinical Prediction Model to Estimate the Probability of Malignancy in Solitary Pulmonary Nodules in Chinese People. *Clinical Lung Cancer*. 2011;12(5):313-9.

[134] Isbell JM, Deppen S, Putnam JB, Jr., et al. Existing general population models inaccurately predict lung cancer risk in patients referred for surgical evaluation. *The Annals of Thoracic Surgery*. Jan 2011;91(1):227-233; discussion 233.

[135] Swensen S, Silverstein M, Edell E, et al. Solitary pulmonary nodules: clinical prediction model versus physicians. *Mayo Clin Proc*. 1999;74:319 - 29.

[136] Croft DR, Trapp J, Kernstine K, et al. FDG-PET imaging and the diagnosis of non-small cell lung cancer in a region of high histoplasmosis prevalence. *Lung Cancer*. 2002;36(3):297-301.

[137] Deppen S, Putnam JB, Jr., Andrade G, et al. Accuracy of FDG-PET to diagnose lung cancer in a region of endemic granulomatous disease. *The Annals of Thoracic Surgery*. 2011 Aug;92(2):428-32; discussion 33.

[138] Sit AK, Sihoe AD, Suen WS, Cheng LC. Positron-Emission Tomography for Lung Cancer in a Tuberculosis-Endemic Region. *Asian Cardiovasc Thorac Ann*. February 1, 2010;18(1):33-8.

[139] Nguyen BD. F-18 FDG PET/CT Imaging of Disseminated Coccidioidomycosis. *Clinical Nuclear Medicine*. 2006;31(9):568-71.

[140] Wiener RS, Schwartz LM, Woloshin S, Welch HG. Population-Based Risk for Complications After Transthoracic Needle Lung Biopsy of a Pulmonary Nodule: An Analysis of Discharge Records. *Annals of Internal Medicine*. 2011 August 2, 2011;155(3):137-44.

[141] Anderson JM, Murchison J, Patel D. CT-guided lung biopsy: factors influencing diagnostic yield and complication rate. *Clin Radiol*. 2003 Oct;58(10):791-7.

[142] Ernst AMD, Eberhardt RMD, Krasnik MMD, Herth FJFMD. Efficacy of Endobronchial Ultrasound-Guided Transbronchial Needle Aspiration of Hilar Lymph Nodes for Diagnosing and Staging Cancer. *Journal of Thoracic Oncology*. 2009;4(8):947-50.

[143] Li H, Boiselle PM, Shepard JO, et al. Diagnostic accuracy and safety of CT-guided percutaneous needle aspiration biopsy of the lung: comparison of small and large pulmonary nodules. *AJR Am J Roentgenol*. 1996 Jul;167(1):105-9.

[144] National Comprehensive Cancer Network. The diagnosis and treatment of lung cancer; NICE CLinical Guideline 121. In: *Excellence NIfHaC*, editor.: National Institute for Health and Clinical Excellence; 2011.

[145] Grogan EL, Jones DR. VATS lobectomy is better than open thoracotomy: what is the evidence for short-term outcomes? *Thorac Surg Clin*. 2008 Aug;18(3):249-58.

[146] Silvestri GA. Screening for Lung Cancer: It Works, but Does It Really Work? *Annals of Internal Medicine*. 2011 September 5, 2011:E-364.

[147] Bach PB. Is our natural-history model of lung cancer wrong? *The Lancet Oncology*. 2008;9(7):693-7.

[148] Bach PB. Inconsistencies in Findings From the Early Lung Cancer Action Project Studies of Lung Cancer Screening. *Journal of the National Cancer Institute*. 2011 July 6, 2011;103(13):1002-6.

[149] Yankelevitz DF, Kostis WJ, Henschke CI, et al. Overdiagnosis in chest radiographic screening for lung carcinoma: frequency. *Cancer*. 2003 Mar 1;97(5):1271-5.

[150] Henschke CI. Survival of patients with clinical stage I lung cancer diagnosed by computed tomography screening for lung cancer. *Clin Cancer Res*. 2007 Sep 1;13(17):4949-50.

In: Lung Cancer: A Comprehensive Overview
Editor: Kathy Gately
ISBN: 978-1-62618-447-3


*Chapter III*

# The Effect of Smoking Habit Intensity, Occupation and Diet on Lung Cancer Risk in Males

*Agustina Bertola Compagnucci*[1,2], *María S Dagatti*[1] *and Stella M Pezzotto*[*1,2]
[1]Instituto de Inmunología, Facultad de Ciencias Médicas, Universidad Nacional de Rosario, Argentina
[2]Consejo de Investigaciones, Universidad Nacional de Rosario, Argentina

## Abstract

Lung cancer is a complex disease with multiple factors involved in the long process of carcinogenesis. Our group has investigated the risk factors that contribute to lung cancer in males living in Rosario, Argentina. This chapter presents the results of a case-control study carried out in this city; which is the third major urban concentration in the country. The city serves as a port for a large agricultural and cattle-raising area, and it also has several metal industries. This study includes 87 newly-diagnosed, histologically-confirmed male lung cancer patients and 153 male controls. These individuals were admitted to the same hospital as the cases with neither neoplasm nor lung diseases, nor their admission being unrelated to smoking or other potential lung cancer risk factors. Their main diagnostic categories were traumatic conditions, and acute surgical conditions. Lung cancer risk was high for heavy smokers (OR=2.5; 95% Cl=1.4–4.5). When comparing with the group unlikely to be exposed to occupational carcinogens, increased risks were observed for mechanics and metallurgic workers (OR=3.9; 95% CI=1.6–9.9), and for farmers (OR=2.6; 95% CI=1.3–5.4). The risk of lung cancer decreased in patients with high intakes of calcium (OR=0.34; 95% CI=0.14–0.84), magnesium (OR=0.23; 95% CI=0.07–0.72), and manganese (OR= 0.35; 95% CI=0.15–

[*] Correspondence to: Stella M. Pezzotto. Instituto de Inmunología, Facultad de Ciencias Médicas; Universidad Nacional de Rosario. Santa Fe 3100. 2000 Rosario, Argentina. E-mail: spezzot@unr.edu.ar. Fax: 00-54-341-4804569.

0.80). Likewise, Vitamins A, C and E showed some protective effect against lung cancer. Subjects in the highest consumption tertile had approximately 60% decrease in lung cancer risk compared with persons in the lowest tertile (A-vitamin: OR=0.42, 95% CI=0.19-0.90; C-vitamin: OR=0.39, 95% CI=0.18–0.84; E-vitamin: OR=0.41, 95% CI=0.18–0.96). There was no relationship between any B-vitamin intake and lung cancer risk. However, lung cancer risk was reduced by 59 percent in those with medium riboflavin intake (OR=0.41; 95% CI=0.18–0.97). No reduction in lung cancer risk was identified with vitamin supplementation. There is no question that tobacco smoking remains the most important modifiable risk factor for lung cancer. However, although more than 80% of lung cancers occur in subjects exposed to tobacco, fewer than 20% of smokers develop this disease. Therefore, the effects of other environmental factors, such as diet and occupational exposure to contaminants may modify the susceptibility of an individual to lung cancer. Lung cancer prevention programs must consider cigarette smoking, occupational exposures, and diet in order to reduce the numbers affected by this disease.

# Introduction

Lung cancer was recognised as a disease by the 19th century; however the link between cigarette smoking and lung cancer was made in the early 20th century. Lung cancer is now the world's leading cause of cancer-related death [1-3]. It is predicted to be a worldwide epidemic in this century producing a high morbi-mortality during the next 25 years [4]. Although more women are diagnosed with breast cancer, and more men with prostate cancer, lung cancer remains the leading cause of cancer deaths for both men and women. Approximately 1 million people worldwide die of this disease each year [5].

It is well known that chronic conditions such as cancer arise from the combination of multiple risk factors, including environmental exposures and genetic susceptibilities [6]. A methodical approach that does not investigate the complex multifactorial effects will unlikely be successful in explaining the occurrence of most common diseases. Most reports on the main factors contributing to lung cancer come from the Northern Hemisphere and there are very few studies published from Latin America. Differences in ethnic composition, socioeconomic profiles, and cultural heritage may also play a role in this disease.

It is almost unthinkable that the cure for lung cancer can be obtained in a short term. Therefore, face of evidence the relationship between this disease and some modifiable risk factors, much suffering and premature deaths could be avoided by strengthening the implementation of preventive measures. So, primary prevention through lifestyle and environmental interventions remains the main way to reduce the burden of this disease [7].

# Risk Factors

Approximately 30% of cancer deaths are due to the five leading behavioral and dietary risk factors including, tobacco use, low fruit and vegetable intake, lack of physical activity, alcohol use, and high body mass index (BMI) [8].

Over the past decades, numerous epidemiological studies have elucidated several important lung cancer risk factors including tobacco smoking, ionizing radiation, occupational exposure to some substances and diet [1, 2]. Moreover, it has been reported that lung cancer risk among men was consistently two to three fold higher in lower socioeconomic classes in developing countries [4], and that heavy alcohol consumption is a lung cancer risk factor among smokers [9].

This chapter provides a summary of the three main modifiable lung cancer risk factors, with an emphasis on issues that are currently relevant to prevention.

## Tobacco Smoking

While tobacco had been extensively used around the world for centuries, the ongoing epidemic of lung cancer followed the introduction of manufactured cigarettes with addictive properties. This has lead to a new pattern of exposure of the lung to inhaled carcinogens [1]. The role of tobacco smoking in increasing the risk of lung cancer is one of the best-known harmful effects of tobacco on human health. It was in 1950 that Doll and Hill in Britain [10] and Wynder and Graham in the United States [11] published their findings about the relationship between lung cancer and cigarette smoking. Since then, the evidence of increased lung cancer risk in smokers has been repeatedly confirmed [12]. Nowadays, tobacco use is the most important risk factor for cancer, causing 22% of global cancer deaths and 71% of global lung cancer deaths [8].

It has been estimated that up to 20% of all cancer deaths worldwide could be prevented by the elimination of tobacco smoking [13]. Nevertheless, the conclusion that cigarette smoking was a major cause of disease had not been easy for some to accept, particularly as it had serious economic implications for a major industry.

In a study about tobacco-attributable cancer burden in the UK in 2010, it was found that about 85% of the lung cancer cases in men are attributable to smoking, and in women the percentage is 80% [14]. The relative risk of lung cancer in long-term male smokers has been estimated as 10 to 20 fold compared with lifetime nonsmokers. The overall relative risk takes into consideration different characteristics of tobacco smoking such as, age at start, duration of the habit, average consumption, and time since quitting [4]. The intensity of the smoking habit is an important risk factor for lung cancer, as the risk increases succesively with the number of cigarettes smoked per day and duration of smoking [15]. When compared with never-smokers, subjects who smoke between 1-14 cigarettes a day have eight times the risk of dying from lung cancer and those who smoke 25 or more cigarettes a day have 25 times the risk. However, the risk is more dependent on duration of smoking habit than consumption: smoking one pack of cigarettes a day for 40 years is more hazardous than smoking two packs a day for 20 years [16].

It is well recognized that the risk of lung cancer declines after giving up smoking, even for people who have been smoking for many years. The extent of the reduction differs among the many reported investigations in a range of approximately 20 to 90 percent. Data from European countries support these results, leading to the conclusion that people who stop smoking, even well into middle age, avoid most of their subsequent risk of lung cancer, and stopping before middle age avoids more than 90% of the risk attributable to tobacco [17, 18]. It has been shown that a lifelong male smoker has a cumulative risk of 15.9% of dying from lung cancer by age 75. However, the cumulative risk of dying from lung cancer falls to 9.9%,

6.0%, 3.0%, and 1.7% for men who quit smoking at ages 60, 50, 40 and 30 years, respectively [17].

Although there is no doubt that tobacco smoking remains the most important risk factor for lung cancer, fewer than 20% of smokers develop the disease, indicating that other factors, such as occupational agents, or dietary habits, may influence the outcome of exposure to chemical carcinogens in tobacco smoke.

## Occupational Exposure

Occupational exposure to some workplace substances are either predicted to be or have been proven to be carcinogens in the lung [19-21]. A total of 29 occupational agents are established human carcinogens, and another 30 workplace substances are suspected carcinogens. The International Agency for Research on Cancer (IARC) has identified arsenic, asbestos, beryllium, cadmium, chloromethyl ethers, chromium, nickel, radon, silica, and vinyl chloride as carcinogens [22-24]. In 2000, an estimated 10% of lung cancer deaths among men and 5% among women worldwide were attributabed to exposure to eight occupational carcinogens, i.e. asbestos, arsenic, beryllium, cadmium, chromium, nickel, silica, and diesel fumes [25]. Furthermore, since these data apply only to known carcinogens, it is possible that the number of lung cancer cases related to occupational exposures is underestimated.

Asbestos exposure has been widely confirmed as an important lung cancer risk factor. It had been estimated that approximately 9000–10000 men develop lung cancer annually in the United States due to past exposure to occupational carcinogens, and more than half of these lung cancers are due to asbestos [26]. It has also been reported that asbestos exposure was associated with a relative risk for lung cancer of 3.5 after adjusting for age, smoking, and vitamin intake [27].

A large number of epidemiological studies have suggested that occupational exposure to formaldehyde may also increase lung cancer risk [28, 29]. However, more recent results about this relationship have been inconsistent [30, 31].

The association between the exposure to diesel exhaust fumes and the risk of lung cancer has been evaluated in many studies since the 1980s [32, 33]. A recent publication showed a strong and consistent relationship between quantitative exposure to diesel exhaust fumes and increased risk of dying from lung cancer, stating that among heavily exposed workers, the risk was approximately three times greater than that among workers in the lowest quartile of exposure [34].

Nickel, chromium, and cadmium have been identified as lung carcinogens in highly exposed cohorts [25, 35]. However, recent population-based case-control studies have found contradictory results [36, 37]. A study carried out in Montreal found that the exposure to these metals did not increase risk among smokers [36], and a study conducted in Central/Eastern Europe and the UK found a weak association for exposure to cadmium fumes. Furthermore, no increased risk was observed for inorganic acid mist, inorganic pigment dust, or nickel, after adjustment for other metal exposure [37]. Another case-control study carried out in New Caledonia found that lung cancer was not associated with any of the exposures related to the nickel industry: nickel compounds, iron and nickel oxides, iron matte, refractory bricks, or silica [38]. They also found no association between exposure to asbestos, arsenic compounds, organic acids, polycyclic aromatic hydrocarbons, or diesel exhaust gas and lung cancer.

The etiological link between lung cancer and occupational exposure to agricultural pesticide has also been widely studied. Exposure to inorganic fertilisers was significantly associated with lung cancer in farm workers [38]. In a case-control study carried out in Germany, a job-related evaluation showed a statistically significant increased odds ratio, adjusted for smoking, among agricultural workers [39]. The large American prospective Agricultural Health Study Exposure examined the relation between 50 widely used agricultural pesticides and lung cancer incidence [40, 41]. They found that exposure to some heavily used herbicides and insecticides were associated with a significant excess lung cancer risk.

The occupational exposure to various carcinogens such as asbestos, coaltar, arsenic and silica remains prevalent, especially in developing countries. Nowadays, there has been an exposure reduction to occupational carcinogens in industrialized countries. However, an effort to avoid occupational carcinogen exposure in developing countries is extremely important.

## Diet

The possibility that diet may have an impact on lung cancer risk was suggested in the 1970s as a result of the observation that, after adjusting for smoking, a low dietary intake of vitamin A was associated with an increased lung cancer risk [42]. Since then, many reports suggest that dietary factors may contribute to the risk of lung cancer [43]. However, this association remains controversial [2, 44-46].

Lung cancer epidemiology agrees with the hypothesis that consumption of fruit and vegetables with high amounts of antioxidants can prevent oxidative DNA damage, and thus prevent cancer development [46-49]. A recent study indicates that high cruciferous vegetable intake was significantly associated with reduction of lung cancer risk among smokers [50]. Consumption of beta-carotene, which is derived almost exclusively from intake of fruits and vegetables, has been associated with a reduced lung cancer risk in smokers. Retrospective observational studies have found that lung cancer patients generally report a lower intake of fruits, vegetables and related nutrients than controls [49, 51]. This apparent relationship may be partly due to residual confounding by smoking, since smokers generally consume less fruits and vegetables than non-smokers, but there may also be some protective effect of these foods. Furthermore, the association of fruits and vegetables with reduced lung cancer risk has been weak in prospective studies [46, 52-54]. The findings from a pooled analysis of seven cohort studies do not support any benefit of higher intake of beta-carotene from dietary sources in the prevention of lung cancer [55]. Moreover, low serum concentrations of antioxidants, such as vitamins A, C, and E, have been associated with lung cancer development [56, 57]. However, the role of these micronutrients in lung cancer prevention is still inconsistent, as observational and experimental studies have generated contradicting results [44]. While there are reports based on observational studies indicating that the consumption of antioxidant vitamins and carotenoids may decrease the risk of lung cancer [53], results are not conclusive. In a review of studies published before 1994, it had been reported that people in the lowest quartile of carotene intake had an increase of about 50% to 100% of lung cancer risk when compared to people in the highest quartile of carotene intake [58]. Subsequently, to confirm this positive association between vitamin supplementation and lung cancer, large-scale intervention studies have been carried out. These studies showed that antioxidant vitamin supplementation have no clear protective effect. In a prospective study conducted to evaluate the association between vitamin C, E, folate and beta-carotene and lung cancer risk while focusing on source-specific effects of dietary and supplemental intake, no protective effect of supplements was found [59]. The association between lung cancer risk and intake of fruit, vegetables, and specific botanical subgroups was also studied in the NIH-AARP Diet and Health study. In this large prospective cohort study, total intake of fruit and vegetables combined or total fruit or total vegetable consumption considered separately were unrelated to lung cancer risk in male current smokers. However, consumption of rosaceae foods (apples, peaches, nectarines, plums, pears, and strawberries) were significantly inversely associated with lung cancer risk in male current smokers, and no relationship was observed between consumption of rutaceae (citrus fruits) and lung cancer risk [60].

It has been established that B vitamins help to maintain DNA integrity and regulate gene expression and may affect cancer risk. However, in a comprehensive investigation of B vitamins in serum samples from the European Prospective Investigation into Cancer and Nutrition (EPIC) cohort study, no beneficial effects of high serum levels of riboflavin on lung cancer risk was found in current smokers [61].

There have been suggestions that low dietary intake of certain minerals, such as magnesium, zinc, copper, and iron, is associated with increased lung cancer risk [62]. However, a recent prospective cohort study observed no significant associations between total mineral intake and lung cancer risk. Nevertheless, total calcium intake (diet + supplement) was protective for current smokers, and dietary magnesium increased risk among men and current smokers [63].

It has been stated that dietary magnesium intake might protect against lung cancer through its role in maintaining genetic stability, regulation and cell proliferation, and protection against inflammation. Low dietary magnesium consumption was associated with poorer DNA repair capacity, increasing lung cancer risk in current smokers [64].

For other nutrients and foods, epidemiological studies have yielded contradictory results. Diets with excess in lipids, red meat, dairy products, and saturated fats seem to influence the development of lung cancer. Case-control studies carried out in Uruguay, had reported an elevated lung cancer risk for those current smokers with a high consumption of red meat and for those with high fat diet [51, 65]. In contrast, a case–control study conducted in Spain found that consumption of meat reduced lung cancer risk, whereas fish consumption increased such risk [66]. In the EPIC study, a multi-center cohort study designed to examine the relationship between diets; lifestyle, environmental factors, and cancer incidence, subjects with high red and processed meat consumption were more likely to be current smokers, and to consume more alcohol and less fruits and vegetables. Their findings do not support the hypothesis that a high intake of meat is a risk factor for lung cancer. Neither red meat nor white meat and fish were significantly associated with lung cancer risk [67].

A study carried out to evaluate the relationship between diet and cancer development proposed that a regular diet based on low vegetables, fruit and fish consumption, high red meat intake, and an imbalance of Omega-3 and Omega-6 fats may contribute to an increase in the risk of cancer [68]. In another study about dietary patterns carried out in Uruguay [69], the high-meat pattern (characterized by the correlated intake of proteins, saturated fats, monounsaturated fats, linoleic acid, alpha-linolenic acid, heterocyclic amines and phosphorus) showed a direct association with lung cancer risk, and the antioxidant pattern (characterized by the correlated intake of high loadings of glucose, fructose, carotenes, vitamin C, vitamin E, folates, flavonoids, phytosterols, reduced glutathione and nitrate) was protective. Moreover, no association was found between the carbohydrate pattern (characterized by high loadings of starch, fiber, thiamine, riboflavin, iron and sodium) and lung cancer risk.

Micronutrient supplements, which are widely used in some populations, are expected to have health-beneficial effects, or at worst to be harmless [70]. Trials on micronutrient supplements and lung cancer [71] have been discouraging, with no beneficial effects found in well-nourished populations [72].

# Case Report

Our group has investigated the risk factors associated with male lung cancer in Rosario, Argentina [15, 19, 43, 73]. Rosario is the third major urban concentration in the country, with almost one million inhabitants. The city serves as a port for a large agricultural and cattle-raising area, and it also has some metal industries.

A retrospective, hospital-based case–control study was carried out in two medical institutions in Rosario, where patients from a wide range of socioeconomic and occupational levels are treated. The purpose of this investigation was to evaluate diet, exposures in working environments as well as cigarette smoking intensity, as possible determinants of primary lung cancer.

# Methods

The study included 87 newly-diagnosed, histological-confirmed male lung cancer patients and 153 male controls. The control patients had no neoplasm or lung disease, and their admission was not related to smoking or other potential lung cancer risk factors. Their main diagnostic categories were traumatic conditions, and acute surgical conditions.

For all patients, information about age, smoking habit, occupation, and diet were recorded. Height and weight at the first consult, as well as weight one and ten years before diagnosis were also recorded.

Since 98% of the cases were smokers, non-smokers were excluded from the study. Years of smoking and number of cigarettes smoked daily were recorded. Patients were classified by the intensity of their smoking habit into two groups: up to 20 cigarettes per day, and more than 20 cigarettes per day (heavy smokers).

Patients were grouped according their lifetime occupational history as follows: not exposed to occupational contaminants (e.g. administrative workers, lawyers) and exposed to contaminants (e.g. workers from the metallurgical industries, and farmers).

To assess individual long-term dietary intake of foods and nutrients, data were collected using a food frequency questionnaire (FFQ) that has been previously validated [74]. The FFQ is a checklist of food and beverages with a frequency response section for subjects to report how often each item was consumed. The FFQ also includes portion size estimates, where respondents are asked to indicate their usual portion size by using photographs. Study participants were asked about their diet during the year prior to diagnosis (cases) and the year prior to enrollment into the study (controls). Although dietary intake data collected through a FFQ will inevitably have some inaccuracies, the FFQ is the most appropriate method for dietary assessment in epidemiological studies because it is practical, inexpensive, and can provide adequate information on long time dietary intake [75]. Calculations for nutrient intake were estimated by multiplying the reported frequency of each item by the amount of nutrient in a serving of that item, using a nutrient database for standard reference [76]. The values obtained were compared with those appointed by the Recommended Daily Allowances (RDA) for Argentina [77].

For statistical analysis, means and standard errors (SE) were computed for each nutrient as well as for total energy intake. Statistically significant differences between cases and controls were evaluated by a covariance analysis model adjusting for energy intake. Differences in distributions for lung cancer cases and controls across the levels of each categorical variable were evaluated using contingency tables, and the chi-square test for independence.

Additionally, multiple logistic regression models were fitted to analyze the effect of macro and micro nutrient intake on the risk of developing lung cancer, adjusting for the potential confounding effect of total energy intake, age, smoking intensity, occupation, and BMI. For this analysis, cases and controls were categorized into 3 groups according to tertile levels of each nutrient intake in the whole studied population: T1 (lowest) to T3 (highest). Association between each nutrient consumption and lung cancer was summarized using odd ratios (OR) and their 95% confidence interval (95% CI), taking the lower tertile consumption level as the reference category. The ORs were calculated for T2 and T3 versus T1. Multiple logistic regression analysis was also applied for the analysis of smoking intensity and occupational categories.

All p-values were two-sided, and the analyses were performed using STATA statistical software (Statistics/Data Analysis. Stata Corporation).

The project was reviewed and approved by the Ethics Committee of the School of Medicine, National University of Rosario. Informed consent was obtained from all participants.

## Results

Although patients' age range for this study was from 30 to 82 years, about 80% of subjects were under 70 years old. There were no statistically significant differences ($p=0.958$) regarding mean age between cases ($59.2\pm10.5$) and controls ($59.1\pm11.8$ years). Table 1 shows cases and controls characteristics' regarding their smoking habit and Table 2 shows the distribution of cases and controls according to their occupation.

The proportion of patients notexposed to occupational contaminants was lower in the lung cancer (cases) group compared to the controls (16.1% versus 38.0%; $p<0.01$), and the proportion of heavy smokers was higher in cases (52.9% versus 32.7%; $p<0.01$).

**Table 1. Distribution of cases and controls according to their smoking habit**

| Characteristic | | Controls | Cases | p-value |
|---|---|---|---|---|
| Smoking history | Current smoker | 51 (43.8%) | 67 (58.6%) | 0.027 |
| | Former smoker | 86 (56.3%) | 56 (41.3%) | |
| Smoking intensity | Up to 20 cigarettes/day | 103 (67.3%) | 41 (47.1%) | 0.002 |
| | More than 20 cigarettes/day (Heavy smokers) | 50 (32.7%) | 46 (52.9%) | |
| Smoking duration ( years) | | 30.4 ±15.2 | 40.5±12.0 | <0.001 |

**Table 2. Distribution of cases and controls according to their occupation**

| Characteristic | | Controls | Cases | p-value |
|---|---|---|---|---|
| Occupation | Mechanics and metallurgic workers | 20 (13.3%) | 18 (20.7%) | 0.002 |
| | Farmers | 73 (48.7%) | 55 (63.2%) | |
| | Non-exposed to occupational contaminants | 57 (38.0%) | 14 (16.1%) | |

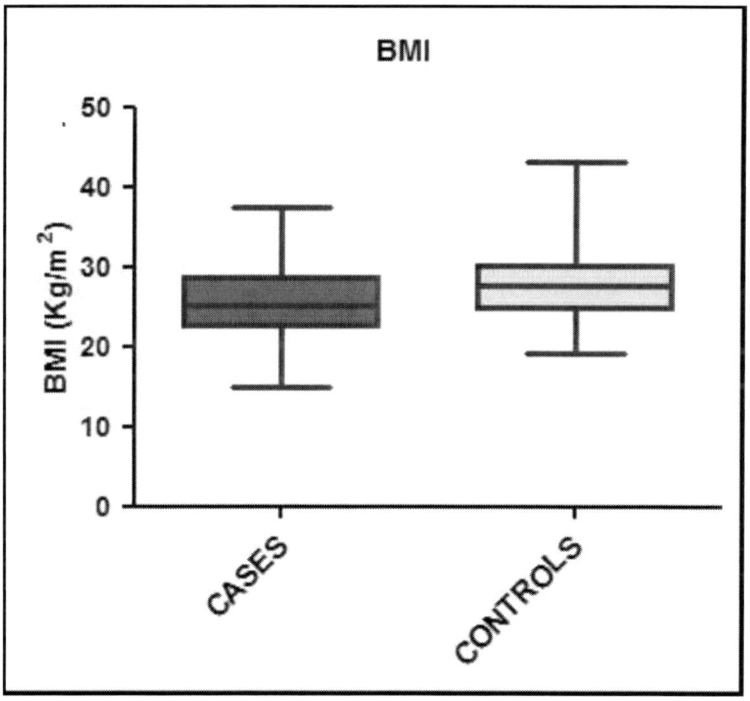


Figure 1. BMI distribution in cases and controls.

Mean BMI (one year before the first visit) was 25.0±5.9 for cases and 27.9±4.5 for controls (Figure 1). Mean BMI, showed significant differences (p<0.001) between cases and controls, whereas there were no significant difference between cases and controls regarding total energy intake.

Mean daily energy intakes were 3952.8±148.5 kcal for cases, and 3881.2±113.1 kcal for controls (p=0.685). Daily mineral intake means adjusted by age, smoking intensity, occupation and energy intake (Kcal) are shown in Table 3. The difference in consumption of these nutrients between cases and controls was statistically significant only for magnesium (p= 0.010) and manganese (p= 0.010) intake. However, both cases and controls largely exceeded the recommended quantities [77].

**Table 3. Daily intake of minerals adjusted by age, smoking intensity, occupation and energy intake (Kcal)**

| Minerals | Controls[a] | % RDA | Cases[a] | % RDA | p-value[b] |
|---|---|---|---|---|---|
| Magnesium (mg) | 511.7 ± 7.0 | 122 % | 481.8 ± 9.2 | 115 % | 0.010 |
| Manganese (mg) | 6.0 ± 0.2 | 260 % | 5.2 ± 0.2 | 226 % | 0.010 |
| Phosphorus (mg) | 2436.8 ± 37.0 | 348 % | 2335.7 ± 49.1 | 334 % | 0.101 |
| Calcium (mg) | 1457.1 ± 53.0 | 121 % | 1336.0 ± 70.3 | 111 % | 0.171 |
| Copper (mg) | 2.3 ± 0.1 | 255 % | 2.2 ± 0.1 | 244 % | 0.170 |
| Iron (mg) | 28.0 ± 0.5 | 350 % | 26.9 ± 0.7 | 336 % | 0.220 |
| Sodium (mg) | 5815.5 ± 185.7 | 447 % | 5486.4 ± 246.3 | 422 % | 0.287 |
| Potassium (mg) | 5497.2 ± 80.9 | 117 % | 5360.9 ± 107.2 | 114 % | 0.311 |
| Zinc (mg) | 27.4 ± 0.5 | 249 % | 27.7 ± 0.7 | 251 % | 0.763 |
| Selenium (μg) | 219.8 ± 4.3 | 339 % | 221.8 ± 5.7 | 403 % | 0.778 |

[a] Data are given as mean ± standard deviation.

[b] Covariance analysis model adjusting for age, BMI, smoking intensity, occupation and energy intake.

Table 4, compares cases and controls according to their average daily vitamin intake. Controls tended to have a higher vitamin C and vitamin A intake than cases but the differences were not statistically significant. Vitamin E consumption was significantly higher in the control group (p= 0.047; Covariance analysis model adjusting for total energy intake). Except for the dietary vitamin E intake in the cases group, the consumption of dietary vitamins in these patients exceeded the recommended minimum in all instances.

**Table 4. Daily intake of vitamins, adjusted by age, smoking intensity, occupation and energy intake (Kcal)**

| Vitamins | Controls[a] | % RDA | Cases[a] | % RDA | p-value[b] |
|---|---|---|---|---|---|
| Vitamin E (mg) | 18.2 ± 0.9 | 121 % | 15.1 ± 1.2 | 100,6 % | 0.047 |
| Vitamin C (mg) | 193.9 ± 11.5 | 215 % | 161.0 ± 15.3 | 179 % | 0.087 |
| Vitamin A (UI) | 20118.6 ± 1402.3 14441402.39853 | 671 % | 16674.6 ± 1859.8 11859.8 1367 | 556 % | 0.141 |
| Tiamina (mg) | 2.6 ± 0.1 | 217 % | 2.6 ± 0.1 | 217 % | 0.387 |
| Riboflavina (mg) | 3.3 ± 0.1 | 254 % | 3.4 ± 0.1 | 261 % | 0.554 |
| Niacina (mg) | 41.4 ± 0.7 | 259 % | 41.3 ± 1.0 | 258 % | 0.913 |

[a] Adjusted by energy intake (Kcal).

[b] Test for estimated marginal means comparison.

The use of multivitamin/mineral supplements was low in cases (9.20%) and in controls (15.69%) p= 0.155). Similar results were found for vitamin A, which was used by 2.30% of cases and 2.61% of controls (p=0.880), and Vitamin C (2.33% and 4.58%, respectively; p=0.381).

There was no difference in daily intake of total lipids, protein, and carbohydrates between cases and controls. However, controls ingested larger quantities of polyunsaturated fatty acids than cases (p=0.042). Daily average consumption was 28.7±1.2 and 24.6±1.6, respectively.

Multivariate analysis adjusting for the effect of confounding is shown in Table 5. As expected, lung cancer risk was high for heavy smokers. When comparing with the group unlikely to be exposed to occupational carcinogens, increased risks were observed for mechanics and metallurgic workers, and also for farmers. The risk of lung cancer decreased in patients with high intakes of calcium, magnesium and manganese. Likewise, high consumptions of dietary vitamin A, vitamin C, and vitamin E were associated with decreases in lung cancer risk. Persons in the highest consumption tertiles had approximately 60% decrease in lung cancer risk compared with persons in the lowest tertiles. There was no relationship between B-vitamins intake and lung cancer risk. However, lung cancer risk was reduced by 59 percent in those with middle riboflavin intake. A reduction in lung cancer risk was not found with vitamin and mineral supplementation consumption.

**Table 5. Lung Cancer according to significant risk factors**

| Risk Factor | OR[a] | 95% CI[a] | p-value |
|---|---|---|---|
| Heavy smokers[b] | 2.5 | 1.4–4.5 | 0.002 |
| Mechanics and metallurgic workers[c] | 3.9 | 1.6–9.9 | 0.004 |
| Farmers[c] | 2.6 | 1.3–5.4 | 0.009 |
| Daily Calcium dietary intake (mg) | | | |
| Medium[d] (962-1544) | 0.34 | 0.16 – 0.72 | 0.005 |
| High[d] (>1544) | 0.34 | 0.14 – 0.84 | 0.020 |
| Daily Magnesium dietary intake (mg) | | | |
| Medium[d] (413-550) | 0.31 | 0.13 - 0.73 | 0.007 |
| High[d] (>550) | 0.23 | 0.07 – 0.72 | 0.012 |
| Daily Manganese dietary intake (mg) | | | |
| Medium[d] (4.5 – 6.0) | 0.58 | 0.28 – 1.20 | 0.143 |
| High[d] (>6.0) | 0.35 | 0.15 – 0.80 | 0.013 |
| Daily Vitamin A dietary intake (IU) | | | |
| Medium[d] (9300-18820) | 0.63 | 0.31 - 1.30 | 0.212 |
| High[d] (>18820) | 0.42 | 0.19 – 0.90 | 0.026 |
| Daily Vitamin C dietary intake (mg) | | | |
| Medium[d] (100 – 190) | 0.57 | 0.28 – 1.16 | 0.122 |
| High[d] (>190) | 0.39 | 0.18 – 0.84 | 0.016 |
| Daily Vitamin E dietary intake (mg) | | | |
| Medium[d] (12.5-17.3) | 0.36 | 0.17 – 0.79 | 0.011 |
| High[d] (>17.3) | 0.41 | 0.18 – 0.93 | 0.032 |
| Daily Rivoflavin dietary intake (mg) | | | |
| Medium[d] (2.71-3.80) | 0.41 | 0.17-0.96 | 0.043 |
| High[d] (>3.80) | 0.84 | 0.26-1.45 | 0.759 |

[a] Odd ratios and Confidence intervals calculated by multivariate logistic regression model, adjusted also by age, BMI, and total energy intake (Kcal).

[b] Compared to non heavy smokers.

[c] Compared to non-exposed to occupational contaminants.

[d] Compared to low intake.

In our study, no beneficial effect of vitamin and mineral supplement consumption was seen. However, our results suggest that high dietary intake of vitamin A, C and E had a protective effect for lung cancer risk. A lower risk for lung cancer was also seen for elevated dietary intake levels of riboflavin. A high dietary consumption of magnesium, manganesium and calcium also has a protective effect. Mean consumption of polyunsaturated fatty acids such as Omega-3 was higher in the control group, but the adjusted odds ratios were not statistically significant. There were no statistically significant differences between cases and controls for the consumption of iron and proteins (the primary source was red meat). Both cases and controls were characterized by a high calorie intake, exceeding the recommendations for total fats consumption as well as for all of the vitamins and minerals.

## Conclusion

Lung cancer research is an area of great interest in medicine and public health because this disease involves expensive treatment and interventions. There is no doubt that the most effective action against lung cancer incidence is the control of modifiable risk factors. While smoking is an important lung cancer risk factor, worsened by occupational contaminants exposure, there is some evidence suggesting that the intake of certain nutrients may decrease lung cancer risk.

## References

[1] Alberg AJ, Samet JM. Epidemiology of Lung Cancer. *Chest* 2003; 123(S):21-49.

[2] Dela Cruz CS, Tanoue LT, Matthay RA. Lung cancer: Epidemilogy, Etiology, and Prevention. *Clin Chest Med* 2011; 32:605–644.

[3] U.S. Cancer Statistics Working Group. United States Cancer Statistics: 1999-2008 Incidence and Mortality Web-based Report. Atlanta (GA): Department of Health and Human Services, Centers for Disease Control and Prevention, and National Cancer Institute, 2012. Available at *http://www.cdc.gov/uscs (accessed Jun 30, 2012).*

[4] Adami HO, Hunter D, Trichopoulos D. *Textbook of Cancer Epidemiology*. Oxford University Press, 2002.

[5] Alberts WM. Lung Cancer Guidelines. Introduction. *Chest* 2003; 123(S):1–2.

[6] Rom WN, Hay JG, Lee TC, et al. Molecular and genetic aspects of lung cancer. *Am J Respir Crit Care Med* 2000; 161:1355–1367.

[7] Danaei G, Vander Hoorn S, Lopez AD, et al. The Comparative Risk Assessment Collaborating Group. Causes of cancer in the world: comparative risk assessment of nine behavioural and environmental risk factors. *The Lancet* 2005; 366(9499): 1784-1793.

[8] Ferlay J, Shin HR, Bray F, et al. Estimates of worldwide burden of cancer in 2008: GLOBOCAN 2008. *Int J Cancer* 2010; 127(12):2893-2917.

[9] Bagnardi V, Randi G, Lubin J, et al. Alcohol Consumption and Lung Cancer Risk in the Environment and Genetics in Lung Cancer Etiology (EAGLE) Study. *Am J Epidemiol* 2010; 171:36–44.

[10] Doll R, Hill AB. Smoking and carcinoma of the lung. Preliminary Report. *Brit Med J* 1950; 2:739-748.

[11] Wynder EL, Graham EA. Tobacco smoking as a possible etiologic factor in bronchiogenic carcinoma. A study of six hundred and eighty four proved cases. *JAMA* 1950; 145: 329-336.

[12] Doll R, Peto P, Boreham J, et al. Mortality in relation to smoking: 50 years' observations on male British doctors. *BMJ* 2004; 328:1519–1527.

[13] Pisani P, Bray F, Parkin DM. Estimates of the world-wide prevalence of cancer for 25 sites in the adult population. *Int J Cancer* 2002; 97(1):72–81.

[14] Parkin DM. Tobacco-attributable cancer burden in the UK in 2010. *Br J Cancer* 2011; 105 (S2):S6-S13.

[15] Pezzotto SM, Mahuad R, Morini JC, et al. Variation in smoking-related lung cancer risk factors by cell type among men in Argentina. A case-control study. *Cancer Causes and Control* 1993; 4:231-237.

[16] Lubin JH, Caporaso NE. Cigarette somoking and lung cancer: modeling total exposure and intensity. *Cancer Epidemiol Biomarkers Prev* 2006; 15(3): 517-523.

[17] Peto R, Darby S, Deo H, et al. Smoking, smoking cessation, and lung cancer in the UK since 1950: combination of national statistics with two case-control studies. *Brit Med J* 2000; 321(5):323-329.

[18] Crispo A, Brennan P, Jöckel K-H, et al. The cumulative risk of lung cancer among current, ex- and never-smokers in European men. *Brit J Cancer* 2004; 91: 1280–1286.

[19] Pezzotto SM, Poletto L. Occupation and histopathology of lung cancer: a case-control study in Rosario, Argentina. *Am J Ind Med* 1999; 36(4):437-443.

[20] Boffetta P. Epidemiology of environmental and occupational cancer. *Oncogene* 2004; 23:6392–6403.

[21] Consonni D, De Matteis S, Lubin JH, et al. Lung Cancer and Occupation in a Population-based Case-Control Study. Am J Epidemiol 2010; 171:323–333.

[22] Cogliano VJ, Baan R, Straif K, et al. Preventable Exposures Associated With Human Cancers. *J Natl Cancer Inst* 2011; 103(24):1827-1839.

[23] IARC. Agents Classified by the IARC Monographs Volumes 1–101. Lyon, France: International Agency for Research on Cancer. Monographs on the Evaluation of Carcinogenic Risks to Humans, 2010. Available at: *http://monographs.iarc.fr/ ENG/Classification/index.php*. (accessed Jun 30, 2012).

[24] Driscoll T, Nelson DI, Steenland K, et al. The global burden of disease due to occupational carcinogens. *Am J Ind Med* 2005; 48(6):419–431.

[25] Fingerhut M, Nelson DI, Driscoll T, et al. The contribution of occupational risks to the global burden of disease: summary and next steps. *Med Lav* 2006; 97(2):313–321.

[26] Steenland K, Loomis D, Shy C, et al. Review of occupational lung carcinogens. *Am J Ind Med* 1996; 29: 474-490.

[27] Weiss W. Asbestosis: a marker for the increased risk of lung cancer among workers exposed to asbestos. *Chest* 1999; 115(2):536–549.

[28] Coggon D, Harris EC, Poole J, et al. Extended follow-up of a cohort of British chemical workers exposed to formaldehyde. *J Natl Cancer Inst* 2003; 95(21):1608–1615.

[29] Sterling TD, Weinkam JJ. Mortality from respiratory cancers (including lung cancer) among workers employed in formaldehyde industries. *Am J Ind Med* 1994; 25(4):593–602.

[30] National Toxicology Program. Final Report on Carcinogens Background Document for Formaldehyde. Rep Carcinog Backgr Doc, 2010; (10-5981):i-512. Available at: *http://www.ncbi.nlm.nih.gov/pubmed/20737003* (accessed Jun 30, 2012).

[31] Alder N, Fenty J, Warren F, et al. Meta-analysis of mortality and cancer incidence among workers in the synthetic rubber-producing industry. *Am J Epidemiol* 2006; 164(5):405–420.

[32] Lipsett M, Campleman S. Occupational exposure to diesel exhaust and lung cancer: a meta-analysis. *Am J Public Health* 1999; 89(7):1009–1017.

[33] Olsson AC , Gustavsson P , Kromhout H , et al. Exposure to diesel motor exhaust and lung cancer risk in a pooled analysis from case-control studies in Europe and Canada. *Am J Respir Crit Care* Med 2011; 183(7): 941–948.

[34] Silverman DT, Samanic CM, Lubin JH, et al. The Diesel Exhaust in Miners Study: A Nested Case – Control Study of Lung Cancer and Diesel Exhaust. *J Natl Cancer Inst* 2012; 104: 855-868.

[35] Lightfoot N, Berriault C, Semenciw R. Mortality and cancer incidence in a nickel cohort. *Occupational Medicine* 2010; 60(3):211–218.

[36] Beveridge R, Pintos J, Parent ME, et al. Lung cancer risk associated with occupational exposure to nickel, chromium VI, and cadmium in two population-based case-control studies in Montreal. *Am J Indl Med* 2010; 53(5):476–485.

[37] Mannetje A, Bencko V, Brennan P, et al. Occupational exposure to metal compounds and lung cancer. Results from a multi-center case-control study in Central/Eastern Europe and UK. *Cancer Causes and Control* 2011; 22(12):1669-1680.

[38] Menvielle G, Luce D, Févotte J, et al. Occupational exposures and lung cancer in New Caledonia. *Occup Environ Med* 2003; 60:584–589.

[39] Bruske-Hohlfeld I, Mohner M, Pohlabeln H, et al. Occupational Lung Cancer Risk for Men in Germany: Results from a Pooled Case-Control Study. *Am J Epidemiol* 2000; 151:384-395.

[40] Purdue MP, Hoppin JA, Blair A, et al. Occupational exposure to organochlorine insecticides and cancer incidence in the Agricultural Health Study. *Int J Cancer* 2007; 120(3):642-649.

[41] Alavanja MCR, Dosemeci M, Samanic C, et al. Pesticides and Lung Cancer Risk in the Agricultural Health Study Cohort. *Am J Epidemiol* 2004; 160(9):876–885.

[42] Bjelke E. Dietary vitamin A and human lung cancer. *Int J Cancer* 1975; 15: 561–565.

[43] Dagatti MS, Wojdyla D, Bertola Compagnucci A, et al. Protective effect of macro and micro nutrients on male lung cancer. A case–control study in Rosario, Argentina. *e-SPEN, the European e-Journal of Clinical Nutrition and Metabolism* 2009; 4:e155–e159.

[44] Key TJ, Schatzkin A, Willett WC, et al. Diet, nutrition and the prevention of cancer. *Public Health Nutrition* 2004; 7(1A): 187–200.

[45] Gallicchio L, Boyd K, Matanoski G, et al. Carotenoids and the risk of developing lung cancer: a systematic review. *Am J Clin Nutr* 2008; 88(2):372-383.

[46] Cranganu A, Camporeale J. Nutrition Aspects of Lung Cancer. *Nutr Clin Pract* 2009; 24: 688-700.

[47] Smith-Warner S, Spiegelman D, Yaun S, et al. Fruits, vegetables and lung cancer: A pooled analysis of cohort studies. *Int J Cancer* 2003; 107:1001–1011.

[48] Linseisen J, Rohrmann S, Miller AB, et al. Fruit and vegetable consumption and lung cancer risk: updated information from the European Prospective Investigation into Cancer and Nutrition (EPIC). *Int. J. Cancer* 2007; 121:1103–1114.
[49] Galeone C, Negri E, Pelucchi C, et al. Dietary intake of fruit and vegetable and lung cancer risk: a case–control study in Harbin, northeast China. *Ann Oncol* 2007; 18:388–392.
[50] Tang L, Zirpoli GR, Jayaprakash V, et al. Cruciferous vegetable intake is inversely associated with lung cancer risk among smokers: a case-control study. *BMC Cancer* 2010; 10:162-170.
[51] De Stefani E, Brennan P, Ronco A, et al. Food groups and risk of lung cancer in Uruguay. *Lung Cancer* 2002; 38:1–9.
[52] Feskanich D, Ziegler RG, Michaud DS, et al. Prospective study of fruit and vegetable consumption and risk of lung cancer among men and women. *J Natl Cancer Inst* 2000; 92:1812–1823.
[53] Voorrips LE, Goldbohm RA, Verhoeven DTH, et al. Vegetable and fruit consumption and lung cancer risk in the Netherlands Cohort Study on diet and cancer. *Cancer Causes and Control* 2000; 11: 101–115.
[54] Riboli E, Norat T. Epidemiologic evidence of the protective effect of fruit and vegetables on cancer risk. *Am J Clin Nutr* 2003; 78 (suppl):559S–569S.
[55] Männistö S, Smith-Warner SA, Spiegelman D, et al. Dietary carotenoids and risk of lung cancer in a pooled analysis of seven cohort studies. *Cancer Epidemiol Biomarkers Prev* 2004; 13(1):40-48.
[56] Lee IM. Antioxidant vitamins in the prevention of cancer. *Proe Assoe Am Phys* 1999; 111:10-15.
[57] Ruano-Ravina A, Figueiras A, Freire-Garabal M, et al. Antioxidant vitamins and risk of lung cancer. *Curr Pharm Des* 2006; 12: 599–613.
[58] Byers TE, Graham S, Haughey BP, et al. Diet and lung cancer risk: findings from the Western New York Diet Study. *Am J Epidemiol* 1987; 125(3): 351–363.
[59] Roswall N, Olsen A, Cristensen J, et al. Source-specific effects of micronutrients in lung cancer prevention. *Lung Cancer* 2010; 67: 275–281.
[60] Wright ME, Park Y, Subar AF, et al. Intakes of fruit, vegetables, and specific botanical groups in relation to lung cancer risk in the NIH-AARP Diet and Health Study. *Am J Epidemiol* 2008; 168: 1024–1034.
[61] Johansson M, Relton C, Ueland PM, et al. Serum B Vitamin Levels and Risk of Lung Cancer. *JAMA* 2010; 303(23): 2377-2385.
[62] Mahabir S, Spitz MR, Barrera SL, et al. Dietary zinc, copper and selenium, and risk of lung cancer. *Int J Cancer* 2007; 120(5):1108–1115.
[63] Mahabir S, Forman MR, Dong YQ, et al. Mineral Intake and Lung Cancer Risk in the NIH-American Association of Retired Persons Diet and Health Study. *Cancer Epidemiol Biomarkers Prev* 2010; 19(8):1976-1983.
[64] Mahabir S, Wei Q, Barrera S, et al. Association between dietary magnesium and DNA repair capacity with lung cancer risk. *Carcinogenesis* 2008; 29: 949–956.
[65] De Stefani E, Ronco AL, Boffetta P, et al. Meat consumption, meat cooking and risk of lung cancer among Uruguayan men. *Asian Pac J Cancer Prev* 2010; 11(6): 1713-1717.

[66] Dosil-Díaz O, Ruano-Ravina A, Gestal-Otero JJ, et al. Meat and fish consumption and risk of lung cancer: a case–control study in Galicia, Spain. *Cancer Lett* 2007; 252:115–122.

[67] Linseisen J, Rohrmann S, Bueno de Mesquita B, et al. Consumption of meat and fish and risk of lung cancer: results from the European Prospective Investigation into Cancer and Nutrition. *Cancer Causes and Control* 2011; 22 (6): 909-918.

[68] Divisi D, Di Tommaso S, Salvemini S, et al. Diet and cancer. *Acta Biomed* 2006; 77:118–123.

[69] De Stefani E, Boffetta P, Ronco AL, et al. Nutrient patterns and risk of lung cancer: A factor analysis in Uruguayan men. *Lung Cancer* 2008; 61, 283—291.

[70] Brower V. An apple a day may be safer than vitamins. *J Natl Cancer Inst* 2008; 100:770–772.

[71] Omenn GS. Chemoprevention of lung cancers: lessons from CARET, the betacarotene and retinol efficacy trial, and prospects for the future. *Eur J Cancer Prev* 2007; 16:184–191.

[72] Kristal AR, Lippman SM. Nutritional prevention of cancer: new directions for an increasingly complex challenge. *J Natl Cancer Inst* 2009; 101: 363–365.

[73] Dagatti MS, Bertola Compagnucci A, Perroud HA, et al. Protective effect of Vitamin A on male lung cancer. In: *Vitamin A: Nutrition, Side Effects and Supplements.* Editor: Lucas P. Scott. Nova Science Publishers, Inc; 2010. ISBN 978-1-61728-915-6.

[74] Navarro A, Osella AR, Guerra V, et al. Reproducibility and validity of a food-frequency questionnaire in assessing dietary intakes and food habits in epidemiological cancer studies in Argentina. *J Exp Clin Cancer Res* 2001; 20(3):365–370.

[75] Willett WC, Hu FB. Not the time to abandon the food frequency questionnaire. *Cancer Epidemiol Biomarkers Prev* 2006; 15:1757–1758.

[76] U.S. Department of Agriculture, Agricultural Research Service, USDA Nutrient Data Laboratory. Composition of Foods. Raw, processed, prepared. *USDA Nutrient Database for Standard Reference*, Release 14; 2001

[77] Lema S, Longo E, Lopresti A, et al. Guías Alimentarias para la población Argentina. 2da ed. *Asociación Argentina de Dietistas y Nutricionistas Dietistas (AADYND).* Buenos Aires, Argentina; 2006.

In: Lung Cancer: A Comprehensive Overview
Editor: Kathy Gately
ISBN: 978-1-62618-447-3


*Chapter IV*

# Lung Cancer: Treatment in Early Stage

***Miriam Méndez*[*,1]*, Ana Custodio*[†2] *and Mariano Provencio*[1]**
[1]Medical Oncology Department,
Hospital Universitario Puerta de Hierro Majadahonda, Madrid, Spain
[2]Medical Oncology Department, Hospital Universitario La Paz, Madrid, Spain

## Abstract

Lung cancer is the most common and deadly tumour worldwide and approximately 1.3 million patients a year die of it. In relation to the treatment, in limited disease (stage I, II, IIIA) patients who undergo surgical resection and the administration of cytostatic treatment achieve a 5-year survival of 51%, with an absolute benefit of 5.4% in 5-year survival, especially in patients with a good performance status. Concurrent chemo-radiotherapy improves overall survival of patients with locally advanced NSCLC, compared with sequential chemo-radiotherapy.

## Introduction

Lung cancer is the most common cancer worldwide, with an estimated 1,600,000 new cases and 1,380,000 deaths in 2008 [1]. In the United States, there will be an estimated 226,000 new cases of lung cancer and 160,000 deaths in 2012 [2]. Almost as many Americans die of lung cancer every year than die of prostate, breast and colon cancer combined.

Around 1953, lung cancer became the most common cause of cancer deaths in men, and in 1985, it became the leading cause of cancer deaths in women. Lung cancer in both genders tops the list on the number of estimated deaths yearly (28% of all cancer deaths for men and 26% of all cancer deaths for women). Lung cancer deaths have begun to decline in men,

* mirimega@hotmail.com.
† These authors contributed equally to this chapter.

reflecting a decrease in smoking [3]. The rise in the death rate in women appears to have reached a plateau, although almost one-half of all lung cancer deaths now occur in women. This chapter will present an overview of treatment options in early stage non-small cell lung cancer

# Adjuvant and Neoadjuvant Therapy for Resectable Non-Small Cell Lung Cancer

Lung cancer is the most common fatal malignancy for both men and women in most countries throughout the world, accounting for 12-13% of all new cancer diagnoses [4]. Non-small cell lung cancer (NSCLC) represents 80-85% of all newly diagnosed cases of lung cancers. The reference treatment for early stage disease (from stage IA to IIB) is surgery. Specific groups of patients with stage III disease may also benefit from pulmonary resection, usually in combination with other treatment modalities. Globally, the proportion of newly diagnosed NSCLC that can benefit from radical resection does not exceed 25% to 30% of the total number of cases.

Despite complete (R0) resection, generally consisting of a lobectomy with adequate mediastinal lymph node dissection, there remains a high risk for developing recurrent disease. The 5-year overall survival (OS) rate changes from 73% for patients with pathological stage IA NSCLC to only 25% for those with stage IIIA disease [5,6].

Over the past few years, one of the most significant advances in NSCLC research is the clear demonstration of longer survival with platinum-based adjuvant chemotherapy (CT) for early-stage disease [7, 8]. However, there is no consensus whether neoadjuvant CT results in improved outcome. We summarize the evidence for adjuvant and neoadjuvant therapy in early-stage NSCLC and opportunities for using clinical and molecular selection criteria to optimize therapeutic benefit.

# Evidence for Adjuvant CT

## Early Studies of Adjuvant CT

The history of adjuvant CT in completely resected NSCLC initiated in the early 1960s and 1970s with trials testing the role of alkylating agents and nonspecific immunotherapies (mainly levamisole and Bacillus Calmette-Guérin) that uniformly failed to demonstrate any survival benefit [9]. Furthermore, adjuvant CT was poorly tolerated during this era, as optimal supportive measures, such as effective antiemetics, were not available. Subsequently, the potential role of cisplatin-based CT was extensively tested in all the stages of resectable NSCLC. All but one of these studies failed to show clinical benefit from adjuvant therapies [10, 11].

Common findings in both of these groups of studies include the overestimation of the potential benefit of adjuvant CT in the calculation of the sample size, the unbalance in patients and treatment characteristics in some trials and, in most of these studies, the impossibility to reach the planned accrual. In addition, dose delivery including dose and dose intensity were very often reported inadequate in most of the trials with an average of 50% of the patients receiving the full course of treatment.

In 1995, the Non-Small Cell Lung Cancer Collaborative Group (NSCLCCG) published a meta-analysis that included data on 4357 patients from 14 randomized trials [12]. It failed to demonstrate a survival advantage for adjuvant CT. In five trials that did not contain cisplatin, patients treated with surgery alone had a survival advantage, and the risk of death was 15% higher among those randomized to adjuvant CT. However, a subset analysis of the eight trials using cisplatin-based regimens suggested that adjuvant CT was associated with a 13% reduction in the risk of death (hazard ratio [HR], 0.87; 95% confidence interval [CI], 0.74-1.02; p=0.08), which translated into a 5% absolute improvement in the likelihood of surviving 5 years, although the difference was not statistically significant.

These findings failed to impact on clinical practice not because the absolute gain was too small, but because such an estimate was still imprecise, ranging from 1% detriment to 10% benefit. In addition, the heterogeneity of surgical procedures, specific CT regimens and difference in the staging modalities limited the applicability of the results of the meta-analysis.

**Table 1. Baseline and treatment characteristics of patients enrolled in platinum-based adjuvant chemotherapy trials**

| | IALT | ANITA | NCIC-BR10 | ALPI | BLT | CALGB 9633[38] |
|---|---|---|---|---|---|---|
| Nº patients enrolled | 1867 | 799 | 450 | 1209 | 381 | 344 |
| CT régimen | Cisplatin + vindesine/ vinblastine/ vinorelbine/ etoposide x 3-4 cycles | Cisplatin+ vinorelbine x 4 cycles | Cisplatin+ vinorelbine x 4 cycles | Cisplatin+ vinblastine +mitomicine x 3 cycles | Cisplatin + vindesine/ vinorelbine/ vindesine/ vinblastine or mytomicin/ ifosfamide x 3 cycles | Carboplatin + paclitaxel x 4 cycles |
| Sequential RT allowed | Yes (27%) | Yes (28%) | No | Yes (43%) | Yes (14%) | No |
| Median age | 59 | 59 | 61 | 61 | 61 | 61 |
| Stage (%) | | | | | | |
| I | 36.5 | 36 | 46 | 39 | 27 | 100 (all IB) |
| II | 24.2 | 24 | 54 | 31 | 38 | |
| IIIA | 39.3 | 39 | NT | 29 | 34 | |
| Histology (%) | | | | | | |
| Squamous | 47 | 59 | 37 | 51 | 48 | 35 |
| Non-squamous | 46 | 40 | 65 | 45 | 52 | NR |
| Pneumonectomy rate (%) | 35 | 38 | 25 | 26 | NR | 11 |

CT: chemotherapy; RT: radiotherapy; NR: not reported; NT: not tested.

## Recent Platinum-Based Adjuvant CT

The aforementioned 1995 meta-analysis strongly supported the planning of several prospective randomized phase III studies evaluating the role of modern platinum-based regimens following complete surgical resection of NSCLC (Tables 1 and 2).

**Table 2. Overall and according to clinical stage survival in platinum-based adjuvant chemotherapy trials**

| Study /year | Treatment arms | DFS | OS | OS according to clinical stage | | |
|---|---|---|---|---|---|---|
| | | | | Stage I | Stage II | Stage III |
| IALT (2010) | Adjuvant CT<br>Observation | NR<br>NR<br>(HR, 0.88; p=0.02) | 54 months<br>45 months<br>(HR, 0.91; p=0.1) | HR, 0.95 (95% CI, 0.74-1.23) | HR, 0.93 (95% CI, 0.72-1.20) | HR, 0.79 (95% CI, 0.66-1.95) |
| ANITA (2006) | Adjuvant CT<br>Observation | 36.3 months<br>20.7 months<br>(HR, 0.76; p=0.002) | 43.7 months<br>65.7 months<br>(HR, 0.80; p=0.017) | HR, 1.14 (95% CI, 0.83-1.57) | HR, 0.67 (95% CI, 0.47-0.94) | HR, 0.60 (95% CI, 0.44-0.82) |
| NCIC-BR10 (2010) | Adjuvant CT<br>Observation | NR<br>NR | 5-year survival 67%<br>5-year survival 56%<br>(HR, 0.78; p=0.04) | HR, 1.03 (95% CI, 0.70-1.52) | HR, 0.68 (95% CI, 0.50-0.92) | Not tested |
| ALPI (2003) | Adjuvant CT<br>Observation | 36.5 months<br>28.9 months<br>(HR, 0.89; p=0.128) | 55 months<br>49 months<br>(HR, 0.96; p=0.59) | HR, 0.97 (95% CI, 0.71-1.33) | HR, 0.80 (95% CI, 0.60-1.06) | HR, 0.79 (95% CI, 0.66-0.95) |
| BLT (2004) | Adjuvant CT<br>Observation | 27 months<br>24.7 months<br>(HR, 0.97; p=0.81) | 33.9 months<br>32.6 months<br>(HR, 1.02; p=0.90) | NR | NR | NR |
| CALGB 9633 (2006) | Adjuvant CT<br>Observation | NR<br>NR<br>(HR, 0.74; p=0.10) | 5-year survival 60%<br>5-year survival 57%<br>(HR, 0.80; p=0.1) | 5-year survival 60%<br>5-year survival 57%<br>(HR, 0.80; p=0.1) | Not tested | Not tested |

CT: chemotherapy; DFS: disease-free survival; OS: overall survival; NR: nor reported; HR: hazard ratio; 95% CI: 95% confidence interval.

Three randomized phase III trials have demonstrated a survival advantage with adjuvant CT: the International Adjuvant Lung Trial (IALT) [13], National Cancer Institution of Canada Cancer Therapeutics Group JBR.10 trial [14], and Adjuvant Navelbine International Trialist Association (ANITA) trial [15]. Although these studies differed in key aspects, such as stage of patients enrolled and the use of adjuvant radiotherapy (RT), they also shared common features. Most importantly, they employed cisplatin-based CT regimens. The largest, platinum-based experience with adjuvant CT comes from the IALT study, in which 1867 patients with resected stage I, II or III NSCLC were randomly assigned to three to four cycles of CT (a doublet of cisplatin plus vinorelbine, vindesine, vinblastine or etoposide) or observation. Postoperative RT was administered to 27% of patients. At a median follow-up of 56 months, the 5-year survival rate was significantly longer in the CT arm (44.5 vs. 40.4 months; HR, 0.86; 95% CI, 0.76-0.98; p=0.03). However, at a subsequent median follow-up of 7.5 years, adjuvant CT was associated with a significant improvement in disease-free survival (DFS) (HR, 0.88; 95% CI, 0.78-0.98; p=0.02) but only a trend toward improved OS that lost significance (HR, 0.91; 95% CI, 0.81-1.02; p=0.10). Some methodological aspects regarding the final analysis of the IALT study raise concerns. The accrual was prematurely interrupted when less than 60% of expected patients had been enrolled and the follow up continued until about only 65% of expected events had been observed. Moreover, there was a significant difference between the results of OS before and after 5 years (HR, 0.86; 95% CI,

0.76-0.97; p=0.01 vs. HR, 1.45; 95% CI, 1.02-2.07; p=0.04, respectively; p value for interaction=0.006). The analysis of non-lung cancer deaths for the whole period showed a HR of 1.34 (95% CI, 0.99-1.81; p=0.06). These results confirmed the efficacy of CT for the first 5 years after surgery. The difference in results between less than and more than 5 years of follow-up may suggest possible late adjuvant CT-related over-mortality.

In the ANITA trial [15], 799 evaluable patients with stage IB, II or IIIA NSCLC were randomly assigned to four cycles of cisplatin (100 $mg/m^2$ on day 1 every four weeks) plus vinorelbine (30 mg/m2 weekly) versus observation. Adjuvant RT was administered to 24% of CT patients and 33% of those assigned to observation. After a median follow-up of 76 months, CT significantly reduced the risk for death (HR, 0.80; 95% CI, 0.66-0.96; p=0.017) with a survival advantage of 8.6% at 5 years (median survival, 65.7 months and 43.7 months in the CT and observation groups, respectively). In contrast with IALT study, the survival advantage in the CT arm was maintained at 7 years (8.4%). Toxicity associated with vinorelbine and cisplatin was manageable. Grade 3 or 4 neutropenia, febrile neutropenia, nausea and vomiting, constipation and peripheral neuropathy were observed in 85%, 9%, 27%, 5%, and 3% of patients, respectively. There were seven CT-related deaths (2%).

A similar degree of benefit for adjuvant CT was reported in another phase III study from the National Cancer Institute of Canada (NCIC), the Intergroup JBR.10 trial, in which 482 patients with completely resected stage IB or II (excluding T3N0) NSCLC were randomly assigned to surgery followed by four cycles of cisplatin (50 $mg/m^2$ days 1 and 8, every four weeks) plus vinorelbine (25 mg/m2 days 1 and 8 weekly for 16 weeks) or surgery alone [24]. Patients did not receive postoperative RT and only 58% of randomized and treated patients (n=231) received three courses of CT. OS was significantly longer in the CT arm (94 vs. 73 months; HR, 0.69; 95% CI, 0.52 to 0.91; p=0.0009), as was DFS (not reached vs. 47 months). Five-year survival rates were 69% and 54%, respectively, with an absolute gain of 15% at 5 years. The updated survival analysis of the JBR.10 trial, presented at the 2009 American Society of Clinical Oncology (ASCO) Annual Meeting, reported an enduring survival advantage for patients treated with adjuvant CT with >9 years of follow-up (5-year survival, 67% vs. 56%; HR, 0.78) [16]. Patients with stage II disease had a significant improvement in 5-year OS (59% vs. 44%). The outcome in patients with stage I NSCLC depended upon the size of the tumor. Overall, there was no benefit (5-year survival, 76 vs. 69%; HR, 1.03). In those with a primary tumor <4 cm, CT was associated with a poorer outcome (73 vs. 79%; HR, 1.73), whereas for those with a primary tumor >4 cm, CT improved survival (79 vs. 59%; HR, 0.68). The most common toxicity was hematologic (grade 3 or 4 neutropenia in 73% of patients, febrile neutropenia in 7%). The most frequent non-hematologic grade 3 or 4 toxicities included fatigue (15%), anorexia (10%), and vomiting (10%). There were two treatment-related deaths. Compared with the IALT study, there was no evidence that adjuvant CT was associated with a significantly higher incidence of non-lung cancer death or secondary malignancies. The impact of adjuvant CT on quality of life (QOL) was assessed in a subset of 359 patients from this trial who completed a baseline assessment. Patients receiving adjuvant CT had transient worsening in QOL due to fatigue, nausea, and vomiting. However, the QOL of patients treated with CT returned to baseline by nine months, except for symptoms of sensory neuropathy and hearing loss. Similarly, an analysis of all 482 patients looking at the quality-adjusted time without symptoms or toxicity found that adjuvant CT improved quality-adjusted survival despite the toxicity associated with treatment.

The survival advantage for adjuvant CT in the described three studies with a positive impact was in the range of 4.1-15%. Why are there such huge differences in survival among these studies? First, there was important differences in the sample size calculations from one trial to another (from less than 500 patients to 3300 according to the planned sample sizes) to assess a similar expected therapeutic effect in a similar patient population. The only two studies designed to observe an estimated survival advantage in an unrestricted population of early-stage patients (stages I to III) in the range of that reported in the 1995 meta-analysis were the Adjuvant Lung Project Italy (ALPI) (17) and the IALT studies that, not surprisingly, demonstrated a survival benefit relatively close to each other (3% for ALPI vs. 4.1% for IALT). Second, in most of the studies no information is available on the proportion of patients who, during surgical resection, underwent systematic lymph node dissection (SND) or mediastinal lymph node sampling (MLS). Third, lung cancer patients frequently suffer from comorbidities, including cardiovascular diseases and chronic obstructive pulmonary disease that were found to affect survival significantly.

Notably, the positive adjuvant therapy trials were preceded by three negative randomized trials completed shortly after the 1995 NSCLCCG meta-analysis, which all failed to show any survival benefit with adjuvant cisplatin-based CT. The North American Eastern Cooperative Oncology Group (ECOG) 3590 study evaluated the efficacy of four cycles of postoperative cisplatin/etoposide plus concomitant thoracic RT in comparison with RT alone in 463 patients with stage II and IIIA NSCLC [18]. No significant differences between the two arms in terms of median time to progression were observed, and the relative likelihood of survival among patients assigned to receive CT plus RT, as compared to those assigned to receive postoperative RT alone, was 0.93 (95% CI, 0.74 to 1.18). The inclusion of adjuvant RT, which has been associated with greater mortality in stage II NSCLC patients [19], may have negated any potential benefit of adjuvant CT. This study was unique in its routine use of postoperative RT. All other studies primarily tested the efficacy of adjuvant CT versus observation alone in completely resected NSCLC, with the optional administration of sequential adjuvant RT in some of them according to an investigator choice [20,21]. A second study, the ALPI trial, randomly assigned 1209 patients with completely resected stage I, II or IIIA NSCLC to observation or three cycles of mitomycin, vindesine and cisplatin (MVP), an antiquated CT regimen [17]. Adjuvant RT was given to 43% of patients according with the policy of individual centers. No significant difference in OS was seen (55 vs. 49 months in the CT and surgery arm, respectively; HR, 0.96). High early death rates and poor compliance with adjuvant CT (only 69% patients completed three cycles with half of those patients requiring dose reduction) were known shortcomings of that study. Finally, the Big Lung Trial (BLT) randomized 381 patients with resected stage I to III NSCLC to three cycles of postoperative CT (doublet of cisplatin with either vindesine or vinorelbine or a triplet with mitomycin and ifosfamide or MVP) or surgery alone. Three cycles of CT were completed in 64% of patients, with 40% of them requiring dose reductions. Adjuvant RT was given to only 14% of cases. No significant differences in terms of survival were seen in the two groups, even if the trial was underpowered to answer the adjuvant CT benefit question, had a short follow-up of 29 months and 15% of patients with incompletely resected disease.

The Cancer and Leukemia Group B (CALGB) 9633 trial is the only large adjuvant CT study utilizing carboplatin rather than cisplatin and focusing exclusively on completely resected stage IB [22]. In this trial, 344 patients were randomly assigned to 4 cycles of adjuvant paclitaxel (200 $mg/m^2$ every 3 weeks) plus carboplatin (area under the concentration x time curve [AUC] 6 every 3 weeks) or observation. The study accrued slowly because of its limited range of eligible patients leading to a reduction in planned overall accrual cohort. A preliminary report presented at the ASCO Meeting in 2004 after a median follow-up time of 34 months detected a 12% absolute improvement in OS at 4 years (71% vs. 59%; HR, 0.62; 95% CI, 0.41-0.95; p=0.028). In accordance with the statistical plan, the trial was stopped early after the planned interim analysis with 90% of patients recruited demonstrating a significant improvement in OS. The delivery of CT was excellent with nearly 85% of patients who received 4 cycles of CT. Toxicity was minimal, with only 36% of patients having grades 3 and 4 myelosuppression. There were no treatment-related deaths. It should be noted, however, that the HR (0.83) was of a magnitude similar to those seen in the IALT (HR, 0.86) and the ANITA trial (HR, 0.80). A number of plausible explanations for the negative results of the CALGB9633 trial can be proposed. The lack of benefit with a carboplatin-based regimen as opposed to a cisplatin backbone is one hypothesis, especially given the cisplatin versus carboplatin meta-analysis demonstrating carboplatin regimens to be inferior to cisplatin-based CT in advanced NSCLC(23). Additional explanations include a true lack of benefit in patients with stage IB disease, because no other positive adjuvant therapy trial has shown a significant survival benefit for this substratum of patients [24] and, finally, a lack of statistical power. The CALGB 9633 trial was initially designed to detect a 13% higher 5-year survival rate (HR, 0.67), with an accrual goal of 500 patients. Because of slow enrollment and early closure, this goal was not reached and the resulting small sample size and low event rate contributed to the inability to detect a statistically significant survival advantage. The 3-year failure-free survival (66% vs. 57%) and 3-year survival (79% vs. 70%; p=0.045) continued to favor the CT group. A subgroup analysis, also presented at the follow-up at ASCO revealed that further dividing patients in CALGB 9633 into those with tumors smaller than 4 cm vs. those greater than or equal to 4 cm identified a higher-risk group for which CT may be beneficial[23]. In an unplanned subset analysis, patients in the CALGB 9633 study with tumors of at least 4 cm (close to 100 patients in each arm) retained an OS advantage (HR, 0.66; p<0.04), whereas the 74 patients in each arm with tumours smaller than 4 cm did not differ in survival (HR, 1.02; p=0.51).

One common feature of most of these studies, with the exclusion of the CALGB 9633, is the less than optima compliance to adjuvant regimens. The feasibility of three cycles of adjuvant CT (including delays and dose reductions) ranged between 58% and 74% of the cisplatin-based studies. Reason for reduced therapeutic compliance may be related to the need of a longer time to fully recover from the surgical procedure itself for lung cancer patients in comparison with that needed for breast or colon cancer patients. For instance, in some of these studies, the pneumonectomy rate was far exceeding that of consecutive surgical series and a specific subset analysis about tolerability of CT in this specific subgroup of patients (ALPI=26%, IALT=45%, ANITA=41%) has not been performed.

The improved survival with adjuvant CT using modern drug regimens was confirmed in the Lung Adjuvant Cisplatin Evaluation (LACE) meta-analysis that combined reported data from the five largest adjuvant clinical trials (ALPI, ANITA, BLT, IALT and JBR.10)[5]. The LACE meta-analysis included 4584 patients and detected a significantly positive effect of CT in terms of OS (HR, 0.89; 95% CI, 0.82-0.96; p=0.005) and DFS (HR, 0.84; 95% CI, 0.78-0.91; p<0.001), with an absolute survival benefit at 5 years of 5.4%. The survival benefit varied according to stage and was most pronounced for patients with stage II and IIIA disease (48.8% vs. 43.3%; HR, 0.83; 95% CI, 0.83-0.95). A small but not significant survival gain was also evident in stage IB (HR, 0.92; 95% CI, 0.78-1.10), but a detrimental effect was seen in stage IA (HR, 1.41; 95% CI, 0.96-2.1). The data were inadequate to establish the optimal cisplatin regimen. An excess of non–lung cancer deaths, primarily resulting from pulmonary/cardio-vascular disease, occurred within 6 months of random assignment (HR, 2.41; 95% CI, 1.64–3.55; p=0.001), but this finding did not extend past this point (HR, 1.06; 95% CI, 0.83–1.37; p=0.001). A subsequent meta-analysis that included individual patient data from these and older trials confirmed the survival benefit seen in the LACE meta-analysis [25]. This analysis provided additional support for the role of adjuvant CT in patients with stage IB disease and, in addition, it provided evidence that adjuvant CT had similar efficacy in patients whose initial treatment included both surgery (5-year survival, 64% vs. 60%; HR, 0.86; 95% CI, 0.81-0.92; p<0.0001) and adjuvant RT (5-year survival, 33% vs. 29%; HR, 0.88; 95% CI, 0.81-0.97; p<0.009).

## Adjuvant Studies with Oral CT Agents

UFT is an orally administered combination of ftorafur (tegafur) plus uracil (UFT), given in a 1:4 molar ratio. Ftorafur is a 5-fluorouracil (5-FU) derivative that is well absorbed orally and is converted into 5-FU *in vivo*. The uracil inhibits degradation of 5-FU, theoretically resulting in sustained tissue levels of the drug. This agent has been extensively studied in Japan as adjuvant single agent or combined with other intravenous agents.

The largest trial of postoperative UFT therapy in resected NSCLC randomly assigned 979 patients with completely resected stage I adenocarcinoma to either oral UFT 250 mg/m$^2$ for 2 years or observation [26]. The OS favored the UFT arm with an HR of 0.71 (95% CI, 0.52-0.98; p=0.04) and a 5-year survival of 88% in the UFT group and 85% in the control group. Subset analysis found the greatest benefit in the T2N0 subgroup (n=263; HR, 0.48; 95% CI, 0.29-0.81; p=0.005) but not in the T1N0 (n=716; HR, 0.97; 95% CI, 0.64-1.46; p=0.87). Compliance was limited at 74% at 12 months and only 61% at 24 months. One questionable point in this trial is the absence of any advantage in DFS for UFT-treated arm, and this clearly contrasts with all the positive, cisplatin-based adjuvant studies (IALT, NCIC-JBR10, ANITA) where improvement in OS for patients receiving adjuvant CT was invariably associated with a similar or greater magnitude in DFS. Results in three other fully studies (27) of adjuvant UFT in smaller sample size of patients were inconsistent with the previously reported study [28,29].

A meta-analysis looked at outcomes in 2003 patients treated with adjuvant UFT as a single agent or in combination with other cytotoxic agents enrolled in six trials with at least five years of follow-up [30]. Ninety-six percent of patients had stage I disease, 84 % had adenocarcinoma and 15% had squamous cell carcinoma. Adjuvant UFT was associated with a significant reduction in mortality compared to surgery alone (HR, 0.74; 95% CI, 0.61-0.88), corresponding to a 4.6% benefit at 5 years (p=0.001) and 7% at 7 years (p=0.001). There was no significant difference according to histologic subtype. The data from that meta-analysis were subsequently reexamined for the 1269 patients with stage IA NSCLC, based upon the 2010 TNM staging system [31]. In this analysis, 5-year OS was significantly improved for patients with T1b (>2 cm to ≤3 cm) primary tumors with adjuvant UFT compared to surgery alone (88 vs. 82%; HR, 0.62; 95% CI, 0.42-0.90), but the difference in 5-year OS was not significantly improved for patients with T1a (≤2 cm) primary tumors (87 vs. 85%; HR, 0.84; 95% CI, 0.58-1.23).

Despite these results, there is no confirmatory data concerning the use of UFT in the adjuvant setting outside Japan. The concept of relatively mild, low-dose continuous adjuvant therapy is attractive, but the absence of confirmatory adjuvant UFT studies outside Japan strongly limits the applicability of these data into clinical practice. Additionally, questions regarding a peculiar genetic sensitivity to UFT in the Japanese population remain unanswered.

## Determinants for Providing Adjuvant CT in Early-Stage NSCLC

Attention has now shifted to developing an approach to select patients most likely to benefit from adjuvant therapy. This approach should incorporate key practical issues such as the stage of disease, patient age and performance status (PS), selection of the appropriate CT regimen, and toxicity risks.

### *Disease Stage*

The adjuvant CT studies discussed above were not uniform in terms of their eligibility criteria for stage of disease, and this variability has contributed to the ongoing debate of determining which early-stage NSCLC patient should be considered for adjuvant CT. However, the available evidence allows for certain conclusions to be made (Table 2).

There is a lack of robust evidence from any of the adjuvant randomized trials or the LACE meta-analysis to advocate adjuvant CT in stage IB NSCLC. Controversy exists as to whether a subset of stage IB patients, defined by tumor size, benefit from this treatment. As discussed above, an unplanned subset analysis of the CALGB 9633 data revealed that, in patients with tumors ≥ 4 cm in diameter, a statistically significant DFS and OS benefit was observed (HR, 0.69; 95% CI, 0.48–0.99; p=0.043)[18]. Updated results of the JBR.10 trial showed that, in a similar subset analysis, patients with stage IB NSCLC and tumors ≥4 cm showed a non-significant trend in favor of adjuvant therapy (HR, 0.66; 95% CI, 0.39–1.14; p=0.13). In the LACE meta-analysis, a non significant survival gain with adjuvant CT was evident in stage IB (HR, 0.92; 95% CI, 0.78-1.10). Although these data suggest clinical benefit with adjuvant CT for tumors ≥ 4 cm, caution should be exercised in placing emphasis on these results, given the nature of unplanned subgroup analyses. The common practice is to consider these patients for adjuvant therapy in an individualized manner, after a thorough discussion of the risks and perceived benefits.

A consistent benefit for adjuvant CT has been established in stage II NSCLC. To date, the JBR.10 trial has shown the most striking survival benefit in this subset of patients (HR, 0.59; 95% CI, 0.42– 0.85; p=0.004), with an absolute 20% higher 5-year survival rate. Similarly, the ANITA trial showed a 13% higher 5-year survival rate (HR, 0.71; 95% CI, 0.49–1.03) and the LACE study revealed a 10% higher 5-year survival rate (HR, 0.83; 95% CI, 0.73–0.95).

For completely resected stage IIIA NSCLC, adjuvant CT is also clearly beneficial. A 16% absolute higher 5-year survival rate was seen in the ANITA trial (HR, 0.69; 95% CI, 0.53-0.90) and in the IALT study, the greatest benefit was observed in stage IIIA patients (HR, 0.79; 95% CI, 0.66–0.95). Finally, the LACE meta-analysis data support the use of adjuvant CT for patients with stage IIIA disease (HR=0.83; 95% CI, 0.72– 0.95), showing a 13% absolute higher 5-year survival rate in those patients receiving adjuvant treatment.

The evidence supporting adjuvant CT in resected NSCLC is derived from trials that staged patients based on the fifth edition of tumor–node–metastasis (TNM) Classification of Malignant Tumors (1997). However, the recently implemented seventh edition contains important changes that are impacting treatment recommendations [32]. Considering that there are no prospectively validated data supporting a survival benefit with adjuvant CT in stage IB patients, the shift of T2 (>5–7 cm)N0 and T2(>7 cm)N0 lesions into the category of stage II disease is potentially problematic. However, by accepting that patients with tumors ≥4 cm benefit from adjuvant CT, then these patients should reasonably be offered this treatment as per other stage II NSCLC patients. The revision to stage based on the location of separate pulmonary nodules is somewhat more challenging. Tumors with satellite nodules within the lobe of the primary tumor previously were classified as T4 lesions and, thus, patients were denoted to have stage IIIB NSCLC. The seventh edition of the TNM classification downstages these lesions to stage IIIA (T3N1 or T3N2) disease. Adjuvant early-stage NSCLC CT trials have all excluded patients with T4 lesions from accrual. Despite the lack of evidence to provide specific recommendations for or against adjuvant therapy in this subset of patients, given the known high risk for recurrence, even with node-negative disease, it is reasonable to offer adjuvant CT for appropriately resected patients.

### *Performance Status (PS)*

It is well recognized that patients enrolled in adjuvant trials are generally those with an excellent PS (ECOG PS score, 0 or 1). For example, the JBR.10 trial excluded patients with a PS score 2 and only 4% of patients had a PS score of 2 in the LACE pooled analysis. Interestingly, a significant interaction between CT effect and PS was seen (test for trend, p=0.009 for OS and p=0.01 for DFS). Adjuvant CT appeared to have a detrimental effect in patients with a PS score of 2. Given these findings, it would be prudent to offer adjuvant CT only to patients with a PS score of 0 or 1.

### *Toxicity and Quality of Life (QOL)*

A complete discussion of NSCLC adjuvant therapy involves a description of not only its benefits but also its potential for harm, such as the risk for death related to treatment, effect of treatment on QOL, and potential for long-term side effects.

The reported toxicity rates from the adjuvant NSCLC clinical trials are highly variable, likely related not only to the patient population studied and CT regimen employed but also to differences in the methods of toxicity surveillance and data collection. The general applicability of the toxicity data is limited, in particular, by the younger population accrued within the clinical trials. The JBR.10 clinical trial was the only adjuvant study formally reporting QOL by implementation of the European Organization for Research and Treatment of Cancer (EORTC) Quality of Life Questionnaire C30 (33). Although patients receiving adjuvant CT reported worsening in certain aspects of QOL from baseline to 3 months of follow-up, likely reflecting the toxicities of treatment, by 9 months, QOL scores were comparable with those of patients in the observation arm. Hearing loss was a notable long-term adverse event and sensory neuropathy could be detected 30 months after randomization. The LACE meta-analysis reported a CT related death rate of 0.9%. There was an excess of non–lung cancer deaths in the first 6 months postrandomization related to CT toxicity and pulmonary/cardiovascular disease. The overall rate of grade 3 or 4 toxicity was 66%, predominantly a result of neutropenia.

*Selection of Adjuvant CT Regimen*

The majority of randomized clinic trials since the 1995 meta-analysis incorporated a cisplatin-based treatment regimen. The three positive trials used cisplatin-doublet CT, and the ANITA and JBR.10 trials specifically used cisplatin plus vinorelbine. The LACE meta-analysis also found a trend for longer survival with cisplatin plus vinorelbine; however, this may be explained by higher number of patients treated with this regimen (1888 patients; HR, 0.80) and to higher cisplatin total doses administered in combination with vinorelbine (320 to 400 mg/m$^2$). Interestingly, no randomized trials have been reported assessing adjuvant CT with a cisplatin doublet combined with a more contemporary cytotoxic agent (gemcitabine, docetaxel, pemetrexed). The prevailing assumption is that the equivalence of modern cisplatin-doublet CT in advanced NSCLC will translate to similar equivalence in the adjuvant setting. Indeed, the current ECOG-sponsored Intergroup trial, ECOG 1505, incorporates standard adjuvant CT regimens of cisplatin combined with vinorelbine, gemcitabine, docetaxel, or pemetrexed. Based strictly on the available evidence, carboplatin plus paclitaxel CT cannot be advocated for routine use in the adjuvant setting. The Cancer Care Ontario/ASCO Joint Expert Panel recommended against the use of carboplatin-based adjuvant regimens, because of the negative CALGB 9633 trial results [34].

## Preoperative CT for Early-Stage NSCLC

Preoperative CT has been assessed as an alternative to adjuvant therapy in a number of trials for patients with resectable NSCLC [37-54]. A meta-analysis based upon seven trials involving 988 patients suggested that neoadjuvant CT improved OS with an HR of 0.82 (5-year survival, 20% vs. 14 % without neoadjuvant CT; 95% CI, 0.69-0.97) [35]. Furthermore, authors found an incremental benefit by stage (stage IA=+4%; stage IB=+6%; stage II to III=+7%), but did not observe any interaction between the kind of platinum-containing regimen or the kind of adjuvant treatment (CT or RT).

The range of results observed with neoadjuvant CT is illustrated by several contemporary phase III trials (Table 3):

In a French trial, 355 patients with NSCLC (188 with stage IB or II, 167 with stage IIIA, including 35% with N2 disease) were randomly assigned to surgery with or without two cycles of preoperative cisplatin-based CT [36]. Responding patients were eligible for postoperative CT, as well. Neoadjuvant CT was associated with a trend toward a longer median DFS (27 vs. 13 months, p=0.15) and, at a median follow-up of 14 years, the 10-year DFS rate was significantly increased with CT plus surgery compared to surgery alone (55% vs. 38%; HR, 0.78; 95% CI, 0.62-0.98) [38]. There was a trend toward increased OS with neoadjuvant CT compared to surgery alone (29% vs. 21%, p=0.12), and the difference was statistically significant when multivariate analysis incorporated age, T stage, and N stage (HR, 0.69; 95% CI, 0.64-0.90).

In the multicenter European Intergroup trial MRC-LU 22 EORT-08012 NVALT-2, 519 patients with resectable NSCLC were randomly assigned to three cycles of platinum-based CT followed by surgery or to immediate surgery [39]. At randomization, 93% of patients had clinical stage I or II disease. Choice of CT regimen was at investigator´s choice, as was the intensity of preoperative staging, resulting in only one fourth of the patients being staged with mediastinoscopy and/or PET. The two most widely used combinations were vinorelbine plus cisplatin and gemcitabine plus cisplatin. Overall, 75% of patients completed all three cycles of CT. The objective response rate (ORR) was 47%. Despite the observed antitumor activity from CT, there was no improvement in PFS with neoadjuvant treatment (2-year DFS, 53% vs. 52% with immediate surgery; HR for recurrence, 0.96, 95% CI, 0.77-1.21). Similarly, there was no improvement in OS with preoperative CT (5-year survival, 44% vs. 45%; HR for death, 1.02; 95% CI, 0.80-1.31). Results were not reported as a function of stage. The negative results in this trial may be attributed to the very high percentage of patients enrolled with stage I disease. This trial also underscores the difficulties in accurately staging patients preoperatively; whereas 18% of the patients who were resected without neoadjuvant CT actually had a lower pathological than clinical stage, 41% were likewise "upstaged".

**Table 3. Contemporary phase III trials or preoperative CT for early-stage NSCLC**

| STUDY/YEAR | Nº PATIENTS/ STAGES | TREATMENT | DFS | OS |
|---|---|---|---|---|
| Westeel (2010) | n=355<br>52.9% IB/II<br>47.5% IIIA<br>(35% N2) | Surgery (n=176) →<br>Cisplatin+mitomicyn+ifosfamide x 2 cycles Surgery (n=178) | Median DFS, 13 months<br>Median DFS, 27 months<br>(p=0.15) | 10-year OS, 20.8%<br>10-year OS, 29.5%<br>(p=0.12) |
| Intergroup MRCLU22/NVALT2/ EORTC08012 (Gilligan, 2007) | n=519<br>61.5% I<br>31.5% II<br>6.8% III | Surgery (n=261) →<br>Cisplatin-based CT x 3 cycles Surgery (n=258) | Median DFS, 25 months<br>Median DFS, 26 months<br>(HR, 0.96; p=0.74) | Median OS, 55 months<br>Median OS, 54 months<br>(HR, 1.02; p=0.86) |
| SWOG 9900 (Pisters 2010) | n=354<br>67% IB/IIA<br>33% IIB/IIIA | Surgery (n=168) →<br>Carboplatin+paclitaxel x 3 cycles Surgery (n=169) | Median DFS, 20 months<br>Median DFS, 33 months<br>(HR,0.80; p=0.10) | Median OS, 41 months<br>Median OS, 62 months<br>(HR, 0.79; p=0.11) |
| NATCH (Felip, 2010) | n=624<br>10.57% IA<br>63.94% IB<br>23.07% II<br>1.44% IIIA (T3N1) | Surgery (n=212) →<br>Carboplatin+paclitaxel x 3 cycles Surgery (n=201) →<br>Surgery<br>Carboplatin+paclitaxel x 3 cycles (n=211) | 5-year DFS, 34.1%<br>5-year DFS, 38.3%<br>(HR,0.92; p=0.17)<br>5-year DFS, 36.6%<br>(HR, 0.96; p=0.74) | 5-year OS, 44%<br>5-year OS, 46.6%<br>(HR,0.88; p=0.31)<br>5-year OS, 45.5%<br>(HR, 1.01; p=0.97) |
| Scagliotti (2012) | n=270<br>53.7% IB/IIA<br>46.7% IIB/IIIA | Surgery (n=141) →<br>Cisplatin+gemcitabine x 3 cycles Surgery (n=129) | Median PFS, 34.8 months<br>Median PFS, 48 months<br>(HR, 0.70; p=0.003) | Median OS, 57.6 months<br>Median OS, 93.6 months<br>(HR, 0.63; p=0.02) |

DFS: disease-free survival; OS: overall survival; HR: hazard ratio.

The Southwest Oncology Group (SWOG) trial 9900 was a phase III trial comparing induction paclitaxel/carboplatin CT for three cycles followed by surgery to surgery alone in clinical stage IB, II and IIIA NSCLC (40). Mediastinoscopy was performed whenever the mediastinal lymph node size exceeded 1 cm and PET imaging was not required. PFS was prolonged with neoadjuvant CT compared to immediate surgery (median, 33 vs. 20 months; HR, 0.80; 95% CI, 0.619-1.04; p=0.10), although differences were not statistically significant. OS was not significantly longer with neoadjuvant CT (median 62 vs. 41 months; HR, 0.79;

95% CI, 0.60-1.06; p=0.11). The trial was terminated prematurely when positive results were obtained in large trials using adjuvant CT.

Neoadjuvant and adjuvant CT were compared to surgery alone in the three-armed NATCH trial [41]. In this trial, 624 patients with IA, IB, II, or III (T3N1) NSCLC were randomly assigned to surgery alone, neoadjuvant CT followed by surgery, or surgery followed by adjuvant CT. CT consisted of three cycles of paclitaxel plus carboplatin. Compliance with CT was significantly higher with neoadjuvant rather than adjuvant treatment (90% vs. 61% receiving three cycles, respectively). Despite this, there were no significant differences in the 5-year DFS rates (34%, 38%, and 37% for surgery alone, neoadjuvant CT, or adjuvant CT, respectively) or five-year OS rates (44%, 47%, and 46 %, respectively).

Finally, a European trial randomly assigned 270 patients to CT with gemcitabine plus cisplatin followed by surgery or to surgery alone [42]. Patients had resectable stage IB, II, or IIIA disease. Enrollment in the trial was terminated prematurely when positive results were obtained in large trials using adjuvant CT. Despite this, there were statistically significant improvements in PFS (3-year rate, 53% vs. 48%; HR, 0.70; p=0.003) and OS (3-year rate, 68% vs. 60%; HR, 0.63; p=0.02).

In summary, the available outcome data trend in favor of neoadjuvant therapy, but the majority of individual trials did not find a statistically significant benefit. The results of these trials and the meta-analysis do not support the use of a neoadjuvant approach rather than immediate surgery with postoperative adjuvant CT for patients with resectable NSCLC [43].

## The Role of Adjuvant RT

The role of adjuvant RT in patients with completely resected NSCLC remains uncertain. Although initial retrospective series suggested improvements in local control, a survival benefit was not confirmed in randomized trials [44]. In a 1998 meta-analysis (PORT) that included 2128 patients enrolled in nine randomized trials evaluating postoperative RT, adjuvant RT was associated with an inferior outcome, with a 21% relative increase in the risk of death, which translated into a 7% absolute reduction in 2-year survival (48% vs. 55% in patients receiving and not receiving adjuvant RT, respectively). However, in subgroup analysis, the detrimental effect on survival was limited to patients with N0 and N1 disease, whereas there was no clear evidence of either an adverse or a beneficial effect for those with N2 disease. These results have been further confirmed by a Cochrane systematic review and meta-analysis originally published in 2000 and substantially updated in 2004 [45]. The results of this recent update indicate a significant adverse effect of adjuvant RT on survival with a HR of 1.18. This is equivalent to an absolute detriment of 6% at 2 years (95% CI, 2-9%) reducing OS from 58% to 52%. Subgroup analysis suggest that this detrimental effect was most pronounced for patients with stage I/II, whereas for patients with stage III, N2, there was no clear evidence of an adverse effect.

The results of these two meta-analysis are subject to several important limitations [46]. For example, older radiation techniques such as cobalt machines, radiation fields inferior to current standards and high overall doses and fraction sizes used in many of the trials are not consistent with current standards. In addition, more than 30% of the patients included in the meta-analysis came from a single study in which large dose fractions (2.5 Gy) and high total doses (up to 60 Gy) were permitted, an approach that may have increased toxicity, thereby biasing the outcome of the meta-analysis [47]. These factors call into question the applicability of the results in a modern setting.

Two subsequent large scale analyses from the Surveillance, Epidemiology and End Results (SEER) database evaluated the role of extent of disease on survival after postoperative RT and the effect of radiation technique on cardiac toxicity [48, 49]. In the first analysis, 7465 patients coded as receiving adjuvant RT or observation with stage II or III NSCLC who underwent a lobectomy or pneumonectomy were selected within the SEER database. Median follow-up time was 3.5 years for patients still alive. Overall, the use of adjuvant RT did not have a significant impact on survival in a multivariate analysis. Exploratory subgroup analysis showed that patients with N0 or N1 disease had a significantly decreased 5-year survival rate with postoperative RT (31% vs. 41% with observation for those with N0 disease; 30% vs. 34% for those with N1 disease), a result consistent with the PORT meta-analysis.

More recently, results from the phase III ANITA trial suggest that the effect of postoperative RT is affected both by the extent of nodal involvement and the use of adjuvant CT [50]. Formal statistical comparisons were not performed because of the nonrandomized nature of this subset analysis. Adjuvant RT was recommended, in a nonrandomized fashion, for patients with node-positive disease but was not mandated by the protocol. If adjuvant RT was used, the recommended dose and fractionation were 45–60 Gy in 2 Gy fractions over 5 weeks. Of the 840 total patients accrued, 232 received adjuvant RT. One third of those were in the observation arm and 21.6% were in the CT arm. For patients with N2 disease, survival was longer in patients who received postoperative RT than in those not given RT (median 47 vs. 24 months in those given adjuvant CT and 23 vs. 13 months in those not given adjuvant CT). In contrast, for those with N1 disease, RT had a negative effect on survival in those given adjuvant CT (47 vs. 94 months) but a positive effect in those not receiving CT (50 vs. 26 months). Although the use of adjuvant RT was not randomized, these findings add to the signal of a potential benefit for adjuvant RT in N2 disease. Furthermore, this benefit was found in the setting of adjuvant CT administration.

To summarize, adjuvant RT has been shown to lead to a lower local recurrence rate, but demonstration of a survival benefit in randomized trials is lacking. Most of the evidence suggesting a potential benefit for adjuvant RT in patients with N2 lymph node involvement is retrospective and nonrandomized.

Based on the current evidence, postoperative RT is commonly used in the following situations:

a. For patients with positive resection margins.
b. For patients with inadequate lymph node sampling in whom mediastinal node involvement was suspected but not confirmed. The use of adjuvant RT in this scenario should not be prioritized over that of adjuvant CT.
c. For patients with involvement of multiple stations of involved N2 lymph nodes.

If RT is planned for the postoperative setting, it should be given after completion of adjuvant CT, since a concurrent approach might compromise the ability to deliver recommended dose and cycles of CT.

However, prospective randomized trials documenting the effectiveness of postoperative RT in these situations are needed. A large multi-institutional European phase III trial, the Lung Adjuvant Radiotherapy Trial (Lung ART), compares three- dimensional conformal adjuvant RT with no RT, and will include patients who have proven N2 disease and a complete resection irrespective of whether adjuvant or neoadjuvant CT was used. Seven hundred patients will be included to show a 10% difference in terms of 3-year DFS, which is the primary end point.

# Future Directions: Targeted Therapies and Genetic Predictive and Prognostic Biomarkers

## Targeted Therapy

Integrating novel biological therapeutics into standard treatment paradigms for advanced NSCLC patients has been successful, and these are now being investigated in the early stage setting within the context of large, phase III, randomized clinical trials.

Epidermal growth factor receptor (EGFR) tyrosine kinase inhibitors (TKI) (erlotinib, gefitinib) have an established role in the treatment of patients with metastatic NSCLC [51, 52] and activating mutations of EGFR and also represents a reasonable therapeutic approach for adjuvant therapy clinical trials. Despite the activity of these EGFR TKI in appropriately selected patients, there is no evidence that these agents have a role in an adjuvant setting. A pivotal Japanese phase III study planned to administer adjuvant gefitinib 250 mg/day or placebo to randomized patients with completely resected NSCLC (stages IB to IIIA) 4 to 6 weeks following surgery, for 2 years or until recurrence/withdrawal [53]. However, recruitment was stopped after the randomization of only 38 patients, because intersticial lung disease-type events were being increasingly reported in Japan in the advanced disease setting leading to safety concerns in this population of potentially cured patients. Safety data for 38 recruited patients (18 gefitinib and 20 placebo) showed no unexpected adverse drug reactions, with the most common being grades 1 and 2 gastrointestinal and skin disorders in 12 and 16 patients receiving gefitinib and in 5 and 6 patients receiving placebo, respectively. In the same patient population, another phase III study from the NCIC, the BR.19, randomly assigned completely resected NSCLC patients to gefitinib vs. placebo between 2002 and 2005 [54].

Adjuvant CT was permitted and patients were stratified based upon whether or not they received such treatment. The trial was closed prematurely after the inclusion of 503 patients as consequence of the negative outcome of other phase III studies (SWOG 0139 in stage IIIB, which tested gefitinib versus placebo in non-progressive patients following concurrent chemoradiotherapy and maintenance docetaxel [55] and a second-line study of gefitinib versus placebo, the ISEL study [56]. A final analysis with a minimum follow-up of four years was presented at the 2010 ASCO meeting. There was a trend toward better OS and DFS in patients assigned to placebo (HR, 1.23; 95% CI, 0.94-1.64 and HR,1.22; 95% CI, 0.93-1.61, respectively). No benefit was observed in subset analyses based upon EGFR mutation status. However, these results must be interpreted with caution, since the number of patients positive for EGFR was limited and the duration of their treatment was highly variable and shorter than planned.

The Randomized Double-Blind Trial in Adjuvant NSCLC with Tarceva (RADIANT) is currently in progress. It is a phase III trial for patients with resected stage IB–IIIA NSCLC who are EGFR+ by immunohistochemistry and/or fluorescent in situ hybridization (FISH). The target accrual is 945 patients, who are being randomized 2:1 to receive erlotinib or placebo for 2 years after surgical resection. Patients may receive up to four cycles of adjuvant CT, but administration of adjuvant CT is not required. Results are not expected until 2014.

**Table 4. Summary of predictive and prognostic biomarkers of benefit from adjuvant chemotherapy**

| MOLECULAR MARKER | BIOLOGICAL ROLE | STUDY | ROLE AS PROGNOSTIC FACTOR | ROLE AS PREDICTOR OF BENEFIT FROM ADJUVANT CT |
|---|---|---|---|---|
| GENE EXPRESSION PROFILES | Angiogenesis, signaling pathways and invasive activity and survival of cancer cells | Potti, 2006 | The lung metagene model for the prediction of recurrence was superior to a predictive model built with clinical data (overall accuracy, 93% vs. 64%). | Gene expression profiles can be useful for selecting high-risk patients to be treated with adjuvant CT |
| | | Chen, 2007 | The patients with a high-risk gene signature had a shorter median RFS (13 months vs. 29 months; p=0.002) and OS (20 months vs. 40 months) than the patients with low-risk gene signature | |
| | | Seike, 2007 | CLASS-11 is and independent prognostic fator for stage I patients (HR for death high risk/low risk, 7.46; p=0.002) | |
| | | Tsao, 2008 | The 15-gene signature separated the 62 observation patients into groups with high and low risk for death (HR, 60.1; p <0.0001) | CT significantly reduced the risk of death in high-risk stage IB (HR, 0.28; p=0.007) and stage II patients (HR, 0.26; p=0.0059), but not in low risk patients (HR, 15.49; p=0.008) |
| ERCC1 | ERCC1 plays a central role in DNA repair pathway by removing cisplatin-induced DNA adducts. It is associated with resistance to platinum-based CT | Olaussen, 2006 | In the control group, the 5-year OS rate was significantly higher among patients with ERCC1-positive tumors than among patients with ERCC1-negative tumors (HR, 0.66; 95% CI, 0.49-0.9; p=0.009). | Adjuvant CT, as compared with observation, significantly prolonged OS among patients with ERCC1 negative tumors (HR, 0.65; 95% CI, 0.50-0.86; p=0.002) but not among patients with ERCC-1 positive tumors (HR, 1.14; 95% CI, 0.84-1.55; p=0.40). |
| RRM1 | RRM1 is involved in carcinogenesis,tu morprogression and the response of NSCLC cells to CT | Zheng, 2007 | High expression of RRM1 is associated with better RFS (HR, 0.46; p=0.004) and OS (HR, 0.61; p=0.02). RRM1 expression correlated with the expression of ERCC1 (p<0.001). The coordinate high expression of RRM1 and ERCC1 defines a subgroup of patients with an excellent outcome. | |

| MOLECULAR MARKER | BIOLOGICAL ROLE | STUDY | ROLE AS PROGNOSTIC FACTOR | ROLE AS PREDICTOR OF BENEFIT FROM ADJUVANT CT |
|---|---|---|---|---|
| BRCA1 | BRCA1 plays an important role in DNA repair and regulates differential sensitivity to different classes of CT agents | Taron, 2004[99] | Patients with low levels of BRCA1 had better median survival (p=0.01). | |
| | | Rosell, 2007 | Patients whose tumors had high BRCA1 expression had significantly worse survival (HR, 1.98; 95% CI, 1.11-6; p=0.02) and should be candidates for adjuvant CT | |
| | | Bartolucci, 2009 | The combination of high BRCA1 and low XPG mRNA expression increases the risk of shorter survival in early NSCLC (p=0.007) | |
| CLASS IIIβ-TUBULIN EXPRESSION (bTubIII) | BTubIII is a component of the mitotic spindle in multiple cell types and it is implicated in clinical resistance to tubulin-binding agents | Sève, 2007 | High bTubIII expression was associated with poorer RFS (HR, 1.92; 95% CI , 1.16-3.18; p=0.01) and OS (HR 1.72; 95% CI 1.02-2.88; p=0.04) in patients treated with surgery alone. | High bTubII patients receiving cisplatin-vinorelbine adjuvant CT had significantly improved RFS (HR, 0.45; 95% CI, 0.27-0.75; p=0.002) and a trend toward improved OS (HR, 0.64; 95% CI, 0.39-1.04; p=0.07) compared with patients in the observation arm. |
| | | Reiman, 2006 | High bTubIII expresion was associated with poorer RFS (HR, 1.9; p=0.01) in patients treated with surgery alone, but not in patients treated with adjuvant CT (HR, 0.45; p=0.002). | High bTubIII expression did not correlate with benefit from adjuvant CT. |
| CELL CYCLE REGULATORS | P53, Ras and p27 play key roles in regulating cell cycle progression, apoptosis, gene transcription, response to stress and DNA repair. Moreover, p27 is a regulator of drug resistance in solid tumors | Tsao, 2007 | In the observation arm, patients with p53 protein overexpression had significantly shorter survival than did those with p53-negative tumors (HR, 1.89; 95% CI, 1.07-3.34; p=0.03) | Patients with p53 protein overexpression derived significant benefit from adjuvant CT (HR, 0.54; 95% CI, 0.32-0.92; p=0.02), while patients with p53-negative tumors had not. |
| | | Filipits, 2007 | Among patients with p27Kip1-negative tumors, cisplatin-based CT resulted in longer OS compared with controls (HR, 0.66; 95% CI 0.50-0.88; p=0.006). In patients with p27Kip1-positive tumors, OS was not different between patients treated with cisplatin-based CT and control (HR, 1.09; 95% CI, 0.82-1.45; p=0.54). | |
| DNA METHYLATION MARKERS | Gene silencing in cancer is associated with hipermethylation of DNA in promoter regions. Epigenetic silencing is involved in the initiation and progression of NSCLC | Brock, 2008 | The methylation of the promoter regions of genes involved in cell-cycle control (p16), invasion and metastasis (CDH13, APC) and RAS signaling (RASSF1A) in a resected NSCLC specimen (tumor, regional and mediastinal lymph nodes) is associated with a significantly increased risk of early recurrences. | |

CT: chemotherapy; RFS: relapse-free survival; OS: overall survival; HR: hazard ratio; CI: confidence nterval; ERCC1: excision repair cross-complementation group 1; RRM1: regulatory subunit of ribonucleotide reductase; BRCA1: breast cancer 1; bTubIII: class III β-tubulin; CDH13: H-cadherin gene; APC: adenomatous polyposis coli gene; RASSF1A: Ras association domain family 1 gene.

On the other hand, the crucial role of angiogenesis in lung cancer development is very well documented. Although other angiogenic factors have been identified, vascular endothelial growth factor (VEGF) is the most potent and specific, with a well-defined role in normal and pathological angiogenesis [57]. VEGF is a strong prognostic indicator in NSCLC and is associated with early postoperative relapse and decreased survival [58]. Bevacizumab, a recombinant, humanized monoclonal antibody against VEGF, inhibits angiogenesis and is the first targeted therapy in NSCLC to improve clinical outcomes when given in combination with CT (59.60). Whether its role is limited to advanced NSCLC or its benefits can extend to earlier stage disease is the focus of an ongoing ECOG adjuvant therapy trial (ECOG 1505). This multicenter phase III trial randomized radically resected stage IB (≥4 cm) to IIIA NSCLC patients to receive adjuvant platinum-based doublet CT (cisplatin/vinorelbine, cisplatin/gemcitabine or cisplatin/docetaxel) with or without bevacizumab. An accrual of 1500 subjects is planned.

Finally, the recombinant melanoma-associated antigen (MAGE)-A3 vaccine is also being investigated in NSCLC. Its immunogenicity has been documented in melanoma and lung cancer, and many CD4 and CD8 T-cell epitopes have been mapped to this target protein (61). Based on encouraging phase II data, a phase III efficacy trial, MAGE-A3 Adjuvant Non-Small Cell Lung Cancer Immunotherapy, was launched for patients with surgically resected stage IB–III NSCLC that expresses MAGE-A3 [62]. It is hypothesized that postoperative MAGE-A3 immunization will result in a longer DFS interval, the primary endpoint of the study.

## Molecular Biomarkers

To individualize, among heterogeneous patient populations, those individuals who are more likely to benefit from adjuvant CT, a better definition of the prognostic or predictive implications of the tumors´ genetic makeup as well as of the tumors´ or patients´ pharmacogenetic variations is needed. Molecular markers may provide additional information about the likelihood of relapse beyond that obtained from pathologic staging. Approaches and specific markers under study include gene expression profiling [63-65] , excision repair cross-complementation group 1 gene (ERCC1) and ribonucleotide reductase M1 (RRM1) expression, , abnormalities in the KRAS oncogene and p53 tumor suppressor gene, β-tubulin expression and DNA methylation markers. Additional studies will be required to determine whether these markers are useful in selecting patients for adjuvant platinum-based CT.

### *Gene Expression Profiling*

Several candidate signatures involving multigene expression profiles have been put forward as predictive of recurrence and survival for resected NSCLC [66]. In one of these studies, researchers looked at 89 patients with early stage NSCLC. Their gene-expression profile (the lung metagene model) predicted recurrence for individual patients significantly better than did clinical prognostic factors, and it was consistent across all early stages of NSCLC. When applied to other two independent cohorts of 25 and 84 patients, the model had an overall predictive accuracy of 72% and 79%, respectively. The predictor also identified a subgroup of patients with stage IA disease who were at high risk for recurrence. As a consequence of these results, the CALGB 30506 study is currently ongoing for patients with resected stage I NSCLC, 2–6 cm in size, who are not candidates for the ECOG 1505 Intergroup trial and who do not routinely receive adjuvant CT. The premise for this trial is founded on a genomics prognostic model known as the lung metagene score (LMS) to select patients for adjuvant CT based on published preliminary data[62]. Low-risk patients will only be observed, whereas high-risk patients will be randomized to either observation, according to standard practice for stage IA NSCLC or receive adjuvant cisplatin-based doublet CT. The key primary objectives of this unique trial are to validate the positive prognostic value for survival of patients with a low LMS, who are believed to be at a low risk for recurrence, and to determine whether a survival advantage is associated with adjuvant CT in patients with an unfavorably high LMS [67].

### *ERCC1, RMM1 and BRCA1 Expression*

The ERCC1 gene encodes an enzyme that is essential for the efficient repair of DNA damage induced by alkylating agents such as platinum compounds [68]. Immunohistochemical detection of ERCC1 expression in a primary NSCLC may be a predictor for lack of benefit from platinum-based adjuvant CT. This was suggested in an analysis of 761 tumors from patients enrolled in the IALT trial (Bio-IALT) [69]. Adjuvant CT resulted in a significant improvement in 5-year survival (47% vs. 39% without CT, HR, 0.65) for patients whose tumors did not express ERCC1. In contrast, CT was associated with a non-significant trend toward worse 5-year survival (40 vs. 46% without CT, HR 1.14) when ERCC1 was expressed on the tumor. At this time, treatment recommendations based on ERCC1 analysis cannot be supported by the available data. Whether these patients would benefit from any form of adjuvant therapy, including non-platinum regimens, is unknown.

Differential expression of RRM1 is also emerging as a promising strategy to molecularly define patients receiving adjuvant CT. RRM1, inhibited by gemcitabine, provides deoxyribonucleotides not only for de novo DNA synthesis but also for DNA repair [70]. In a retrospective study, RRM1 and ERCC1 expression as evaluated through a recent innovation in methodology for quantitative protein expression (automated quantitative analysis) was found to have a prognostic impact on survival after surgical treatment of early stage NSCLC (71). The OS was more than 120 months for patients with tumours with high expression of RRM1 vs. 60 months for those with low expression of RRM1. Among these 187 patients, the survival advantage was limited to the 30% for patients with tumours that had a high expression of both RMM1 and ERCC1.

The ongoing SWOG 0720 clinical trial is evaluating the prognostic and predictive role of ERCC1 and RRM1 in selecting patients with stage I (primary tumor ≥2 cm) NSCLC for adjuvant platinum based CT. In that trial, patients with completely resected stage IA–IB NSCLC with high expression levels of ERCC1 and RRM1 are assigned to observation alone, because of a good prognosis, whereas those with low levels of either biomarker are assigned to cisplatin–gemcitabine adjuvant therapy, given the poorer expected prognosis and predicted benefit of platinum-based CT [72]. The primary objective is to test the feasibility of such an approach, defined by the percentage of patients who can be assigned to treatment appropriately, reflecting the adequacy of tumor specimen collection and analysis.

Breast cancer 1 (BRCA1) also plays a crucial role in DNA repair and it is implicated in transcription-coupled nucleotide excision repair (TC-NER). Modulation of its expression leads to modification of TC-NER and hence to radio and chemoresistance [73,74]. Rosell and colleagues found that the overexpression of BRCA1 mRNA was strongly associated with poor survival in early-stage (IA-IIIA) NSCLC patients. Patients whose tumours had high BRCA1 expression (HR for death; 1.98; p=0.02) had significantly worse survival and should be candidates for adjuvant CT. In addition, xeroderma pigmentosum group G (XPG) RNA expression levels also modulate prognosis in resected NSCLC in conjunction with BRCA1 expression. High BRCA1 mRNA expression confers poor prognosis in early NSCLC, and the combination of high BRCA1 and low XPG expression still further increases the risk of shorter survival. These findings can help optimize the customization of adjuvant CT [75].

Many European groups are focusing on biomarker-driven adjuvant therapy in order to move toward personalized care. In an ongoing phase III International Tailored Chemotherapy Adjuvant trial (ITACA), patients with completely resected stage II–III NSCLC are treated with standard adjuvant CT or a tailored regimen based on thymidylate synthase and ERCC1 gene expression levels. The TAilored Post-Surgical Therapy in Early Stage (TASTE) trial is randomizing patients with stage II–IIIA (non-N2) resected nonsquamous NSCLC to a non-customized adjuvant CT arm and a genotypic arm, in which patients with known EGFR-activating mutations receive erlotinib for 1 year, while those who have wild-type EGFR receive CT based on the level of ERCC1 expression. Finally, the Spanish Customized Adjuvant Trial (SCAT) is looking at assigning adjuvant CT after determining the level of BRCA1 mRNA expression, which predicts response or lack of response to cisplatin and docetaxel, in surgically resected stage II–IIIA NSCLC patients, compared with a standard arm of cisplatin plus docetaxel for all patients.

### *KRAS and P53*

Both the KRAS oncogene and the p53 tumor suppressor gene have been implicated in the pathogenesis of NSCLC [76,77]. Abnormalities in these genes were studied in a subset of 253 patients from the JBR.10 adjuvant CT trial[75]. Patients with mutations in KRAS in their tumor did not appear to benefit from adjuvant CT, while those with wild-type KRAS did significantly better. Overexpression of the p53 gene as assessed by immunohistochemistry was associated with a significantly poorer prognosis compared to patients who were negative for p53 overexpression, but the benefit from adjuvant CT was greater among those with p53 overexpression. Patients with mutations in p53 did not appear to benefit from adjuvant CT.

### *B-Tubulin Expression*

Overexpression of class I and class III β-tubulin play a significant role in the acquisition of paclitaxel resistance [78]. Class III β-tubulin expression is also correlated with patient outcome in NSCLC patients treated with vinorelbine-based regimens [79,80]. The role of class III β-tubulin was assessed in the NCIC-BR10 study on 265 out of 482 patients enrolled in the trial. Overexpression of class III β-tubulin was associated with worse OS in the observation arm (HR, 1.72; 95% CI, 1-02-2.88; p=0.04) but not in the CT arm. A greater benefit from adjuvant CT was seen in patients with high expression of class III β-tubulin, whereas in the setting of advanced disease, the opposite was evident. Such data need larger confirmatory studies.

### *DNA Methylation Markers*

Methylation of the promoter region of four genes thought to be important in the pathogenesis of lung cancer (p16, CDH13, APC, and RASSF1A) has been associated with a significantly increased risk of recurrent NSCLC [81]. In a study of 167 patients who underwent potentially curative resection of stage I NSCLC, including 51 who relapsed within 40 months after surgery, the absence of promoter methylation correlated with higher rates of subsequent DFS (77%, 51%, and 30 % at five years in those with none, one or two, and three or four methylated genes, respectively). As with other molecular markers, these results require confirmation in a larger prospective study before they can be used to select patients for adjuvant therapy.

## Conclusion

Multiple phase III randomized trials have conclusively demonstrated that adjuvant CT using modern cisplatin-based regimens has a positive impact on DFS and OS in carefully selected patients with NSCLC. These benefits have been confirmed in a meta-analysis of trials based upon individual patient data using modern CT regimens[21]. The survival advantage is most pronounced for those with stage II and IIIA disease, but some patients with stage IB may benefit as well.

Guidelines from the ASCO and Cancer Care Ontario and from the National Comprehensive Cancer Network (NCCN) [82] recommend adjuvant systemic CT with a cisplatin-based regimen for patients with completely resected stage II or IIIA NSCLC. A reasonable option is the combination of vinorelbine plus cisplatin as used in the JBR.10 and ANITA trials, although other modern cisplatin-based regimens may be equally effective. The role of carboplatin-based combinations as an adjuvant remains uncertain. For patients with stage IB NSCLC, the evidence from individual trials is conflicting, although the LACE meta-analysis provides additional support for this approach. The ASCO Cancer Care Ontario guidelines do not endorse adjuvant CT for routine use because the lack of definitive evidence establishing improved survival. The NCCN guidelines consider either observation or adjuvant CT appropriate options for patients with resected stage IB NSCLC depending on risk factors for recurrence. For patients with resected stage IA NSCLC, guidelines do not recommend using adjuvant CT except in the context of a clinical trial because of the favorable prognosis and absence of data supporting a benefit.

Despite all these promising data, considerable gains have yet to be made. The landscape for treating NSCLC patients is in flux and the identification of predictive biomarkers and the development of genomic and pharmacogenomic models to "personalize" the adjuvant treatment of early-stage NSCLC patients is an active area of current, and undoubtedly, future research. Moreover, as research efforts continue to unravel the molecular pathways behind lung tumorigenesis, novel targets are being exposed, forming the rationale for modern adjuvant therapy clinical trials integrating biological agents such as bevacizumab and erlotinib. Whether these approaches will substantially improve upon the current standard of adjuvant cisplatin-based doublet CT remains to be seen.

## References

[1] Jemal A, Bray F, Center MM, et al. Global cancer statistics. *CA Cancer J Clin* 2011; 61:69.

[2] Siegel R, Naishadham D, Jemal A. Cancer statistics, 2012. *CA Cancer J Clin* 2012; 62:10.

[3] Jemal A, Thun MJ, Ries LA, et al. Annual report to the nation on the status of cancer, 1975-2005, featuring trends in lung cancer, tobacco use, and tobacco control. *J Natl Cancer Inst* 2008; 100:1672.

[4] Siegel R, Naishadham D, Jemal A. Cancer statistics, 2012. *CA Cancer J Clin* 2012; 62:10-29.

[5] Goldstraw P, Crowley J, Chansky K, et al. The IASLC Lung Cancer Staging Project: Proposals for the revision of the TNM stage groupings in the forthcoming (seventh) edition of the TNM Classification of malignant tumours. *J Thorac Oncol* 2007;2:706-714.

[6] Besse B, Le Chevalier T. Adjuvant or induction cisplatin-based chemotherapy for operable lung cancer. *Oncology* (Williston Park) 2009;23:520-527.

[7] Arriagada R, Dunant A, Pignon JP, et al. Long-term results of the International Adjuvant Lung Cancer Trial evaluating adjuvant cisplatin-based chemotherapy in resected lung cancer. *J Clin Oncol* 2010;28:35-42.

[8] Pignon JP, Tribodet H, Scagliotti GV et al. Lung adjuvant cisplatin evaluation: A pooled analysis by the LACE Collaborative Group. *J Clin Oncol* 2008;26:3552–3559.

[9] Wagner H Jr, Bonomi P. Preoperative and postoperative therapy for non-small cell lung cancer. In: Roth JA, Ruckdeschel JC, Weisenburger TH, eds. *Thoracic Oncology. 2nd ed.* Philadelphia: WB Saunders 1995: 147-163.

[10] Niiranen A, Niitamo-Korhonen S, Kouri M, et al. Adjuvant chemotherapy after radical surgery for non-small-cell lung cancer: a randomized study. *J Clin Oncol* 1992; 10:1927-1932.

[11] Dautzenberg B, Chastang C, Arriagada R, et al. Adjuvant radiotherapy versus combined sequential chemotherapy followed by radiotherapy in the treatment of resected non-small cell lung carcinoma. A randomized trial of 267 patients. GETCB (Groupe d'Etude et de Traitement de Cancers Bronchiques). *Cancer* 1995; 76: 779-786.

[12] Non-Small Cell Lung Cancer Collaborative Group. Chemotherapy in non-small-cell lung cancer: A meta-analysis using updated data on individual patients from 52 randomised clinical trials. *BMJ* 1995; 311:899-909.

[13] Arriagada R, Bergman B, Dunant A, et al. Cisplatin-based adjuvant chemotherapy in patients with completely resected non-small-cell lung cancer. *N Engl J Med* 2004;350:351-360.

[14] Winton T, Livingston R, Johnson D et al. Vinorelbine plus cisplatin vs. observation in resected non-small-cell lung cancer. *N Engl J Med* 2005;352: 2589-2597.

[15] Douillard JY, Rosell R, De Lena M, et al. Adjuvant vinorelbine plus cisplatin versus observation in patients with completely resected stage IB-IIIA non-small-cell lung cancer (Adjuvant Navelbine International Trialist Association [ANITA]): A randomised controlled trial. *Lancet Oncol* 2006;7:719-727.

[16] Butts CA, Ding K, Seymour L, et al. Randomized phase III trial of vinorelbine plus cisplatin compared with observation in completely resected stage IB and II non-small cell lung cancer: Updated survival analysis of JBR.10. *J Clin Oncol* 2010;28:29-34.

[17] Scagliotti GV, Fossati R, Torri V, et al. Randomized study of adjuvant chemotherapy for completely resected stage I, II, or IIIA non-small-cell lung cancer. *J Natl Cancer Inst* 2003;95:1453-1461.

[18] Keller SM, Adak S, Wagner H, et al. A randomized trial of postoperative adjuvant therapy in patients with completely resected stage II or IIIA nonsmall-cell lung cancer. Eastern Cooperative Oncology Group. *N Engl J Med* 2000;343:1217–1222.

[19] PORT Meta-analysis Trialists Group. Postoperative radiotherapy in non-small-cell lung cancer: Systematic review and meta-analysis of individual patient data from nine randomised controlled trials. *Lancet* 1998;352:257–263.

[20] Waller D, Peake MD, Stephens RJ, et al. Chemotherapy for patients with non-small cell lung cancer: The surgical setting of the Big Lung Trial. *Eur J Cardiothorac Surg* 2004;26:173-82.

[21] Strauss GM, Herndon JE 2nd, Maddaus MA, et al. Adjuvant paclitaxel plus carboplatin compared with observation in stage IB non-small-cell lung cancer:CALGB9633 with the Cancer and Leukemia Group B, Radiation Therapy Oncology Group, and North Central Cancer Treatment Group Study Groups. *J Clin Oncol* 2008;26:5043–5051.

[22] Strauss G, Herndon J, Maddaus M, et al. Adjuvant chemotherapy in stage IB non-small cell lung cancer (NSCLC): Update of Cancer and Leukemia Group B (CALGB) protocol 9633. *J Clin Oncol* 2006;24:18s (Abstr 7007).

[23] Ardizzoni A, Boni L, Tiseo M et al. Cisplatin- versus carboplatin-based chemotherapy in first-line treatment of advanced non-small-cell lung cancer: An individual patient data meta-analysis. *J Natl Cancer Inst* 2007;99:847–857.

[24] Pignon JP, Tribodet H, Scagliotti GV et al. Lung adjuvant cisplatin evaluation: A pooled analysis by the LACE Collaborative Group. *J Clin Oncol* 2008;26:3552–3559.

[25] Arriagada R, Auperin A. NSCLC Meta-analyses Collaborative Group. Adjuvant chemotherapy, with or without postoperative radiotherapy, in operable non-small-cell lung cancer: two meta-analyses of individual patient data. *Lancet* 2010; 375: 1267-1277.

[26] Kato H, Ichinose Y, Ohta M, et al. A randomized trial of adjuvant chemotherapy with uracil-tegafur for adenocarcinoma of the lung. *N Engl J Med* 2004; 350: 1713-1721.

[27] Wada H, Hitomi S, Teramatsu T, et al. The West Japan Study Group for Lung Cancer Surgery. Adjuvant chemotherapy after complete resection in non-small-cell lung cancer. *J Clin Oncol* 1996; 14: 1048-1054.

[28] Endo C, Saito Y, Iwanami H, et al. A randomized trial of postoperative UFT therapy in p stage I, II non-small cell lung cancer: Northest Japan Study Group for Lung Cancer Surgery. *Lung Cancer* 2003; 40: 181-186.

[29] Imaizumi M. Postoperative adjuvant cisplatin, vindesine, plus uracil tegafur chemotherapy increased survival of patients with completely resected p-stage I non-small cell lung cancer. *Lung Cancer* 2005; 49: 85-94.

[30] Hamada C, Tanaka F, Ohta M, et al. Meta-analysis of postoperative adjuvant chemotherapy with tegafur-uracil in non-small-cell lung cancer. *J Clin Oncol* 2005; 23: 4999-5006.

[31] Hamada C, Tsuboi M, Ohta M, et al. Effect of postoperative adjuvant chemotherapy with tegafur-uracil on survival in patients with stage IA non-small cell lung cancer: an exploratory analysis from a meta-analysis of six randomized controlled trials. *J Thorac Oncol* 2009: 4: 1511-1516.

[32] Fleming ID, Cooper JS, Hensen DE, et al., eds. *AJCC Cancer Staging Manual, Fifth Edition*. Philadelphia: Lippincott-Raven, 1997:1–294.

[33] Edge SB, Byrd DR, Compton CC et al., eds. *AJCC Cancer Staging Manual, Seventh Edition.* New York: Springer, 2010:1-730.

[34] Bezjak A, Lee CW, Ding K, et al. Quality-of-life outcomes for adjuvant chemotherapy in early-stage non-small-cell lung cancer: Results from a randomized trial, JBR.10. *J Clin Oncol* 2008;26:5052-5059.

[35] Pisters KM, Evans WK, Azzoli CG, et al. Cancer Care Ontario and American Society of Clinical Oncology adjuvant chemotherapy and adjuvant radiation therapy for stages I-IIIA resectable non small-cell lung cancer guideline. *J Clin Oncol* 2007;25:5506-5518.

[36] Burdett S, Stewart LA, Rydzewska L. A systematic review and meta-analysis of the literature: chemotherapy and surgery versus surgery alone in non-small cell lung cancer. *J Thorac Oncol* 2006; 1:611-621.

[37] Depierre A, Milleron B, Moro-Sibilot D, et al. Preoperative chemotherapy followed by surgery compared with primary surgery in resectable stage I (except T1N0), II, and IIIa non-small-cell lung cancer. *J Clin Oncol* 2002; 20:247-253.

[38] Westeel V, Milleron BJ, Quoix EA, et al. Long-term results of the French randomized trial comparing neoadjuvant chemotherapy followed by surgery versus surgery alone in resectable non-small cell lung cancer. *J Clin Oncol* 2010; 28:15s (Abstr 7003).

[39] Gilligan D, Nicolson M, Smith I, et al. Preoperative chemotherapy in patients with resectable non-small cell lung cancer: results of the MRC LU22/NVALT 2/EORTC 08012 multicentre randomised trial and update of systematic review. *Lancet* 2007; 369:1929-1937.

[40] Pisters KM, Vallières E, Crowley JJ, et al. Surgery with or without preoperative paclitaxel and carboplatin in early-stage non-small-cell lung cancer: Southwest Oncology Group Trial S9900, an intergroup, randomized, phase III trial. *J Clin Oncol* 2010; 28:1843-1849.

[41] Felip E, Rosell R, Maestre JA, et al. Preoperative chemotherapy plus surgery versus surgery plus adjuvant chemotherapy versus surgery alone in early-stage non-small-cell lung cancer. *J Clin Oncol* 2010; 28:3138-3145.

[42] Scagliotti GV, Pastorino U, Vansteenkiste JF, et al. Randomized phase III study of surgery alone or surgery plus preoperative cisplatin and gemcitabine in stages IB to IIIA non-small-cell lung cancer. *J Clin Oncol* 2012; 30:172-178.

[43] Bradbury PA, Shepherd FA. Chemotherapy and surgery for operable NSCLC. *Lancet* 2007; 369:1903-1904.

[44] Sawyer TE, Bonner JA, Gould PM, et al. Effectiveness of postoperative irradiation in stage IIIA non-small cell lung cancer according to regression tree analyses of recurrence risks. *Ann Thorac Surg* 1997; 64:1402-1407.

[45] PORT Meta-analysis Trialist Group. Postoperative radiotherapy in non-small-cell lung cancer. Cochrane Database of Systematic Reviews 2000; Issue 2. In *The Cochrane Database of Systematic Reviews 2007 Issue 4,* 2007 The Cochrane Collaboration. Published by John Wiley and Sons, Ltd. DOI:10.1002/14651558. CD002142.pub

[46] Bonner JA, Spencer SA. Postoperative radiotherapy in non-small-cell lung cancer warrants further exploration in the era of adjuvant chemotherapy and conformal radiotherapy. *J Clin Oncol* 2006; 24:2978-2980.

[47] Dautzenberg B, Arriagada R, Chammard AB, et al. A controlled study of postoperative radiotherapy for patients with completely resected nonsmall cell lung carcinoma. Groupe d'Etude et de Traitement des Cancers Bronchiques. *Cancer* 1999; 86:265-73.

[48] Lally BE, Zelterman D, Colasanto JM, et al. Postoperative radiotherapy for stage II or III non-small-cell lung cancer using the surveillance, epidemiology, and end results database. *J Clin Oncol* 2006; 24:2998-3006.

[49] Lally BE, Detterbeck FC, Geiger AM, et al. The risk of death from heart disease in patients with nonsmall cell lung cancer who receive postoperative radiotherapy: analysis of the Surveillance, Epidemiology, and End Results database. *Cancer* 2007; 110:911-917.

[50] Douillard JY, Rosell R, De Lena M, et al. Impact of postoperative radiation therapy on survival in patients with complete resection and stage I, II, or IIIA non-small-cell lung cancer treated with adjuvant chemotherapy: the adjuvant Navelbine International Trialist Association (ANITA) Randomized Trial. *Int J Radiat Oncol Biol Phys* 2008; 72:695-701.

[51] Shepherd FA, Rodrigues Pereira J, Ciuleanu T, et al. Erlotinib in previously treated non-small-cell lung cancer. *N Engl J Med* 2005; 353:123-132

[52] Rosell R, Carcereny E, Gervais R, et al. Erlotinib versus standard chemotherapy as first-line treatment for European patients with advanced EGFR mutation-positive non-small-cell lung cancer (EURTAC): a multicentre, open-label, randomised phase 3 trial. *Lancet Oncol* 2012; 13:239-246.

[53] Tsuboi M, Kato H, Hagai K, et al. Gefitinib in the adjuvant setting: safety results from a phase III study in patients with completely resected non-small-cell lung cancer. *Anticancer drugs* 2005; 16: 1123-1128.

[54] Goss GD, Lorimer I, Tsao MS, et al. A phase III randomized, double-blind, placebo-controlled trial of the epidermal growth factor receptor inhibitor, gefitinib, in completely resected stage IB-IIIA non-small-cell lung cancer (NSCLC), NCIC CTG BR.19. *J Clin Oncol* 2010; 28

[55] Kelly K, Chansky K, Gaspar LE, et al. Updated analysis of SWOG 0023: a randomized phase III trial of gefitinib versus placebo maintenance after definitive chemoradiation followed by docetaxel in patients with locally advanced stage III non-small cell lung cancer. *J Clin Oncol* 2007; 25 (suppl): 388s (abstr 7513).

[56] Thatcher N, Chang A, Pariskh P, et al. Gefitinib plus best supportive care in previously treated patients with refractory advanced non-small-cell lung cancer: results from a randomised, placebo-controlled, multicentre study (Iressa Survival Evaluation in Lung Cancer). *Lancet* 2005; 366: 1527-1537.

[57] Ferrara N. VEGF-A: a critical regulator of blood vessel growth. *Eur Cytokine Netw* 2009; 20:158-163.

[58] Yuan A, Yu CJ, Kuo SH, et al. Vasxular endotelial growt factor 189 mRNA isoform expression specifically correlates with tumor angiogenesis, patient survival, and postoperative relapse in non-small-cell lung cancer. *J Clin Oncol* 2001; 19: 432-441.

[59] Sandler, Gray R, Perry MC, et al. Paclitaxel-carboplatin alone or with bevacizumab for non-small-cell lung cancer. *N Engl J Med* 2006; 355: 2542-2550.

[60] Reck M, von Pawel J, Zatloukal P, et al. Phase III trial of cisplatin plus gemcitabine with either placeno or bevacizumab as first-line therapy for nonsquamous non-small-cell lung cancer: AVAIL. *J Clin Oncol* 2009; 27: 1227-1234.

[61] Romero P. Current state of vaccine therapies in non-small-cell lung cancer. *Clin Lung Cancer* 2008;9 (suppl 1):S28 –S36.

[62] Vansteenkiste J, Zielinski M, Linder A et al. Final results of a multi-center, double-blind, randomized, placebo-controlled Phase II study to assess the efficacy of MAGE-A3 immunotherapeutic as adjuvant therapy in stage IB/II non-small cell lung cancer (NSCLC). *J Clin Oncol* 2007; 25:18s(abstr 7554).

[63] Potti A, Mukherjee S, Petersen R, et al. A genomic strategy to refine prognosis in early stage non-small cell lung cancer. *N Engl J Med* 2006; 355: 570-580.

[64] Chen HY, Yu SL, Chen CH, et al. A five-gene signature and clinical outcome in non-small-cell lung cancer. *N Engl J Med* 2007; 356:11-20.

[65] Seike M, Yanaihara N, Bowman ED, et al. Use of a cytokine gene expression signature in lung adenocarcinoma and the surrounding tissue as a prognostic classifier. *J Natl Cancer Inst* 2007; 99:1257-1269.

[66] Lau SK, Boutros PC, Pintilie M, et al. Three-gene prognostic classifier for early-stage non small-cell lung cancer. *J Clin Oncol* 2007; 25:5562-5569.

[67] Wakelee H, Langer C, Vokes E, et al. Cooperative group research efforts in lung cancer: Focus on early-stage non-small-cell lung cancer. *Clin Lung Cancer* 2008; 9: 9-15.

[68] Reed E. ERCC1 measurements in clinical oncology. *N Engl J Med* 2006; 355:1054-1055.

[69] Olaussen KA, Dunant A, Fouret P, et al. DNA repair by ERCC1 in non-small-cell lung cancer and cisplatin-based adjuvant chemotherapy. *N Engl J Med* 2006; 355:983-991.

[70] Bepler G, Kusmartseva I, Sharma S, et al. RRM1-modulated in vitro and in vivo efficacy of gemcitabine and platinum in noin-small-cell lung cancer. *J Clin Oncol* 2006; 24:4731-4737.

[71] Zheng Z, Chen T, Li X, et al. DNA synthesis and repair genes RRM1 and ERCC1 in lung cancer. *N Engl J Med* 2007; 356: 800-808.

[72] Gautschi O, Mack PC, Davies AM; et al. Pharmacogenomic approaches to indivisulaizing chemotherapy for non-small-cell lung cancer: Current status and new directions. *Clin Lung Cancer* 2008; 9 (suppl 3): S129-S138.

[73] Taron M, Rosell R, Felip E, et al. BRCA1 mRNA expression levels as an indicator of chemoresistance in lung cancer. *Human Molecular Genetics* 2004; 13: 2443-2449.

[74] Rosell R, Skrzypski M, Jassem E, et al. BRCA1: A novel prognostic factor in resected non-small-cell lung cancer. *PloS ONE* 2007; 2: e1129.

[75] Bartolucci R, Wei J, Sanchez JJ, et al. XPG mRNA expression levels modulate prognosis in resected non-small-cell lung cancer in conjunction with BRCA1 and ERCC1 expression. *Clin Lung Cancer* 2009;10:47-52.

[76] Tsao MS, Aviel-Ronen S, Ding K, et al. Prognostic and predictive importance of p53 and RAS for adjuvant chemotherapy in non small-cell lung cancer. *J Clin Oncol* 2007; 25:5240-247.

[77] Filipits M, Pirker R, Dunant A, et al. Cell cycle regulators and outcome of adjuvant cisplatin-based chemotherapy in completely resected non-small-cell lung cancer: the International Adjuvant Lung Cancer Trial Biologic Program. *J Clin Oncol* 2007; 25: 2735-2740.

[78] Kamath K, Wilson L, Cabral F, et al. β III-tubulin induces paclitaxel resistance in association with reduced effects on microtubule dynamic instability. *J Biol Chem* 2005; 280:12902-12907.
[79] Sève P, Isaac S, Tredan O, et al. Expression of class III β-tubulin is predictive of patients outcome in patients with non-small cell lung cancer receiving vinorelbine-based CT. *Clin Cancer Res* 2005; 11: 5481-5486.
[80] Reiman T, Sève P, Vataire A, et al. Prognostic value of class III β-tubulin (TUBB3) in operable non-small-cell lung cancer (NSCLC) and predictive value for adjuvant cisplatin-based chemotherapy (CT): A validation study on three randomized trials. *J Clin Oncol* 2008; 26: 20s (Abstr 7506).
[81] Brock MV, Hooker CM, Ota-Machida E, et al. DNA methylation markers and early recurrence in stage I lung cancer. *N Engl J Med* 2008; 358:1118-1128.
[82] National Comprehensive Cancer Network (NCCN) guidelines. Available at: *www.nccn.org*.

In: Lung Cancer: A Comprehensive Overview
Editor: Kathy Gately
ISBN: 978-1-62618-447-3


*Chapter V*

# Lung Cancer: Treatment in Advanced Stages

***Miriam Méndez*[*1], Ana Custodio[2] and Mariano Provencio[1]***
[1]Medical Oncology Department,
Hospital Universitario Puerta de Hierro Majadahonda, Madrid, Spain
[2]Medical Oncology Department, Hospital Universitario La Paz, Madrid, Spain

## Abstract

Lung cancer is the leading cause of cancer-related mortality worldwide. In North America and in Europe, an estimated 40% of all newly diagnosed non-small-cell lung cancer (NSCLC) patients present with advanced-stage disease [1]. Moreover, a significant number of patients who present with early stage NSCLC will eventually relapse with extrathoracic metastases.

Current practice for the treatment of patients with metastatic disease includes the addition of cisplatin to new cytostatic agents such as vinorelbine, gemcitabine, paclitaxel or docetaxel, although none of the combinations has stood out over the others as the reference standard. With the new combinations like cisplatin/pemetrexed survival is reaching means that oscillate between 8.4 and 14.2 months. The addition of bevacizumab to chemotherapy was shown to produce a benefit in chemotherapy-naïve, advanced, non-squamous non-small-cell lung cancer (NSCLC) patients. The other monoclonal antibody for which phase III date exist in NSCLC is cetuximab, the addition of this drug modestly improved survival.

Determination of EGFR mutation status for upfront tyrosine-kinase inhibitors (TKI) is standard for treatment of adenocarcinoma, so erlotinib provides significant benefits over first line chemotherapy in EGFR mutation positive disease. Anaplastic lymphoma kinase (ALK) is one of the newest tyrosine-kinase targets in NSCLC. In a recent phase 1 clinical trial, crizotinib (inhibitor of ALK) showed marked antitumor activity in patients with advanced ALK-positive NSCLC.

[*] mirimega@hotmail.com. These authors contributed equally to this chapter.

# Introduction

Locally advanced, unresectable non-small cell lung cancer constitutes 35-40% of all newly diagnosed cases of NSCLC. During the past two decades, the management of these patients has undergone considerable change. Whereas radiotherapy as a sole treatment modality was standard treatment prior to 1990, current management combines radiotherapy with chemotherapy in patients with good performance status. On occasion, surgical resection may be beneficial. Progress in the management of locally advanced NSCLC came about in part due to the recognition that cisplatin-based chemotherapy yields a modest survival benefit even in patients with far advanced disease. With current combination chemotherapy regimens containing vinorelbine, gemcitabine, paclitaxel or docetaxel, additional modest survival gains have been achieved due to either these agents or improved selection of patients. However, improving local and systemic tumor control will be key to optimizing survival.

Patients with limited-stage disease are likely to be treated with multimodality regimens aimed at acure, but those with poor prognostic features or extensive-stage disease can gain substantial benefits, in terms of both symptom relief and linger survival, from less-intensive treatment. Chemotherapy agents have reached a plateau of efficacy and are associated with significant toxicity; thus, newer approaches for the treatment of advanced lung cancer are emerging, based on our growing understanding of the biology and genetics of the disease.

# Treatment of Stage III Non-Small Cell Lung Cancer (NSCLC)

Historically stage III lung cancer was defined as locoregionally advanced disease due to primary tumor extension into extrapulmonary structures (T3 or T4) or mediastinal lymph node involvement (N2 or N3) without evidence of distant metastases (M0). With the 2009 revisions to the TNM staging system, stage III lung cancers now include T3 tumors greater than 7 cm in size and T3 tumors with multiple nodules in the same lobe, when associated with N1 involvement.

Patients with stage III disease are stratified clinically into those with bulky or nonbulky mediastinal lymph node disease. The definition of bulky mediastinal lymphadenopathy varies in the literature, but a reasonable definition is lymph nodes >3 cm, groupings of multiple smaller lymph nodes, or involvement of more than two lymph node stations [2]. The distinction between nonbulky and bulky stage IIIA and IIIB disease is primarily useful in selecting appropriate patients for surgical resection after neoadjuvant therapy.

At diagnosis, at least 40% of patients are already at an advanced stage and a third have locally advanced disease. In the past, radiotherapy treatment was considered standard for patients at stages IIIA and IIIB, but with very low survival, poor local control and early development of disease at distance. Patients with inoperable stage III treated only with thoracic radiotherapy had mean survival of 9-11 months, 2-year survival of 10-20% and 3-year survival of 5-10%.

## Resected Stage IIIA Disease

Patients with tumors involving the chest wall or proximal airways (within 2 cm of the carina) with hilar, but not mediastinal, lymph node involvement are classified as stage IIIA (T3 N1) [3]. The appropriate initial management of these patients involves surgical resection, if technically feasible, followed by adjuvant chemotherapy for those with completely resected disease.

With improvement in surgical techniques and in surgical care, however, carefully selected patients with carinal involvement, superior vena caval or vertebral body involvement may benefit from surgery in the context of a multimodality approach. Survival rates up to 50 percent at five years have been reported [4]. As a result, patients with T4N0-1 lesions have been reclassified as stage IIIA tumors in the 7th edition of the TNM system.

Patients with completely resected stage III NSCLC are at a high risk for both local and distant failure, providing a rationale for postoperative RT and adjuvant chemotherapy.

### *Adjuvant Radiotherapy*

Although survival is often limited by the development of distant metastatic disease, postoperative RT may prevent locoregional recurrence and may improve survival in patients with N2 lymph node involvement. An analysis of 7465 patients with stage II or III NSCLC between 1988 and 2002 found that patients with N0 or N1 disease had a significantly decreased five-year survival rate with postoperative RT (31 versus 41 percent with observation for those with N0 disease; 30 versus 34 percent for those with N1 disease). In contrast, patients with N2 lymph node involvement had a significantly improved five-year survival rate with adjuvant RT (27 versus 20 percent, $p = 0.0077$).

Results from the phase III ANITA trial, which evaluated adjuvant chemotherapy in patients with completely resected stage IB-IIIA NSCLC, suggest that the effect of postoperative RT is affected both by the extent of nodal involvement and the use of adjuvant chemotherapy [5]. For patients with N2 disease, survival was longer in patients who received Postoperative Radiation Treatment (PORT) than in those not given RT (median 47 versus 24 months in those given adjuvant chemotherapy and 23 versus 13 months in those not given adjuvant chemotherapy). In contrast, for those with N1 disease, RT had a negative effect on survival in those given adjuvant chemotherapy (47 versus 94 months) but a positive effect in those not receiving chemotherapy (50 versus 26 months).

An analysis of the Surveillance Epidemiology and End Results (SEER) database showed no evidence of overall survival benefit with use of PORT. This analysis also showed survival detriment with use of PORT in patients with N0-N1 disease. However, the SEER analysis showed a survival benefit with use of PORT in patients with N2 disease [6].

A recent analysis of patients enrolled in the Eastern Cooperative Oncology Group (ECOG) 3590 showed that the risk of death from intercurrent disease (DID) in patients with resected stage II or IIIA NSCLC was not increased with use of PORT alone or use of concurrent chemotherapy and PORT [7]. Another study of patients with NSCLC treated with resection and postoperative radiation showed no increase in risk of DID with use of modern radiation [8].

Currently, PORT may be considered for patients with stage III disease who have inadequate mediastinal lymph node evaluation, multistation disease, or extracapsular nodal extension in order to reduce local-regional recurrence. The radiation should be given sequentially following adjuvant chemotherapy since there is no evidence that concurrent treatment is beneficial in resected stage III patients [9].

These data suggest that careful interpretation of the available data in the context of an individual patient is necessary to make clinical decisions regarding postoperative radiation treatment at this time. Further research is necessary to define the exact role of postoperative radiation treatment in patients with resected NSCLC.

### *Adjuvant Chemotherapy*

Adjuvant chemotherapy has been extensively evaluated in an attempt to decrease the incidence of distant metastases and improve long-term survival. Three separate meta-analyses suggested that systemic treatment following surgery for stage I to III NSCLC produced a 4 to 5 percent absolute improvement in five-year survival. More recent clinical trials utilizing modern platinum-based doublet regimens have confirmed a survival benefit and suggested that the magnitude of benefit may be even larger than suggested in the meta-analyses. Although results have differed according to stage in various trials, the weight of evidence suggests that adjuvant chemotherapy benefits patients with completely resected stage II and III disease.

In the last 10 years, the results from a new generation of adjuvant trials have been reported. In general these trials had more consistent surgical staging and have usually employed platinum based chemotherapy (Table 1).

**Table 1. Recent platin-based adjuvant trials and 5-year survival**

| Trial | Patients | Stage | Chemotherapy | 5-year survival |
|---|---|---|---|---|
| INT 0115[117] | 488 | II-IIIA | Cis, VP16 | 33 vs 39 % |
| BLT [44] | 381 | I-III | Cis-based | 58 vs 60% |
| ALPI1209 [41] | 1209 | I-IIIA | MVP | HR 0.06 |
| IALT [31] | 1867 | I-IIIA | Cis-based | 44.5 vs 40.4 % |
| NCIC | 482 | IB-II | Cis, Vnr | 69 vs 54 % |
| ANITA 840 [39] | 840 | IB-IIIA | Cis, Vnr | 8.6% improved |
| CALGB | 344 | IB | Pac, Carbo | 64 vs 61% |

Carbo: carboplatin, Cis: cisplatin, HR: hazard ratio, MVP: mitomycin, vindesine, cisplatin, Vnr: vinorelbine.

The first reported study was the North American Intergroup Trial (INT0115, ECOG 3590) [10]. Patients with stages II and IIIA NSCLC were randomized to receive radiotherapy or concurrent chemoradiotherapy after surgery. This trial was unique in that all patients received postoperative radiotherapy and the adjuvant chemotherapy was delivered concurrent with the radiation. There were no differences between the patient groups with regard to survival and patterns of recurrence. There was more toxicity on the concurrent arm of the study, which may have accounted for the lack of efficacy on this trial particularly for the stage II.

The Adjuvant Lung Project Italy (ALPI) was probably the first adequately powered trial enrolling over 1200 participants [11]. Patients with stages I-IIIA were randomized to receive

MVP (mitomycin, vindesine, cisplatin) or observation. Postoperative radiotherapy was allowed. There was no significant difference in overall survival between the study arms (HR 0.96, 95% CI: 0.81-1.13, p=0.589). Problems with chemotherapy delivery and toxicity may have accounted for the lack of benefit for the adjuvant chemotherapy.

The Big Lung Trial (BLT) evaluated cisplatin based chemotherapy in a number of treatment situations [12]. Patients with stages I-IIIA NSCLC were randomly assigned to cisplatin-based neoadjuvant/adjuvant chemotherapy or surgery alone. There was no difference in overall survival between the study arms but this trial was not designed to specifically evaluate adjuvant chemotherapy, therefore it was underpowered to detect a significant survival difference.

The International Adjuvant Lung Cancer Trial (IALT) was a landmark study that initially justified the use of adjuvant chemotherapy in resected NSCLC [13]. Over 1800 patients with stages I-IIIA resected NSCLC received three to four cycles of cisplatin-based chemotherapy or observation. The 5-year survival (44.5% versus 40.4%, HR 0.86, p<0.03) and disease-free survival (p<0.003) was significantly higher for the patients treated with chemotherapy. The toxicity was acceptable and benefit was seen for all disease stages with the most survival advantage being in stage IIIA.

The Adjuvant Navelbine International Trialist Association (ANITA) reported a randomized trial in patients with resected stages IB-IIIA NSCLC [14]. The chemotherapy employed was cisplatin and vinorelbine. Postoperative radiation was allowed. For the patients treated with chemotherapy there was a significant improvement in overall survival (65.7 versus 43.7 months, HR 0.80, p=0.017). Survival at 5 years improved by 8.6% with chemotherapy and was maintained at 7 years.

The second issue has to do with the choice of the platinum (cisplatin or carboplatin) for treatment in the adjuvant situation. The CISCA meta-analysis evaluated cisplatin versus carboplatin- based chemotherapy in advanced NSCLC [15]. There was a slight survival benefit for cisplatin-based chemotherapy which became significant in patients treated with nonsquamous histology and those treated with third-generation chemotherapeutic agents. Although this analysis was in advanced NSCLC the demonstration of a slight survival advantage for cisplatin may be of more importance in a curative situation, that is, adjuvant chemotherapy.

For all, adjuvant cisplatin-based chemotherapy is now considered the standard of care for patients with completely resected stage II and III NSCLC [16].

## Neoadjuvant Therapy

Induction (neoadjuvant) therapy refers to the use of chemotherapy and/or RT prior to surgery. This approach carries several theoretical advantages: a decrease in tumor volume resulting in better local control with subsequent treatment, relatively high response rates to chemotherapy in patients with stage III as compared to those with stage IV NSCLC, earlier treatment of micrometastatic disease and better tolerance of and compliance with preoperative chemotherapy compared with adjuvant chemotherapy after surgery.

Early phase 2 trials of neoadjuvant chemotherapy using mitomycin, vinblastine, and cisplatin performed at the Memorial Sloan-Kettering Cancer Center and the University of Toronto demonstrated improved survivals of 20% in patients with preoperatively identified

N2 disease [17, 18]. Similar results were seen in early phase 2 studies performed combining radiation (3000–4500 cGy) with platinum-containing chemotherapy [19].

In 1994 small phase 3 trials demonstrated improved survival with induction chemotherapy followed by surgery compared with surgery alone. In this trial, patients underwent induction therapy with a combination of cyclophosphamide, etoposide, and cisplatin, followed by surgery and then 3 additional cycles postoperatively. Thirty-five percent of the patients had a major clinical response, and their 2-year and 3-year survivals were 60% and 50% compared with the surgery-alone group (25% and 15%) [20]. In the trial from Barcelona patients were treated with induction mitomycin, ifosfamide, and cisplatin followed by surgery and postoperative radiation in comparison with surgery and radiation. The 2-year and 5-year survivals were 29% and 17% in the chemotherapy/surgery/radiation arm, and 5% and 0% in the surgery/radiation arm [21].

In 1989 the Cancer and Leukemia Group B (CALGB) designed a multi-institutional phase 2 trial of high-intensity trimodality therapy for patients with surgically staged IIIA-N2 non–small cell lung cancer, and published these results in 1995 (CALGB 8935A). The trial combined 2 cycles of neoadjuvant cisplatin and vinblastine with surgical resection and radical lymphadenectomy, followed by 2 additional cycles of adjuvant chemotherapy followed by radiation therapy (5400–6000 cGy). This study was performed by 30 separate teams. Their definition for a complete resection was defined as all margins negative as well as the highest lymph node resected. The operative mortality was 3.2% and the morbidity 30%. However, only 31% of the patients had an R0 resection by their criteria. Nonetheless, the study was important because it demonstrated that an aggressive approach that included induction therapy could be delivered with a then relatively low treatment-related mortality of 5.4%. The study also demonstrated the importance of an R0 resection. These patients had a 3-year survival of 46% compared with 21% for those having an incomplete resection and 0% for unresectable patients [22].

In 1995 the mature results of Southwest Oncology Group (SWOG) 8805 were published. This phase 2 trial evaluated the impact of induction chemotherapy and concomitant radiotherapy on survival in 126 patients with stage IIIA/B non–small cell lung cancer. All patients had biopsy-proven N2 or N3 disease or T4 lesions. The induction regimen consisted of 2 cycles of cisplatin and etoposide with concurrent radiation to 4500 cGy. Seventy-five patients had stage IIIA-N2 and 51 patients had stage IIIB disease. Twenty-seven of the patients with stage IIIB disease were N3. Operation consisted of resection and lymph node sampling. Unresectable patients or patients with positive nodes received additional chemotherapy and radiation postoperatively. In this study 85% of patients with stage IIIA-N2 and 80% of patients with stage IIIB were resected. There were 10% treatment-related deaths. With this aggressive induction approach, 21% of patients had a complete pathologic response and 37% had only residual microscopic disease. There was no difference in the survival of patients with stage IIIA and stage IIIB disease. The 2-year survivals were 37% and 39% and the 3-year survivals 27% and 24%, respectively. However, this study demonstrated the importance of downstaging on survival, and the strongest predictor of survival was an absence of tumor in the mediastinal lymph nodes. The median and 5-year survivals for these patients were 30 months and 44% versus 10 months and 18% for patients with residual nodal disease [23].

In 2001 Rusch and colleagues published the initial results of SWOG 9416, which adopted the protocol of 8805 and applied it to superior sulcus tumors. Eighty T3 and 31 T4 patients were enrolled. The resection rate was 91% for T3 tumors and 87% for T4 tumors. Once again the impact of the induction regimen on downstaging was impressive, with 28 patients having a complete pathologic response and only 26 patients having microscopic residual disease [24]. The long-term results of this study, published in 2007, demonstrated a 54% survival for patients undergoing a complete resection [25].

In 2005 Albain and colleagues reported the initial results of a randomized trial of definitive chemoradiotherapy (194 patients) versus induction chemoradiotherapy followed by surgical resection (202 patients) for patients with stage III-N2 non–small cell lung cancer (RTOG 9309, Intergroup Trial 0139). All patients received 2 cycles of chemotherapy with cisplatin and etoposide. Both groups received concomitant radiation. However, the radiation doses were significantly different between the two groups. The patients randomized to go onto surgical resection received a total dose of 4500 cGy and the patients randomized to definitive radiation received a total dose of 6100 cGy. The mature results of this trial were reported in 2009. Although all patients were to receive 2 additional cycles of chemotherapy, this was only accomplished in 55% of the surgical group and 74% of the nonsurgical group. While there was a difference in the progression-free survival between the two groups (12.8 months in the surgical group vs 10.5 months in the nonsurgical group; P = 0.017), there was no difference in the overall survival (23.6 months vs 22.2 months; P = 0.24). However, the operative mortality for patients undergoing pneumonectomy was 26%. In the lobectomy group there was a difference in survival (33.6 months vs 21.7 months in a matched chemotherapy-radiation group; P=0.002). However, despite these results many centers have considered patients with N2 disease inoperable. Surgery, however, was not the only variable in this study, as there is a significant difference in the biological effectiveness between 4500 and 6000 cGy of radiation [26].

Several reports from both multi-institutional and single-institution studies using neoadjuvant chemotherapy or chemoradiotherapy show that the percentage of patients undergoing an R0 resection is approximately 10% to 20% lower than the percentage of patients resected. Many of these trials include adjuvant therapy in their protocols, but in virtually all of these studies patients undergoing an incomplete resection do significantly poorer. It is also unclear whether radiation added to the induction regimen improves the resectability rate. The study by Thomas and colleagues, reporting the results of a randomized trial of the German Lung Cancer Cooperative Group in 481 patients, demonstrated only a 5% difference in resectability between patients receiving induction chemotherapy and those receiving induction chemotherapy followed by concurrent chemotherapy and radiation, favouring the group that did not receive the radiation [27].

**Table 2. Trials demonstrating survival with and without nodal downstaging**

| Authors | Year | Resected patients | Nodal dowstaging (%) | Survival of node postive | Survival or node negative | P value |
|---|---|---|---|---|---|---|
| Mathisen | 1996 | 35 | 40 | 26 months | Not reached | 0.04 |
| Bueno | 2000 | 103 | 52 | 15.9 months | 21.3 months | 0.02 |
| Rice | 1998 | 40 | 31 | 33% 2 years | 83% 2 years | 0.01 |
| Granetzny | 2003 | 26 | 38 | 11.4 months | 34.7 months | 0.01 |

Achieving a complete pathologic response with induction therapy is variable, but overall appears to be higher in those patients receiving neoadjuvant chemotherapy and concurrent high-dose radiation as opposed to chemotherapy alone or chemotherapy and lower doses of radiation. The significance of this ultimately remains to be determined, although it has been suggested that patients who achieve a complete pathologic response have a survival advantage [28]. A more important determinant of survival has been the downstaging of involved mediastinal lymph nodes from N3 or N2 to N0 or N1, and this finding has been consistently demonstrated in multiple studies (Table 2).

The only study using high-dose radiation in the neoadjuvant protocol and limited to patients with N2 disease was published by Cerfolio and colleagues [29]. This retrospective study demonstrated higher mediastinal nodal downstaging in patients receiving high-dose radiation (83%) than in those receiving low-dose radiation (median 4500 cGy; 74%). Consistent with other studies, there was an increase in the disease-free survival in the high-dose radiation group compared with the low-dose radiation group (estimated 3-year survival 65% vs 30%; P =0 .047). Overall, patients receiving high-dose radiation have a higher rate of nodal downstaging than those in studies using either chemotherapy alone or chemotherapy and lower doses of radiation in the induction protocol, as well as significant survival.

Reports of one large randomized phase III trial have not confirmed a significant survival advantage for surgery following induction chemotherapy. EORTC 08941 was a phase III trial investigating the role of surgery versus RT after induction chemotherapy, 579 patients with biopsy-proven unresectable stage IIIA-N2 NSCLC received three cycles of platinum-based chemotherapy. Nonprogressors were then randomized to surgery (n = 167) or thoracic RT (n = 165). Median survival and five-year overall survival rates were similar (16.4 versus 17.5 months and 16 versus 14 percent for the surgery and RT groups, respectively; HR 1.06, 95% CI 0.84-1.35). A major criticism of this trial is that only 50 percent of patients randomized to surgical resection achieved a complete resection. The operative mortality of patients who underwent pneumonectomy after induction chemotherapy however was much more acceptable at 7 percent [30].

There are several points not fully clarified today. The first controversy is whether patients with N2 disease should be operated on at all. This controversy is primarily based on the early results of the Intergroup 0139 study that showed no difference in the overall survival of patients undergoing neoadjuvant chemoradiotherapy followed by surgery versus definitive chemoradiotherapy. The more mature results of this study, however, do show a difference for patients undergoing lobectomy [25]. The poor results in the pneumonectomy group are largely due to the high operative mortality of 26% in these patients. When one looks at the number of patients with residual disease in the primary tumor who have been resected after high-dose radiation and concurrent chemotherapy it is likely that 50% of patients will ultimately fail locally if they do not succumb to metastases. Thus, the rationale for surgery in non–small cell lung cancer after treatment with concurrent chemotherapy and high-dose radiation is local control [31].

The second controversy is whether patients with gross mediastinal nodal disease, multistation mediastinal nodal disease, or even residual nodal disease after induction therapy should be offered resection. While it is intuitive that patients with gross or multistation N2 disease are more likely to do poorly with any treatment algorithm, this is not universally accepted [32]. In most studies of patients with stage III-N2 disease, survival is significantly compromised when residual nodal disease is present after induction therapy, and they might do as well overall without surgery. However, the authors have seen a median survival of 41 months in patients with residual nodal disease with an induction regimen that includes high-dose radiation, and continue to offer these patients resection.

The most significant controversy is whether pneumonectomy should be offered to patients undergoing resection after induction therapy particularly when radiation is included in the induction regimen, and some surgeons omit radiation when pneumonectomy is contemplated. Unfortunately, many of these patients have advanced disease and the incidence of pneumonectomy in these patients is relatively high [33]. The operative mortality rate in several recent series is significant, and in several recent large series has varied from 6% to 12% with 90-day mortalities significantly higher [34]. On the other hand, the recent study by Weder and colleagues reported that the 90-day mortality rate was only 3% [35]. Even so, these patients tend to have a shorter survival than a comparable group of patients undergoing lobectomy, likely due to both their more advanced disease and the physiologic consequences of the resection. Patients who required a pneumonectomy in the Intergroup 0139 study had an unacceptable mortality following induction chemoradiotherapy. Although some centers have reported less surgery-related mortality, consideration of pneumonectomy in this setting should generally be recommended to surgeons in centers of excellence [36].

## Inoperable Stage III

There are various therapeutic options for the treatment of locally advanced NSCLC. The choice of which will depend on the patient´s clinical situation, closely linked to their general situation, how far advanced the tumor is on diagnosis, and the experience at the hospital.

The use of induction chemotherapy treatment began after a series of clinical trials in the mid 1980s [37]. In 1995, a meta-analysis based on individual data from 3,033 patients showed that combining chemotherapy and radiotherapy gave a statistically significant benefit [38]. This difference was greater in those trials that had used platinum treatment, with a hazard ratio of 0.87 ($p<0.005$) in favour of combined chemotherapy and radiotherapy treatment.

From that time, various therapeutic designs have been investigated in the search for the best treatment sequence. We briefly explain here the main studies and their findings on each of the various types of treatment.

### *Sequential Chemotherapy SND Radiotherapy vs Exclusive Radiotherapy*

Three trials and two meta-analyses established that sequential chemotherapy followed by RT improved survival compared with definitive RT alone (Table 3). RT without chemotherapy remains the preferred approach for poor-risk patients who are not candidates for combined modality therapy. The benefits of RT include palliation of tumor-related symptoms, local control of tumor growth, and possibly a survival advantage

The pivotal trial was performed by the Cancer and Leukemia Group B (CALGB) 8433 [39]. 155 patients with stage III NSCLC were randomly assigned to RT alone (60 Gy over six weeks) or two cycles of cisplatin-based chemotherapy followed by the same RT. With seven-year follow-up, the addition of chemotherapy was associated with significantly better median and five-year survival (14 versus 10 months and 17 versus 6 percent).

A three arm confirmatory study was conduced by the Radiation Therapy Oncology Group (RTOG), Southwest Oncology Group (SWOG) and ECOG [40]. This trial randomly assigned 452 patients with stage III disease to conventional RT (60 Gy in 30 daily fractions) hyperfractionated RT (69.6 Gy in 58 fractions of 1.2 Gy each, given twice daily), or chemotherapy (vinblastine plus cisplatin) followed by conventional RT. The overall survival with sequential chemotherapy and RT was significantly better than with either conventional or hyperfractionated RT alone (median survival, 13.2 versus 11.4 and 12 months, respectively). The observed differences in survival rates were greater at two years (32 versus 19 and 24 percent, respectively) than at five years (8, 5, and 6 percent, respectively) with sequential chemoradiotherapy, conventional RT alone, and hyperfractionated RT alone, respectively.

**Table 3. Studies of chemotherapy followed by radiotherapy vs radiotherapy alone**

| Authors | Nº patients | Treatment | Median survival (months) | Overall 5 year survival |
|---|---|---|---|---|
| Dillman [146] | 155 | Cisplatin/Vinblastine+ Rt<br>Rt | 13.8<br>9.7 | 19%<br>7% |
| Sause [147] | 458 | Cisplatin/Vinblastine+Rt<br>Cisplatin/Vinblastine+hyperfractionated Rt<br>Rt | 13.2<br>12<br>11.4 | 8%<br>6%<br>5% |
| Le Chevalier [148] | 353 | Cisplatin/Vindesine/Cyclophos /Lomustine+Rt<br>Rt | 12<br>10 | 12%<br>4% |

A third study with 353 patients compared three induction chemotherapy cycles (cisplatin, vindesine, cyclophosphamide and lomustine) followed by radiotherapy and three more cycles, vs exclusive radiotherapy [41]. With an average follow-up of 40 months, two year survival of the radiotherapy group was 14% vs 21% for the combination arm (p=0.08). A second analysis with a mean follow-up of 61 months, found statistically significant benefit in overall survival, at 3 years of 12% vs 4% (p=0.004).

Two meta-analyses of trials comparing sequential chemoradiotherapy versus RT alone or chemotherapy alone also concluded that one- and two-year survival rates were better with the combined approach, but that this short-term survival benefit did not translate into better long-term outcomes [42].

### *Concurrent Chemo-Radiotherapy vs Exclusive Radiotherapy*

Various phase III trials compared concurrent chemo-radiotherapy treatment vs exclusive radiotherapy. One of these was conducted by the European Organization for Research and Treatment of Cancer (EORTC). Time to relapse (p=0.015) and 3-year survival were significantly greater in patients receiving daily chemotherapy with cisplatin vs those with radiotherapy alone (16% vs 2%; p=0.09).

Two other trials analyzed the efficacy of concurrent treatment based in carboplatin plus etoposide. The group of patients with concurrent treatment showed a significant improvement in mean (22 months vs 14 months) and 4-year survival (23% vs 9%; p=0.021) [43].

These trials indicate that concurrent chemo-radiotherapy clearly improves local control of the disease, which is translated into greater survival. It should also be noted that the chemotherapy doses used in these trials were lower than the doses normally used to treat systemic disease.

### *Sequential vs Concurrent Chemo-Radiotherapy*

The superiority of concurrent chemoradiotherapy compared with sequential chemotherapy and RT has been demonstrated in two large, multicenter, randomized phase III trials.

Radiation Therapy Oncology Group (RTOG) trial 9410, a three-arm trial which included 610 patients with unresected stage III disease, compared sequential cisplatin plus vinblastine for two cycles followed by conventional RT (60 Gy in 30 fractions) with two cycles of the same regimen administered concurrently with conventional RT. A third study arm evaluated concurrent cisplatin plus etoposide with twice daily RT to a total dose of 69.6 Gy. Concurrent chemoradiotherapy with conventional RT fractionation was superior to sequential chemoradiotherapy (median survival 17.0 versus 14.6 months, hazard ratio for death 0.81, 95% CI 0.663-0.996). The difference between the conventional fractionation chemoradiotherapy and twice daily regimen was not statistically significant (median survival 17.0 versus 15.6 months) [44].

The West Japan Lung Cancer Group randomized 320 patients with unresectable stage III NSCLC to either concurrent chemotherapy (two cycles of cisplatin, mitomycin, and vindesine) plus split-course thoracic RT (two courses of 28 Gy in 2 Gy daily fractions, separated by ten days) or to two cycles of the same chemotherapy regimen followed by a single course of RT (56 Gy in 28 fractions). Despite the use of a split-course RT schedule, concurrent therapy was associated with a significantly better response rate (84 versus 66 percent), median survival (17 versus 13 months), and two- and five-year survival rates (35 versus 27 percent and 16 versus 9 percent, respectively) [45].

A phase II trial randomized 102 stage IIIA and B patients to receive concurrent or sequential treatment with chemotherapy based on cisplatin and vinorelbine. Median survival was greater in the concurrent arm (16.6 vs 12.9 months; $p=0.023$) and 3-year survival was 18.6% for concurrent treatment vs 9.5% but the treatment arms were not well-balanced to the detriment of the sequential treatment group [46].

The French group randomized 212 patients to receiving sequential treatment with two cycles of cisplatin and vinorebline, followed by radiotherapy vs cisplatin and etoposide concurrent with radiotherapy. Median survival was 14.5 months for the sequential arm vs 16.3 months for the concurrent treatment arm ($p=0.24$) [47].

A review of various trials published between 2000 and 2005 concluded that 5-year survival for inoperable stages IIIA and B increased from the 7% obtained with radiotherapy alone to 10% to sequential treatment, and as much as 15% for concurrent treatment [48]. A meta-analysis of 12 clinical trials with 1921 patients at various stages analyzed the role of chemotherapy based on cisplatin associated with radiotherapy and concluded that the addition of cisplatin to radiotherapy improves survival, with absolute benefit of 4% at 2 years ($p=0.02$), and that the combination of cisplatin and etoposide is more effective than cisplatin alone [49].

In an attempt to unify criteria, a meta-analysis was published to clarify whether concurrent or sequential treatment is better. This included 1205 patients with a 6-year follow-up, and demonstrated that concomitant treatment contributed absolute benefit on overall survival at 5 years of 4.5% (15.1% vs 10.5%) over sequential treatment. This was statistically significant (HR=0.84, p=0.004), but at the cost of increasing toxicity in the form of degree 3-4 esophagitis from 3 to 18% (p<0.0001). Grade 3-4 bone marrow toxicity increases with concurrent treatment, depending on the type of chemotherapy and the timing of control blood counts, with a range extending from 20% to 90% [50]. Even in groups of patients with higher comorbidity, concurrent treatment is considered feasible and maintains its effectiveness [51].

### *Role of Induction Chemotherapy Prior to Concurrent Therapy*

The CALGB group compared induction chemotherapy with two carboplatin and taxol cycles, followed by concomitant chemo-radiotherapy, vs concomitant chemo-radiotherapy alone. Median survival in the chemo-radiotherapy arm was 11.4 months vs 14 in the induction arm (p=0.154), with one-year survival of 48% and 54% respectively [52].

The LAMP (Locally Advanced Multimodality Protocol) phase-II randomized study compared 276 stage IIIA and B patients, who were randomized to receive induction chemotherapy followed by radiotherapy, induction chemotherapy followed by concurrent chemo-radiotherapy or concurrent chemo-radiotherapy followed by chemotherapy. The chemotherapy was with carboplatin and paclitaxel. However, the trial was closed down early due to poor recruitment without reaching sufficient statistical power for the direct comparison of the three arms. This, with the bias of patients who experienced weight loss, the small number of samples and the phase II design, makes it hard to interpret the study findings. Median survival, after a follow-up or 39.6 months, was higher in the arm receiving concurrent chemo-radiotherapy followed by chemotherapy, with a median survival of 16.3 months, vs 13 months in the sequential arm and 12.7 months for induction chemotherapy followed by concurrent chemo-radiotherapy [53]. All this leads to the conclusion that the most usual treatment option, as recommended by international guidelines, is definitive concomitant chemo-radiotherapy, although other options are admitted, among which are those including induction chemotherapy.

## Treatment of Metastasic Non-Small Cell Lung Cancer

Palliative systemic therapy is the standard of care for patients with advanced NSCLC. Generally, treatment should be initiated after interdisciplinary discussion, ideally at a tumour-board involving different specialists (medical and radiation oncologist, pneumologist, thoracic surgeon, radiologist and pathologist). Systemic treatment should be guided by an experienced medical oncologist and selection of agents should take into account the patient´s situation, the treatment goal and potential adverse events.

The initial management of patients with advanced NSCLC depends upon the patients´s age, performance status, comorbidities and patient´s preferences. Moreover, therapy should be individualized based upon the presence or absence of characteristic molecular and histologic features of the tumor. If feasible, patients should have tumor tissue assessed for the presence of a somatic mutation in the epidermal growth factor receptor (EGFR), which confers sensitivity to EGFR tyrosine kinase inhibitors (TKI) [54,55], and for the anaplastic lymphoma kinase (ALK) fusion oncogene, which confers sensitivity to crizotinib [56]. Patient management can then be dictated by the results of these molecular studies:

- Patients with an EGFR mutation are managed with an EGFR TKI (gefitinib or erlotinib).
- Those with an ALK fusion oncogene in their tumor are preferentially treated with crizotinib.
- For patients without a mutation in the EGFR or when the EGFR status is unknown, chemotherapy (CT) is the foundation for initial treatment.

The approach to systemic therapy for patients who present with advanced NSCLC and for those who relapse after initial definitive therapy is reviewed.

# Initial Systemic Therapy for Advanced NSCKC without an EGFR Mutation or the ALJ Fusion Oncogene

## Platinum-Based CT

In multiple clinical trials that compared regimens incorporating a platinum compound with best supportive care (BSC), systemic CT increased survival without compromising quality of life (QOL) [57,58]. A number of new cytotoxic agents, including vinorelbine, paclitaxel, docetaxel, gemcitabine and pemetrexed, have been found to possess single-agent activity in advanced NSCLC. Third generation platinum-based doublets represent the current standard of care in patients with advanced NSCLC and good performance status (PS) (PS 0 to 1). With the new combinations, survival is reaching means that oscillate between 8.4 and 14.2 months and, in some cases, 1 year survival reaches 54%.[59,60]. Although there are some modest differences in the activity and toxicity among these regimens, no truly clinically relevant survival differences have emerged and none of the combinations have stood out over the others as the reference standard. Moreover, although treatment intensification by adding a third drug to a two drug combination improves response rates (RR), the impact on survival is inconsistent and toxicity is clearly increased [61,62].

Carboplatin is often substituted for cisplatin in combination regimens for patients with advanced NSCLC due to its more favorable toxicity profile. Overall, the evidence suggests that cisplatin gives a higher ORR than carboplatin, although the survival benefit is small and may not be clinically meaningful [63,64]. In a meta-analysis that included individual patient data from 2968 patients in nine trials, substitution of cisplatin for carboplatin was associated with a significantly lower RR (24 vs. 30%, odds ratio [OR], 1.37; 95% confidence interval [CI], 1.16-1.61) and a statistically non-significant shortening of survival (median, 8.4 vs. 9.1 months; HR for death,1.07; 95% CI, 0.99-1.15). In subset analyses, the difference in survival was statistically significant when the analysis was restricted to patients with non-squamous cancers and when the platinum compound was combined with a third generation chemotherapy agent [65].

Non-platinum-based combinations of third-generation agents can be considered if platinum therapy is contraindicated. Most trials show lower RR for non-platinum combinations but similar survival rates [66,67]. A meta-analysis that included 4792 patients treated in 17 randomized trials found that the use of a platinum-based doublet regimen was associated with a slightly higher survival at one year (relative risk [RR] of survival 1.08; 95% CI, 1.01-1.16) [68]. When the trials were analyzed according to the platinum compound used, cisplatin was associated with a significantly high 1-year survival compared to non-platinum regimens (RR of survival 1.16; 95% CI, 1.06-1.27). In contrast, carboplatin-based regimens were not better than non-platinum regimens (RR of survival, 0.95; 95% CI, 0.85-1.07).

In addition, although early studies failed to demonstrate a difference in outcome with different regimens based upon histologic subtypes, histology has become an important factor affecting sensitivity with some contemporary agents. In the largest phase III trial to compare two CT regimens, 1725 previously untreated patients with stage IIIB or IV NSCLC were randomly assigned to cisplatin plus pemetrexed or cisplatin plus gemcitabine [69]. Overall, there was no difference in median overall survival (OS) (10.3 months with both regimens; hazard ratio [HR], 0.94; 95% CI, 0.84-1.05). However, in a preplanned subset analysis, survival in the 847 patients with adenocarcinoma was significantly prolonged with cisplatin plus pemetrexed compared to cisplatin plus gemcitabine (median, 12.6 vs. 10.9 months). Conversely, cisplatin plus gemcitabine was superior to cisplatin plus pemetrexed in the 473 patients with squamous cell carcinoma (median, 10.8 vs. 9.4 months). Based upon these results, approval of pemetrexed in advanced NSCLC has been restricted to patients with non-squamous histology.

## CT Plus Bevacizumab

Vascular endothelial growth factor (VEGF) is a potent endothelial-specific angiogenic factor that is expressed in a wide array of tumors. In NSCLC, high levels of VEGF expression are associated with a poor prognosis, suggesting that treatment targeted toward this pathway might be useful therapeutically. One of the most promising approaches to blocking the VEGF pathway is the administration of bevacizumab, a recombinant humanized monoclonal antibody (mAb) that binds VEGF, thereby preventing its interaction with the VEGF receptor [70,71]. To date, first-line bevacizumab combined with standard platinum-based CT has demonstrated clinical activity in a phase II trial and in two phase III trials in patients with advanced NSCLC [72]. In the phase II trial, 99 patients were randomized to carboplatin/paclitaxel every 3 weeks (n=32), carboplatin/paclitaxel with bevacizumab 7.5 mg/Kg (n=32) or 15 mg/Kg (n=35) every 3 weeks. The combination of bevacizumab 15 mg/Kg with CT increased RR (31.5% vs. 18.8%) and prolonged time to progression[18] (median, 7.4 vs. 3.2 months; HR, 0.54; p=0.023). With bevacizumab 7.5 mg/Kg, there was a modest increase in RR (28.1% vs. 18.8%) but no difference in TTP (median, 4.3 vs. 3.2 months). Further analysis excluding patients with squamous histology suggested that both doses of bevacizumab improved survival compared with CT alone and with only a small increased risk of bleeding (~4%).

Based on the positive results of this phase II trial, a phase III trial of bevacizumab-based first-line therapy, the ECOG 4599 trial, randomized 878 patients with recurrent or advanced

NSCLC (stage IIIB or IV) to bevacizumab 15 mg/Kg with carboplatin/paclitaxel (n=434) or carboplatin/paclitaxel alone (n=444) every 3 weeks. The 15 mg/Kg dose was chosen based on its activity in the phase II trial. The primary end point was OS. Patients receiving CT plus bevacizumab had significant increases in the overall response rate (ORR) (35% vs. 15% with paclitaxel plus carboplatin alone), OS (median, 12.3 vs. 10.3 months; HR for death, 0.79; 95% CI 0.67-0.92; p=0.003), 1-year and 2-year survival rates (51% vs. 44% and 23% vs. 15%, respectively), and PFS (6.2 vs. 4.5 months; HR, 0.66; p<0.001). In a combined analysis from the phase II and phase III trials, the only clinical risk factor for pulmonary hemorrhage identified in a subsequent analysis of patients with severe hemorrhage was the presence of tumor cavitation prior to bevacizumab treatment [73]. In addition, grade 3 or 4 hypertension was significantly more common in patients treated with bevacizumab compared to placebo (7.0% vs. 0.7%). A subsequent analysis of patients in this trial suggested that the onset of hypertension after treatment with CT plus bevacizumab was associated with a better response to therapy compared to the response in patients treated with bevacizumab but not developing hypertension [74]. Moreover, in a pre-planned subset analysis of patients with adenocarcinoma histology, bevacizumab-based therapy extended median OS to 14.2 months compared with 10.3 months for CT alone (HR, 0.69) [75]. CT plus bevacizumab was also associated with a significantly higher incidence of grade 3 to 5 toxicities than paclitaxel/carboplatin (61% vs. 87%; p<0.001) [76].

The improved outcome for bevacizumab-based first-line therapy in NSCLC has recently been confirmed in a second randomized phase III trial of bevacizumab in combination with cisplatin and gemcitabine. In the AVAiL trial (Avastin in Lung Cancer), 1043 patients with advanced non-squamous NSCLC were randomly assigned to cisplatin (80 mg/m$^2$ on day 1) and gemcitabine (1250 mg/m$^2$ on days 1 and 8) every three weeks plus either bevacizumab (7.5 mg/kg), bevacizumab (15 mg/kg), or placebo on day 1 every three weeks. The cisplatin plus gemcitabine was continued for a maximum of six cycles, while the bevacizumab or placebo was continued as maintenance until there was evidence of progressive disease. Median PFS for bevacizumab 7.5 mg/Kg and 15 mg/Kg vs. placebo was 6.7 vs. 6.1 months (HR, 0.75; p=0.003) and 6.5 vs. 6.1 months (HR, 0.82; p=0.003), respectively. ORR was increased with both doses of bevacizumab (34%, 30%, and 20%, for the 7.5 mg/kg, 15 mg/kg, and placebo, respectively). In a subsequent report with a median follow-up of 13 months, the benefit in terms of ORR and PFS was maintained, but did not translate into a significant OS benefit, possibly due to the high use of efficacious second-line therapies [77]. Median OS for bevacizumab 7.5 mg/Kg and 15 mg/Kg vs. placebo was 13.6 months vs. 13.1 months (HR, 0.93; p=0.420) and 13.4 vs. 13.1 months (HR, 1.03; p=0.761), respectively. The majority of adverse events were grade 1 or 2 and the incidence of grade ≥3 toxicity was similar across arms. The adverse event fatality rate from any cause was similar across treatment groups (4%, 4% and 5%, respectively). As referred above, pemetrexed is being widely used in platinum-based combinations because of its selective activity in patients with non-squamous NSCLC. A phase II study have demonstrated the feasibility and potential benefit of combining bevacizumab with carboplatin plus pemetrexed followed by maintenance pemetrexed and bevacizumab [78]. A phase III trial (the PointBreak trial) is comparing this regimen with the bevacizumab plus carboplatin-paclitaxel regimen used in the ECOG 4599 study [79].

In addition to the two phase III trials, ECOG 4599 and AVAiL, the clinical activity and safety of bevacizumab-based therapy is being investigated in two large phase IV, open-label studies, the Safety of Avastin in lung (SAiL) trial in European population [80], and the

ARIES trial in American institutions [81]. Both trials have been conducted to generate further safety and efficacy data for bevacizumab combined with a range of standard first-line CT regimens in a broad "real-life" clinical population of patients with advanced non-squamous NSCLC. SAiL is a large, single-arm study that included 2122 patients with advanced NSCLC receiving bevacizumab. Although patients with known brain metastases were excluded, 281 individuals were diagnosed with brain metastases during the course of the study. In this subset, five (2%) had central nervous system bleeding.

## CT Plus Cetuximab

Epidermal-growth factor receptor (EGFR) expression is detected in up to 85% of NSCLC patients and has been shown to be associated with tumor growth, invasion, metastasis and poor prognosis. Thus EGFR blockade may improve outcome in patients with advanced NSCLC [82]. Strategies to block EGFR function have focused on the use of EGFR-directed mAb [83, 84] or tyrosine kinase inhibitors (TKIs). The mAb binds to the surface of the EGFR, thereby, competitively blocking the binding of epidermal growth factor (EGF). Antibody receptor complexes are internalized and degraded. This then results in the down-regulation of the EGFR on the surface of tumor cells. The mAb may also act via immunological mechanisms such as antibody-dependent cellular cytotoxicity.

Several EGFR-directed mAbs have been evaluated in clinical trials. Among them, cetuximab is by far the most studied antibody and its impact on outcome of palliative platinum-based standard CT has already been studied in combination with different CT regimens in both phase II [85, 86] and phase III trials in patients with advanced NSCLC (Table 4).

Two randomized phase II trials then suggested improved efficacy of CT plus cetuximab compared to CT alone. The Lung Cancer Cetuximab Study (LUCAS) compared cisplatin/vinorelbine plus cetuximab to CT alone in 86 chemo-naïve patients with advanced EGFR-positive NSCLC. ORR was 35% and 28%, respectively.

Median PFS (5.0 vs. 4.6 months) and median OS (8.3 vs. 7.3 months) also favored the combination arm. The HR was 0.71 (0.4–1.2), representing a trend towards longer PFS favoring the cetuximab-containing regimen. Skin toxicity grade 3–4 occurred in 10% of the patients.

Development of skin rash was associated with higher RR. The second randomized phase II trial evaluated platin plus gemcitabine with and without cetuximab in patients with advanced NSCLC independent of EGFR expression. ORR was 28% and 18% and median PFS times were 5.1 and 4.2 months in the cetuximab arm and CT-alone arm, respectively.

A meta-analysis then confirmed the benefit of cetuximab when added to standard first-line platin-based CT compared to CT alone [87]. This meta-analysis included 2018 patients from two randomized phase II trials and the two phase III trials. The CT protocols included cisplatin plus vinorelbine, platin plus gemcitabine, and carboplatin plus a taxane. The benefit was seen for OS (HR, 0.878; 95% CI, 0.795–0.969; p= 0.01), PFS (p=0.036) and ORR (p=0.001). The results of this meta-analysis also suggest a survival benefit irrespective of the type of CT protocol used.

**Table 4. Summary of phase II and III data for bevacizumab- and cetuximab-based therapy**

| STUDY/YEAR | TREATMENT | ORR (%) | PFS (months) | OS (months) |
|---|---|---|---|---|
| CT+bevacizumab | | | | |
| Phase II (Johnson, 2004) | Carboplatin+paclitaxel (Cb+P)(n=32) Cb+P+Bevacizumab 7.5 mg/Kg(n=32) C+P+Bevacizumab 15 mg/Kg (n=35) | 18.8 28.1 (p=NR) 31.5 (p=NR) | 4.2 4.3 (p=NS) 7.4 (p=0.023) | 14.9 11.6 (p=0.84) 17.7 (p=0.63) |
| ECOG 4599 (Sandler, 2006) | Carboplatin+paclitaxel (Cb+P) (n=444) Cb+P+Bevacizumab 15 mg/Kg (n=434) | 15% 35% (p<0.001) | 4.5 6.2 (HR, 0.66; p<0.001) | 10.3 12.3(HR, 0.79; p=0.003) |
| AVAIL (Reck, 2009-10) | Cisplatin+gemcitabine (C+G) (n=347) C+G+Bevacizumab 7.5 mg/Kg (n=345) C+G+Bevacizumab 15 mg/Kg (n=351) | 20.1 34.1 (p<0.0001) 30.4 (p=0.0023) | 6.1 6.7 (HR, 0.75; p=0.003) 6.5 (HR,0.85; p=0.045) | 13.7 14.1 (HR, 0.94; p=0.553) 14.5 (HR,0.97; p=0.750) |
| CT+cetuximab | | | | |
| LUCAS (Rosell, 2008) | Cisplatin+vinorelbine (C+V) (43) C+V+Cetuximab (43) | 28 35 (p=NR) | 4.6 5 (HR,0.71, p=NS) | 7.3 8.3 (HR,0.71; p=NS) |
| Phase II (Butts, 2010) | Platinum+gemcitabine (C/Cb+G) (66) C/Cb+G+Cetuximab (65) | 18.2 27.7 (p=NR) | 4.21 5.9 (p=NR) | 9.26 11.99 (p=NR) |
| FLEX (Pirker, 2009) | Cisplatin+vinorelbine (C+V) (568) C+V+Cetuximab (557) | 29 36 (p=0.01) | 4.8 4.8 (HR,0.94; p=NS) | 10.1 11.3 (HR,0.87; p=0.044) |
| BMS099 (Lynch, 2010) | Carboplatin+paclitaxel (Cb+P) (338) C+P+Cetuximab (338) | 17.2 25.7 (p=0.0066) | 4.24 4.40 (HR,0.902; p=0.235) | 9.69 8.38 (HR,0.89; p=0.168) |

CT: chemotherapy; ORR: overall response rate; PFS: progression-free survival; OS: overall survival; HR: hazard ratio; NR: not reported; NS: not significative.

Finally, current research focuses on the characterization of biomarkers which predict benefit from EGFR-directed mAbs [88, 89]. Suggestive results from phase II studies suggested that EGFR gene copy number might be useful in predicting benefit from cetuximab in patients with metastatic NSCLC. However, a subset analysis of the BMS-099 trial found no correlation between abnormalities in EGFR or KRAS in terms of either PFS or OS [90]. Similarly, a molecular analysis of the Fracture Intervention Trial Long-Term Extension (FLEX) trial did not find any predictive value for EGFR mutations, KRAS mutations or expression of KRAS by FISH [91].

A recent retrospective analysis of the FLEX trial, however, found that patients with the highest expression of EGFR on the tumor, as measured by the EGFR score, which is a product of the percentage of cells stained (0-100) and the intensity of the staining (0-3), had a significantly improved OS when cetuximab was added to CT compared with CT alone (median survival, 12.0 vs. 9.6 months). No benefit was observed in those with limited expression of EGFR, defined as those with a score less than 200 (median 9.8 vs. 10.3 months) [92].

Whether this method is superior than other biomarkers, and more importantly, whether the EGFR score is ready to be used in clinical practice to select patients who benefit from the addition of cetuximab, remains unclear. Further studies are needed to confirm these observations.

## Maintenance Therapy for Patients with Advanced NSCLC Who Respond to Initial Therapy

Although second-line treatment has been shown to improve survival and palliated symptoms, only approximately 50% of the patients will be able to receive this treatment, mainly because of the worsening of clinical condition. One of the strategies that has been extensively investigated in recent years in order to improve current clinical results in advanced NSCLC is the maintenance therapy. Approximately 40% to 60% of patients with advanced NSCLC complete 4 cycles of platinum-based CT without progression or unacceptable toxicity [94]. For these patients, the options to continue treatment after first-line induction include 1) continuing induction therapy for a fixed number of additional cycles over the standard or, when possible, until progression; 2) continuing only the third-generation non-platinum compound used in the induction regimen; 3) switching to a different agent after induction therapy.

### *Continuing First-Line Induction Therapy*

Initial trials addressing the question of duration of combination CT failed to show any response, survival or QoL benefit for the prolonged administration over a fixed number of cycles with an increased risk for cumulative toxicity [95, 96]. As a consequence the American Society of Clinical Oncology (ASCO) changed its recommendations regarding the appropriate duration of therapy in 2003, stating that treatment should have been stopped at four cycles for non responders patients and no more than six cycles should have been administered for any patient [97]; no major changes for this specific issue were reported in the ASCO guideline update in 2009 [98].

### *Continuation-Maintenance Therapy*

In patients responding or stable after the induction, a maintenance strategy should be to continue the same therapy withholding platinum, in an attempt to consolidate disease control and increasing survival, maintaining tolerability within acceptable limits. In three multicenter trials, positive results were seen when the maintenance therapy agent had been a component of the original CT regimen (Table 5) [99-101].

In the French phase III trial (IFCT-GFCP 0502), 834 patients with previously untreated, advanced NSCLC were treated with cisplatin and gemcitabine and the 464 patients with non-progressive disease after four cycles of CT were randomly assigned to observation, gemcitabine maintenance or erlotinib maintenance. PFS by independent review, the primary endpoint of the study, was significantly prolonged by gemcitabine (3.8 vs. 1.9 months; HR, 0.55; $p<0.001$) vs. observation. The OS data are not mature, but no significant difference in OS has been observed with 69.6% of events having occurred (12.1 vs. 10.7 months; HR, 0.86; 95% CI, 0.66 to 1.12) (207).

In the phase III PARAMOUNT trial, 939 patients were treated with cisplatin plus pemetrexed for advanced, non-squamous NSCLC (208). The 539 patients who did not progress after four cycles of treatment were randomly assigned (2:1 ratio) to pemetrexed (500 $mg/m^2$ every three weeks) or placebo, plus BSC. Among the 359 patients randomised to continuation maintenance with pemetrexed, there was a significant reduction in the risk of disease progression over the placebo group (HR, 0.62; 95% CI, 0.49-0.79; p<0·0001). The median PFS, measured from randomisation, was 4.1 months for pemetrexed and 2.8 months for placebo.

**Table 5. Summary of phase III trials evaluating maintenance therapy strategies**

| STUDY/YEAR | INDUCTION THERAPY | MAINTENANCE THERAPY | PFS (months) | OS (months) |
|---|---|---|---|---|
| CONTINUATION MAINTENANCE THERAPY | | | | |
| IFCT-GFCP 0502 (Perol, 2010) | Cisplatin+gemcitabine x 4 cycles (n=834) | Observation (n=152)<br>Gemcitabine (n=155) | 1.9<br>3.8 (HR, 0.55; p<0.001) | 10.7<br>12.1 (HR, 0.86; p=NS) |
| PARAMOUNT (Paz-Ares, 2012) | Cisplatin+pemetrexed x 4 cycles (n=979) | Placebo + BSC (n=180)<br>Pemetrexed + BSC (n=359) | 2.8<br>4.1 (HR, 0.62; p<0.001) | NR<br>NR |
| AVAPERL (Barlesi, 2011) | Cisplatin+pemetrexed +bevacizumab x 4 cycles (n=376) | Bevacizumab (n=125)<br>Pemetrexed+Bevacizumab (n=128) | 3.7<br>7.4 (HR, 0.62; p<0.0001) | NR<br>NR |
| SWITCH MAINTENANCE THERAPY | | | | |
| Immediate vs. delayed docetaxel (Fidias, 2009) | Cisplatin+gemcitabine x 4 cycles (n=566) | Immediate docetaxel (n=153)<br>Delayed docetaxel (n=309) | 5.7<br>2.7 (p<0.001) | 12.3<br>9.7 (p=0.00853) |
| JMEN (Ciuleanu, 2009) | Platinum-based doublet x 4 cycles (n=745) | BSC (n=222)<br>BSC + pemetrexed (n=441) | 2.6<br>4.3 (HR, 0.50; p<0.001) | 10.6<br>13.4 (HR,0.79; p=0.012) |
| SATURN (Cappuzo, 2009) | Platinum-based doublet x 4 cycles (n=1949) | Placebo (n=451)<br>Erlotinib (n=437) | 2.75<br>3.07 (HR,0.71; p<0.001) | 11<br>12 (HR,0.81; p=0.0088) |
| IFCT-GFCP 0502 (Perol, 2010) | Cisplatin+gemcitabine x 4 cycles (n=834) | Observation (n=152)<br>Erlotinib (n=153) | 1.9<br>2.9 (HR, 0.82; p=0.002) | 10.7<br>11.8 (HR, 0.86; p=NS) |
| WJTOG 0203 (Takeda, 2010) | Platinum-based doublet x 4-6 cycles (n=604) | Observation (n=298)<br>Gefitinib (n=300) | 4.3<br>4.6 (HR, 0.68; p<0.001) | 12.9<br>13.7 (HR, 0.86; p=0.11) |
| EORTC 08021-ILCP 0103 (Gaafar, 2010) | Platinum-based doublet x 4 cycles (n=173) | Observation (n=86)<br>Gefitinib (n=87) | 2.9<br>4.1 (HR, 0.61; p=0.0015) | 9.4<br>10.9 (HR, 0.81; p=0.204) |

CT: chemotherapy; PFS: progression-free survival; OS: overall survival; HR: hazard ratio; BSC: best supportive care; NR: not reported.

In the AVAPERL trial, 376 patients with previously untreated advanced non-squamous NSCLC were treated with four cycles of cisplatin plus pemetrexed plus bevacizumab (209). The 253 patients with an objective response or SD by RECIST criteria and without severe bevacizumab toxicity were randomly assigned to continuation maintenance with either bevacizumab alone or bevacizumab plus pemetrexed. Although the AVAPERL trial demonstrated the superiority of pemetrexed plus bevacizumab over bevacizumab alone, the trial does not address whether that combination is superior to continuation with pemetrexed alone.

### *Switch-Maintenance Therapy*

According to the Goldie-Coldman hypothesis, showing that even the smallest detectable cancers contain at least one drug resistant clone and that increasing numbers of resistant clones emerge as tumors grow and progress [102], a rational strategy would be to use all effective drugs as early as possible in the treatment program. Different non-cross-resistant agents have been used as a maintenance strategy after a defined number of induction cycles with a platinum-based regimen in several randomized clinical trials [103,104].

The strategy of early switch-maintenance therapy has also been tested for targeted therapies [105,106]. The EGFR TKIs, gefitinib and erlotinib, represent the most studied agents in this setting. In the SATURN trial, 1949 patients with previously untreated advanced NSCLC were treated with four cycles of platinum-based doublet CT. The 889 patients who had not experienced PD were then randomly assigned to treatment with erlotinib or placebo. Patients assigned to erlotinib experienced a statistically significant improvement in PFS in both the intent-to treat (median, 12.3 vs. 11.1 weeks; HR, 0.71; 95% CI, 0.62-0.82; $p < 0.0001$) and the EGFR IHC positive patient populations (HR, 0.69, 95% CI, 0.58-0.82; $p < 0.0001$). The improvement in PFS was seen both in patients with adenocarcinoma and squamous carcinoma. Based on this trial, maintenance erlotinib was recently approved by the Food and Drug Administration (FDA) in all patients who do not experience disease progression after platinum-based therapy. The European Medicines Agency (EMA) approved maintenance erlotinib only for patients with SD after 4 cycles of standard platinum-based first-line therapy.

The ATLAS study is a second phase III trial designed to build on the use of bevacizumab as maintenance therapy for patients treated with an induction containing the same mAb together with a platinum-based treatment. Specifically, the ATLAS study sought to determine whether the addition of erlotinib to bevacizumab could be more effective than bevacizumab alone when used in the maintenance setting. A total of 1,160 patients were enrolled and, after completion of four induction cycles, non-progressing patients (n=768, 66%) were randomized to receive bevacizumab 15 mg/Kg alone or in combination with erlotinib. This trial was stopped after a planned interim efficacy analysis, reaching an improvement in PFS, the primary end point. Patients receiving erlotinib and bevacizumab experienced a superior PFS compared to bevacizumab alone (median PFS, 4.8 vs. 3.7 months; HR, 0.71; 95% CI, 0.58-0.86; $p = 0.006$). Post-study therapy was at the discretion of the investigator, and the rates of subsequent therapies on the erlotinib/bevacizumab and bevacizumab arms were 50.3% and 55.5%, respectively. Pre-planned subgroup analysis showed that the PFS benefit with bevacizumab+erlotinib maintenance therapy was seen regardless of age, gender, ethnicity, smoking habit or histology.

The European Organization for the Research and Treatment of Cancer (EORTC) 08021-ILCP trial was similar in design to the SATURN study. Initially, all patients with advanced NSCLC, not-progressing after 4 cycles of platinum-based CT were randomized to receive either gefitinib 250 mg/day or matched placebo until progression or unacceptable toxicity. Initially all stable and responding patients were eligible for the study, which was then amended to require also evidence of EGFR protein expression by IHC. After inclusion of 173 patients and based on 149 of the required 514 deaths, PFS was significantly different in favor of gefitinib (4.1 vs. 2.9 months; HR, 0.61; 95% CI 0.45-0.83; p=0.0015), but no difference in OS could be detected (median OS, 10.9 vs. 9.4 months; HR, 0.83; 95% CI, 0.60-1.15; p=0.204).

# Initial Treatment with Targeted Agents

## Initial Systemic Therapy for Advanced NSCLC with a Mutation in the Epidermal Growth Factor Receptor

EGFR inhibitors have proven effective in some patients with advanced NSCLC. The EGFR TKIs gefitinib and erlotinib first demonstrated clinical activity in patients who had been previously treated with cytotoxic CT [107,108]. After encouraging results of EGFR TKI as second line therapy, it was natural to test these agents in the initial management of patients with advanced NSCLC. Multiple clinical and molecular markers are useful in predicting which patients are most likely to benefit from therapy with this class of agent, both for the initial and second-line therapy in patients with advanced NSCLC.

**Table 6. Summary of phase III studies with EGFR TKI in previously untreated patients with sensitizing mutations in EGFR**

| STUDY/YEAR | POPULATION | TREATMENT | PFS (months) | OS (months) |
|---|---|---|---|---|
| IPASS (Mok, 2009) | 1217 patients Asian, adenocarcinoma, never/former smokers 261 patients with EGFR mutations | Carboplatin+paclitaxel (n=608) Gefitinib (n=609) | Longer PFS for gefitinib Overall population: HR, 0.74; p<0.001 EGFR mutations: HR, 0.48; p<0.001 | 17.4 18.1 (HR, 0.91; p=NS) |
| WJTOG 3405 (Mitsudomi, 2010) | 177 patients with EGFR mutations Asian population | Cisplatin+docetaxel (n=86) Gefitinib (n=86) | 6.3 9.2 (HR, 0.48; p<0.001) | NR NR |
| NEJ 002 (Maemodo, 2010) | 230 patients with EGFR mutations Asian population | Carboplatin+paclitaxel (n=114) Gefitinib (n=114) | 5.4 10.8 (HR, 0.30; p<0.001) | 23.6 30.5 (p=0.31) |
| OPTIMAL (Zhou, 2011) | 154 patients with EGFR mutations Asian population | Carboplatin+gemcitabine (n=82) Erlotinib (n=83) | 4.6 13.1 (HR, 0.16; p<0.001) | NR NR |
| EURTAC (Rosell, 2012) | 174 patients with EGFR mutations European population | Cisplatin/carboplatin+ docetaxel/gemcitabine (n=87) Erlotinib (n=86) | 5.2 9.7 (HR, 0.37; p<0.0001) | 10.3 19.5 (p=NS) |

CT: chemotherapy; PFS: progression-free survival; OS: overall survival; HR: hazard ratio; NR: not reported; NS: not significative.

### *Single Agent Therapy*

Several prospective phase II clinical trials with erlotinib and gefitinib have shown ORR in the range from 55% to 82% and median time to progression from 8.9 to 13.3 months when patients with NSCLC were selected based upon molecular criteria [109].

The impressive findings from phase II clinical trials has prompted the initiation of multiple phase III trials comparing initial treatment with an EGFR TKI and cytotoxic CT in previously untreated patients with sensitizing mutations in EGFR (Table 6) [110-112].

The most extensive data come from the Iressa Pan-Asian Study (IPASS), in which 1217 CT-naïve patients were randomly assigned to either gefitinib or CT with carboplatin plus paclitaxel. For the entire cohort, first-line gefitinib proved superior to paclitaxel and carboplatin, which 25% vs. 7% of the respective treatment groups progression free at 1 year (HR for progression or death, 0.74). However, the difference in OS was not statistically significant (median, 18.8 vs. 17.4 months; HR, 0.90; 95% CI, 0.79-1.02). In the subgroup of patients who were positive for EGFR gene mutations, PFS was significantly longer among those who received gefitinib than among those who received carboplatin-paclitaxel therapy (median, 9.5 vs. 6.3 months; HR 0.48). However, OS was not increased with gefitinib (median, 22 months in both groups, HR 1.00). It could be explained because, among mutation positive patients who initially received carboplatin plus paclitaxel, 64% subsequently were treated with an EGFR TKI. Based upon the results of the IPASS trial, the EMA approved gefitinib for the initial treatment of patients with advanced NSCLC and activating mutations of the EGFR tyrosine kinase.

The potential benefit of erlotinib compared with first-line CT in patients harbouring EGFR mutations have also been assessed in phase III trials. In the OPTIMAL trial from China, 154 patients with known EGFR mutations and measurable disease were randomly assigned to erlotinib or up to four cycles of carboplatin plus gemcitabine. Median PFS, the primary end point of the study, was significantly longer in erlotinib-treated patients than in those on CT (13.1 vs. 4.6; HR, 0.16; 95% CI, 0.10-0.26; $p<0.0001$). Similarly, the ORR was significantly improved with erlotinib (83 vs. 36%). CT was associated with more grade 3 or 4 toxic effects than was erlotinib and with increased treatment-related serious adverse events. The most common grade 3 or 4 toxic effects with erlotinib were increased alanine aminotransferase concentrations (4%) and skin rash (2%).

The phase III EURTAC trial have confirmed the efficacy of erlotinib compared with standard CT for first-line treatment of European patients with advanced EGFR-mutation positive NSCLC (163). A total of 174 patients were randomly assigned to receive oral erlotinib or 3 week cycles of standard intravenous CT with cisplatin plus docetaxel or gemcitabine. At a median follow-up of 19 months for the erlotinib group and 14 months for those assigned to CT, PFS, the primary endpoint of the trial, was significantly increased with erlotinib compared with CT (median, 9.7 vs. 5.2 months; HR, 0.37, 95% CI 0.25-0.54; $p<0.0001$). There was no significant difference in OS (median, 19.3 and 19.5 months, respectively).

In contrast to these results, the use of an EGFR TKI for initial therapy of advanced NSCLC in an unselected population appears to be less effective than initial treatment with cytotoxic CT. In the phase III TORCH trial, patients were randomly assigned either to gemcitabine plus cisplatin or erlotinib. Patients were crossed over to the opposite regimen upon disease progression [(113]. The trial was stopped prematurely after enrolling 760 patients because of poorer OS in those who initially received erlotinib (median, 10.9 vs. 7.7 months; HR, 1.40; 95% CI, 1.13-1.73).

### *EGFR TKI Plus CT*

Another clinical question that is being evaluated is the impact of CT in addition to EGFR TKI for previously untreated patients with advanced NSCLC that were not selected on the basis of EGFR mutation status. Two randomized phase III trials, each including over 1000 patients, did not demonstrate a benefit in outcome when erlotinib was combined with either carboplatin plus paclitaxel (TRIBUTE) [114] or cisplatin plus gemcitabine (TALENT) (115). Similarly, two phase III trials in which gefitinib was combined with these same CT doublets (INTACT 1 [116] and INTACT 2 [117]) failed to show any improvement in survival compared with CT alone.

In summary, the addition of combination CT to an EGFR TKI did not lead to a significant improvement in survival in patients whose tumors express an EGFR mutation, lending support for the use of an EGFR TKI monotherapy in these patients.

### *Predictors of Responsiveness*

Clinical correlation studies have found that specific activating mutations in the TK domain of the EGFR (exon 19 deletions, L858R point mutation in exon 21) are associated with increased responsiveness to EGFR TKIs [118,119]. One study that included 197 patients with EGFR mutations found that deletions in exon 19 are associated with a significantly higher response rate compared to the L858R point mutation (odds ratio 3.08, 95% CI 1.63-5.81) [120]. Among patients with adenocarcinoma histology, the incidence of activating mutations decreases with an increasing history of tobacco use. In a series of 2142 patients, mutations were present in 52% of never smokers, and the frequency of such mutations decreased progressively to less than 10% in those with 25 or more pack years of cigarettes smoked. Although mutations were significantly more common in females than males (26 vs. 19%), this difference was not statistically significant when never smokers and smokers were analyzed separately [121].

Preexisting somatic mutations in KRAS are associated with primary resistance to EGFR TKI. Furthermore, mutations in KRAS only rarely occur in conjunction with mutations in EGFR [122,123].

### *Anaplastic Lymphoma Kinase (ALK) Fusion Gene Positive Advanced NSCLC*

A group of patients with NSCLC have tumors that contain an inversion in chromosome 2 that juxtaposes the 5' end of the echinoderm microtubule-associated protein-like 4 (EML4) gene with the 3' end of the anaplastic lymphoma kinase (ALK) gene, resulting in the novel fusion oncogene EML4-ALK [124]. The resulting chimeric protein, EML4-ALK, contains an N-terminus derived from EML4 and a C-terminus containing the entire intracellular tyrosine kinase domain of ALK. Since the discovery of this fusion oncogene in 2007 by Soda and colleagues [125], multiple variants of EML-ALK have been reported, all of which encode the same cytoplasmic portion of ALK but contain different truncations of EML4 [91, 126]. For EML4-ALK, the EML4 fusion partner mediates ligand-independent dimerization and/or oligomerization of ALK, resulting in constitutive kinase activity. This fusion oncogene rearrangement possesses potent oncogenic activity both *in vitro* and *in vivo* [127] and defines a distinct clinicopathologic subset of NSCLC.

### *Clinic Pathological Characteristics of ALK-Mutated NSCLC Patients*

In unselected NSCLC populations, the ALK rearrangement is a relatively rare event. In the initial report, 5 of 75 lung tumors (7%) demonstrated expression of the fusion transcript. The overall incidence of ALK gene rearrangements in subsequent series has been about 4% [128, 129]. Except in rare cases, the presence of ALK gene rearrangements in NSCLC is a molecular alteration mutually exclusive with other common mutations such as EGFR or KRAS mutations.

Current available data confirm that the majority of NSCLC tumours harbouring ALK alterations have been diagnosed as adenocarcinomas on histological examination. In addition, signet-ring cells are frequently seen and more than 90% of patients are never smokers or former light smokers (≤10 packs/year) [130, 131]. Curiously, these two features are shared by EGFR-mutated NSCLC. However, in the ALK-mutated population, patients tend to be younger than the average age of diagnosis for patients with lung cancer, without any gender difference.

In one study in which patients were selected for genetic screening based on clinical features commonly associated with EGFR mutation, including never/light smoking status and adenocarcinoma histology, 13% harbored the ALK fusion oncogene. Within the group of never or light smokers in this study, the frequency of ALK positivity was 22%, and among never or light smokers who did not have an EGFR mutation, the frequency was 33%. These findings suggest that in NSCLC patients with clinical characteristics associated with EGFR mutation but with negative EGFR testing, as many as one in three may harbor the ALK fusion oncogene [132].

### *Diagnosis*

There are three methods that can be used to identify ALK gene rearrangements: IHC, reverse transcription polymerase chain reaction of cDNA (RT-PCR), and FISH.

The gold standard assay for diagnosing ALK-positive NSCLC is FISH [133]. In fact, clinical trials to test the effectiveness of crizotinib in ALK-positive patients established FISH as the method of choice. Arbitrarily, crizotinib trials established that a patient is "ALK-positive" when there is at least 15% dissociation of the signal in at least 60 cells. However, it is not known if tumours with inferior results and less strict ALK definition may be sensitive to crizotinib. In addition, FISH requires sufficient material, usually obtained by biopsy, lacking a clear validation in cytological specimens.

### *Crizotinib*

In the same year that Soda *et al.* found the potential oncogenic activity of ALK rearrangements in NSCLC, it was demonstrated that the aminopyrimidine PF-02341066, crizotinib, inhibits the tyrosine phosporylation induced by ALK at nanomolecular concentrations and reduces tumour proliferation [134]. Crizotinib is an oral multitargeted small molecule TKI, which was originally developed as an inhibitor of mesenchymal epithelial transition growth factor (c-MET). It is also a potent inhibitor of ALK phosphorylation and signal transduction. This inhibition is associated with G1-S phase cell cycle arrest and induction of apoptosis in positive cells *in vitro* and *in vivo*.

The antitumor efficacy of crizotinib was demonstrated in an open-label, multi-centre, two-step phase I trial. The first part of the study enrolled patients with any solid tumor refractory to standard therapy in a dose-escalation fashion to determine toxic effects and the maximum tolerated dose. Doses of 200 mg or higher twice daily resulted in a mean concentration higher than 120 ng/ml, the preclinical predictive effective concentration.

Indirect evidence of the impact of crizotinib on survival of patients comes from a nonrandomized, retrospective analysis of the patients enrolled in the phase I study. The one and two-year survival rates for patients treated with crizotinib were 74 and 54%, respectively, with a median follow-up of 18 months. In a cohort of 36 patients with the ALK fusion oncogene who were not treated with crizotinib, the survival rates at one and two year rates were 44 and 12%, respectively. A comparison with a larger cohort of patients with wild-type tumors did not identify a difference compared with those with the ALK rearrangement not treated with crizotinib, suggesting that the presence of ALK rearrangement was not prognostically significant.

Based on this data, crizotinib was approved by the US FDA in August 2011. This approval is independent of whether or not the patient has received previous treatment for advanced NSCLC and it was based upon RR rather than survival data.

In addition, two ongoing phase III trials are exploring the role of crizotinib in the treatment of ALK-positive NSCLC. One trial randomizes ALK-positive patients with progressive, metastatic NSCLC who have received one prior, platinum-based CT regimen to either crizotinib or single-agent docetaxel or pemetrexed (NCT00932893). A second trial is randomly assigning patients to crizotinib or CT with pemetrexed plus a platinum compound (either cisplatin or carboplatin) in the first-line setting (NCT01154140). Patients assigned to CT can crossover to crizotinib when progressive disease is documented. The primary endpoint for the trial is PFS.

# Second Line Therapy

Cytotoxic CT and/or molecularly targeted agents may delay disease progression and prolong survival in patients with advanced NSCLC. For patients with disseminated metastatic disease who have progressed after an initial treatment regimen, second-line systemic therapy (CT or small molecule EGFR TKI) provides palliation and increases survival in selected patients [135,136].

## Cytotoxic Chemotherapy

Second-line cytotoxic CT for advanced NSCLC should be considered in patients with a good PS after progression initial CT or treatment with a targeted agent. Both docetaxel and pemetrexed have been approved by the US FDA for second-line monotherapy. Other cytotoxic agents that are active as initial therapy may also have utility, but these have not been compared with either BSC or the approved agents in randomized trials in previously treated patients (Table 7).

### *Docetaxel*

The potential benefits of administering second-line CT were first shown in the TAX 317 trial. This was a randomized phase III trial of docetaxel vs. BSC for stage IIIB/IV NSCLC patients, PS 0 to 2, who had previously been treated with one or more platinum-based CT regimens. Patients were randomized to docetaxel 100 mg/m$^2$ (49 patients) or 75 mg/m$^2$ (55 patients) every 3 weeks until disease progression or unacceptable toxicity or BSC. Of 84 patients with measurable lesions, six (7.1%) achieved partial responses (three patients at each dose level). PFS was longer for docetaxel patients than for BSC patients (10.6 vs. 6.7 weeks, respectively; P<.001), as was median OS (7.0 vs. 4.6 months; p =0.047). The difference was more significant for docetaxel 75 mg/m$^2$ patients, compared with corresponding BSC patients (median, 7.5 vs. 4.6 months; p=0.010; 1-year survival, 37% vs. 11%; p=0.003). In a subsequent analysis from the same study, patients receiving docetaxel had improved pain control and significantly less deterioration in quality of life compared to those receiving BSC, in whom pain control worsened over the course of the study [137].

Supportive evidence that docetaxel is an effective second-line therapy for patients with NSCLC comes from the TAX 320 trial reported by Fossella *et al* [138]. In this trial, patients with PS 0 to 2 were randomly assigned to docetaxel (100 mg/m$^2$ every three weeks), docetaxel (75 mg/m$^2$ every three weeks) or a control arm with vinorelbine (30 mg/m2 weekly) or ifosfamide (2 g/m2 daily for three days, every three weeks). Both docetaxel groups had a significantly higher RR than the control group (10.8%, 6.7% and 0.8% in the docetaxel 100, docetaxel 75 y the control arm, respectively). The median time to progression was similar among the three groups.

The trials by Shepherd *et al.* and Fossella *et al.* established docetaxel 75 mg/m$^2$ administered every 21 days as the standard of care for second-line therapy for NSCLC.

### *Pemetrexed*

Based on the phase II activity of pemetrexed, Hanna *et al.* conducted a phase III trial (JMEI study) of second-line therapy in NSCLC comparing a standard arm of docetaxel 75 mg/m$^2$ every 21 days with pemetrexed 500 mg/m$^2$ every 21 days until PD or unacceptable toxicity. The study was designed to show that OS of patients randomized to pemetrexed was non-inferior to that of docetaxel. Five hundred and seventy-one patients were randomized (283 pemetrexed, 288 docetaxel). The ORR (9.1% vs. 8.8%) was almost identical for pemetrexed and docetaxel, respectively. There were no differences in the PFS of pemetrexed compared with docetaxel (median PFS, 2.9 for both groups; HR, 0.97; 95% CI, 0.82-1.16) and median OS (8.3 months vs. 7.9 months) and 1-year survival with pemetrexed was not statistically different to that of docetaxel (HR, 0.99; 95% CI, 0.8-1.20). Although there were no differences in any of the efficacy parameters, pemetrexed was associated with significantly less grade 3 or 4 neutropenia (5 vs. 40%), febrile neutropenia (2 vs. 13%), use of granulocyte colony-stimulating factor support (3 vs. 19%) and hair loss (6 vs. 38%). Interestingly, despite these differences in toxicity, there were no differences in QOL between the two treatment groups [139].

A further retrospective analysis of the JMEI trial suggested that there may be a difference in the effectiveness of pemetrexed compared with docetaxel based on histology [140].

Pemetrexed was more active than docetaxel in patients with non-squamous tumors (median OS, 9.3 vs. 8.0 months; HR, 0.78; 95% CI, 0.61-1.00). In contrast, pemetrexed was less effective than docetaxel in patients with squamous carcinomas (median OS, 6.2 vs. 7.4 months; HR, 1.56; 95% CI 1.08-2.26). Based upon these results, the FDA has restricted the approval of pemetrexed in advanced NSCLC to patients with non-squamous histology.

**Table 7. Summary of phase II/III studies evaluating chemotherapy and targeted agents in second-line therapy**

| STUDY/YEAR | TREATMENT | ORR (%) | PFS (months) | OS (months) |
|---|---|---|---|---|
| SECOND-LINE CT | | | | |
| TAX 317 (Shepherd, 2000) | Docetaxel 75 mg/m$^2$/3 weeks (n=55)<br>Docetaxel 100 mg/m$^2$/3 weeks (n=49) | 7.1<br>7.1 (p=NR) | 2.65 (p=0.004)<br>2.65 (p=0.037) | 7.5 (p=0.01)<br>5.9 (p=0.78) |
| TAX 320 (Fosella, 2000) | Vinorelbina/Ifosfamida (n=123)<br>Docetaxel 75 mg/m$^2$/3 weeks (n=125)<br>Docetaxel 100 mg/m$^2$/3 weeks (n=125 | 0.8<br>6.7 (p=0.036)<br>10.8 (p=0.001) | 1.67<br>2.1 (p=0.044)<br>2.1 (p=0.093) | 19<br>32 (p=0.025)<br>21 (p=NS) |
| DISTAL 01 (Gridelli, 2004) | Docetaxel 75 mg/m$^2$/3 weeks (n=110)<br>Docetaxel 33.3 mg/m$^2$/weekly (n=110) | 2.7<br>5.5 (p=0.50) | NR<br>NR | 7.25<br>6.25 (p=0.80) |
| JMEI (Hanna, 2004) | Docetaxel 75 mg/m$^2$/3 weeks (n=288)<br>Pemetrexed 500 mg/m2/3 weeks (n=283) | 8.8<br>9.1 (p=NS) | 2.9<br>2.9 (HR,0.97; p=NS) | 7.9<br>8.3 (HR,0.99, p=NS) |
| Smit (2009) | Pemetrexed 500 mg/m$^2$/3 weeks (n=119)<br>Carboplatin+pemetrexed (n=121) | 4<br>9 (p=NR) | 2.8<br>4.2 (HR,0.67; p=0.005) | 7.6<br>8 (p=NS) |
| SECOND-LINE TARGETED AGENTS | | | | |
| BR.21 (Shepherd, 2005) | Placebo (n=243)<br>Erlotinib (n=488) | <1<br>9 (p<0.001) | 1.8<br>2.2 (HR,0.61, p<0.001) | 7.6<br>8 (p=NS) |
| TITAN (Ciuleanu, 2012) | Pemetrexed/Docetaxel (n=221)<br>Erlotinib (n=203) | 6.3<br>7.9 (p=NS) | 2.07<br>1.57 (p=NS) | 5.5<br>5.3 (p=0.73) |
| ISEL (Thatcher, 2005) | Placebo (n=563)<br>Gefitinb (n=1229) | 1<br>8 (p<0.0001) | 2.6<br>3 (HR,0.82; p=0.006) | 5.1<br>5.6 (HR,0.89; p=0.087) |
| INTEREST (Douillard, 2010) | Docetaxel (n=773)<br>C+P+Cetuximab (n=773) | 42.1<br>21.2 (p=0.04) | 4.1<br>7 (HR,0.16; p=0.001) | 14.2<br>16.6 (HR,0.83; p=0.6) |

CT: chemotherapy; ORR: overall response rate; PFS: progression-free survival; OS: overall survival; HR: hazard ratio; NR: not reported; NS: not significative; BSC: best supportive care.

## EGFR TKI

In phase III trials, erlotinib increased survival compared to BSC. Based upon a comparison with results from other trials, the prolongation of survival appeared to be similar to that with second-line chemotherapeutic drugs. In contrast, the data with gefitinib are conflicting [141,142].

### *Erlotinib*

The clinical activity of erlotinib as a second- or third-line therapy for NSCLC was evaluated in a phase III trial conducted by the National Cancer Institute of Canada Clinical Trials Group (BR.21). A total of 731 patients who had received one or two prior CT regimens and were not considered for further CT were randomized in a 2:1 ratio to erlotinib (n=488) or placebo (n=243). Erlotinib significantly improved the ORR (9% vs. <1% with placebo), PFS (2.2 months vs. 1.8 months; HR, 0.61; 95% CI, 0.51-0.74) and OS (6.7 months vs. 4.7 months; HR, 0.70; 95% CI, 0.58-0.85) compared with placebo. An increase in OS in the subset of patients ≥70 years of age was equivalent to that seen in younger patients. However, severe toxicities were more common in the elderly (35 vs. 18% in younger patients) and required discontinuation of treatment more frequently (12 vs. 3%) [143]. QOL analyses demonstrated that patients randomized to erlotinib experienced improved QoL and significantly longer time to deterioration in cough, dyspnea and pain compared with the placebo group [144].

Erlotinib was also compared to CT in the TITAN trial, in which 424 patients were randomly assigned to erlotinib or CT with either pemetrexed or docetaxel, according to the investigators discretion, until PD or unacceptable toxicity [145]. All patients had PD following a single platinum-based CT regimen. With a median follow-up of 27.9 months in the erlotinib group and 24.8 months in the placebo group, there was no significant difference in OS, the primary endpoint of the trial, between erlotinib and CT (median, 5.3 vs. 5.5 months; HR, 0.96; p=0.73). Similarly, there was no significant difference in either ORR (7.9% vs. 6.3%) or median PFS (6.3 vs. 8.6 weeks). The adverse-event profile of each group was in line with previous studies.

## Bevacizumab

The role of bevacizumab in previously treated patients remains uncertain. A randomized phase II trial found a trend toward improved PFS when bevacizumab was added to either CT (HR, 0.66; 95% CI, 0.38-1.16) or erlotinib (HR, 0.72; 95% CI, 0.42-1.23) [146]. However, in a much larger phase III trial, 636 patients were randomly assigned to erlotinib plus bevacizumab or erlotinib alone in patients who had progressed after standard first-line CT [147]. OS, the primary end-point of the study, did not differ between 317 controls and 319 patients in the bevacizumab group (HR, 0.97; 95% CI, 0.80-1.18, p=0·7583). Although PFS seemed to be longer in the bevacizumab group (3.4 months) than in the control group (1.7 months) (HR, 0.62; 95% CI, 0.52-0.75) and ORR suggested some clinical activity of bevacizumab and erlotinib, median OS, the primary end-point of the study, did not differ between 317 controls and 319 patients in the bevacizumab group (median OS, 9.3 months vs. 9.2 month, respectively; HR, 0.97; 95% CI, 0.80-1.18; p=0·7583).

# Conclusion

The initial management of patients with advanced NSCLC depends upon the presence or absence of characteristic molecular abnormalities, as well as the patient's age, functional status, comorbidities, and prior therapy. Patients should have tumor tissue assessed for the presence of a somatic mutation in EGFR, which confers sensitivity to EGFR TKI, and for the ALK fusion oncogene, which confers sensitivity to crizotinib.

Cytotoxic CT is the primary treatment for patients with advanced NSCLC who have neither an activating mutation of EGFR nor an ALK fusion oncogene. Platinum-based combination CT using doublets of contemporary drugs can prolong survival compared to either BSC or less intense single-agent CT, and control symptoms in patients with a good PS. Recommended third-generation agents include vinorelbine, gemcitabine, taxanes and pemetrexed (non-squamous histology only). Pemetrexed is preferred to gemcitabine in patients with non-squamous histology according to a survival benefit demonstrated in a pre-planned subgroup analysis of one large randomized trial. Several meta-analyses showed higher RR for cisplatin combinations when compared with carboplatin combinations. OS was significantly superior for cisplatin in the subgroup on non-squamous histologies treated with third-generation regimens in one meta-analysis.

According to two randomized clinical trials, bevacizumab may be added to a combination regimen of carboplatin-paclitaxel or cisplatin-gemcitabine in patients with tumours of non-squamous histology and PS 0-1. Prolongation of survival has only been demonstrated with carboplatin-paclitaxel combination. In addition, one large randomized clinical trial showed a survival benefit when cetuximab is combined with cisplatin-vinorelbine CT in EGFR-protein-expressing patients with PS 0-2 independent of histology.

Palliative first-line treatment CT should be initiated while the patient is in good PS. In most patients four cycles should be administered and in responding patients, a maximum of six cycles should not be exceeded. The role of maintenance therapy with a cytotoxic CT agent or an EGFR TKI is evolving and may provide an option for patients with a response or SD after their initial course of treatment. Survival benefits were observed in phase III trials for pemetrexed (non-squamous histologies) and erlotinib. The superiority of immediate maintenance therapy versus delayed therapy is not proven.

First-line treatment with an EGFR TKI (erlotinib and gefitinib) is an option in patients with tumours harbouring an activating EGFR mutation in exon 19 and/or 21. For patients whose tumors contain a characteristic ALK fusion oncogene, treatment with the ALK inhibitor crizotinib is strongly recommended. Second-line therapy can improve both survival and QOL after failure of an initial cytotoxic CT regimen or after progression on an EGFR TKI in carefully selected NSCLC patients. The choice of treatment depends upon the previous therapy administered. For patients who have progressed after an initial CT regimen, treatment with either an EGFR TKI or single-agent cytotoxic CT is a reasonable option. The standard CT options include pemetrexed (non-squamous histology) and docetaxel. For patients who have progressed after treatment with an initial EGFR TKI, cytotoxic CT rather than additional molecularly targeted therapy is suggested. The reintroduction of the EGFR TKI, in conjunction with cytotoxic CT, can slow this progression. In addition, second generation TKI or c-Met inhibitors have now entered clinical trials and have further improved the prognosis of patients with EGFR TKI resistant NSCLC. Despite all these results, outcome in NSCLC patients remain poor. Therefore, there is a critical need for development of prognostic and predictive biomarkers of efficacy and toxicity to optimize the selection of treatment. In addition, several therapeutic approaches that target specific molecular abnormalities which characterize NSCLC, such as small molecule inhibitors, immunotherapy, antisense oligonucleotides and gene therapy, are currently under active investigation. The optimal way to integrate these targeted therapies will be a major focus of future trials.

# References


[1] Siegel R, Naishadham D, Jemal A. Cancer statistics, 2012. *CA Cancer J Clin* 2012; 62:10-29.

[2] Robinson LA, Ruckdeschel JC, Wagner H Jr, et al. Treatment of non-small cell lung cancer-stage IIIA: ACCP evidence-based clinical practice guidelines (2nd edition). *Chest* 2007; 132:243S.

[3] Harpole DH Jr, Healey EA, DeCamp MM Jr, et al. Chest wall invasive non-small cell lung cancer: patterns of failure and implications for a revised staging system. *Ann Surg Oncol* 1996; 3:261.

[4] de Perrot M, Fadel E, Mussot S, et al. Resection of locally advanced (T4) non-small cell lung cancer with cardiopulmonary bypass. *Ann Thorac Surg* 2005; 79:1691.

[5] Douillard JY, Rosell R, De Lena M, et al. Impact of postoperative radiation therapy on survival in patients with complete resection and stage I, II, or IIIA non-small-cell lung cancer treated with adjuvant chemotherapy: the adjuvant Navelbine International Trialist Association (ANITA) Randomized Trial. *Int J Radiat Oncol Biol Phys* 2008; 72:695.

[6] Lally BE, Zelterman D, Colasanto JM, et al. Postoperative radiotherapy for stage II or III non-small-cell lung cancer using the surveillance, epidemiology, and end results database. *J Clin Oncol* 2006;24:2998–3006.

[7] Wakelee HA, Stephenson P, Keller SM, et al. Post-operative radiotherapy (PORT) or chemoradiotherapy (CPORT) following resection of stages II and IIIa non-small cell lung cancer (NSCLC) does not increase the expected risk of death from intercurrent disease (DID) in Eastern cooperative oncology group (ECOG) trial e3590. *Lung Cancer* 2005;48:389–397.

[8] Machtay M, Lee JH, Shrager JB, et al. Risk of death from intercurrent disease is not excessively increased by modern postoperative radiotherapy for high-risk resected non-small-cell lung carcinoma. *J Clin Oncol* 2001;19:3912–3917.

[9] Wozniak AJ, Gadgeel SM. Adjuvant therapy for resected non-small cell lung cancer. *Ther Adv Med Oncol.* 2009 Sep;1(2):109-18.

[10] Keller, S.M., Adak, S., et al. A randomized trial of postoperative adjuvant therapy in patients with completely resected stage II or III non-small cell lung cancer. *N Engl J Med* 2000; 343: 1217-1222

[11] Scagliotti, G.V., Fossati, R., et al. Randomized study of adjuvant chemotherapy for completely resected stage I, II or IIIA non-small cell lung cancer. *J Natl Cancer Inst* 2003; 95: 1453-1461.

[12] Waller D, Peake M.D, et al. Chemotherapy for patients with non-small cell lung cancer. The surgical setting of the Big Lung Trial. *Eur J Cardio Thorac Surg* 2004; 26: 173-182.
[13] The International Adjuvant Lung Cancer Trial Collaborative Group. Cisplatin-based adjuvant chemotherapy in patients with completely resected non-small-cell lung cancer. *N Engl J Med* 2004; 350: 351-360.
[14] Douillard JY, Rosell R, et al. Adjuvant vinorelbine plus cisplatin versus observation in patients with completely resected stage IB-IIIA nonsmall- cell lung cancer (Adjuvant Navelbine International Trialist Association [ANITA]): a randomized controlled trial. *Lancet Oncol* 2006;7: 719-727.
[15] Ardizzoni A, Boni L, et al. Cisplatin versus carboplatin-based chemotherapy in first-line treatment of advanced non-small-cell lung cancer: An individual patient data meta-analysis. *J Natl Caner Inst* 2007; 99: 847-857.
[16] Le Péchoux C, Dunant A, Pignon JP, et al. Need for a new trial to evaluate adjuvant postoperative radiotherapy in non-small-cell lung cancer patients with N2 mediastinal involvement. *J Clin Oncol* 2007; 25:e10.
[17] Martini N, Kris M, Flehinger BJ, et al. Preoperative chemotherapy for stage IIIa (N2) lung cancer: the Sloan-Kettering experience with 136 patients. *Ann Thorac Surg* 1993;55:1365–73.
[18] Burkes RL, Ginsberg RJ, Sheperd FA, et al. Induction chemotherapy with mitomycin, vindesine, and cisplatin for Stage III unresectable non-small cell lung cancer; results of the Toronto phase II trial. *J Clin Oncol* 1992;10:580–6.
[19] Ginsberg RJ. Neoadjuvant (induction) treatment for non-small cell lung cancer. *Lung Cancer* 1995;12:S33–40
[20] Roth JA, Fosella F, Komaki R, et al. A randomized trial comparing perioperative chemotherapy and surgery with surgery alone in resectable Stage IIIA nonsmall cell lung cancer. *J Natl Cancer Inst* 1994;86:673–80.
[21] Rosell R, Gomez-Codina J, Camps C, et al. A randomized trial comparing preoperative chemotherapy plus surgery with surgery alone in patients with non-small cell lung cancer. *N Engl J Med* 1994;330:153–8.
[22] Sugarbaker DJ, Herndon J, Kohman LJ, et al. Cancer and Leukemia Group B Thoracic Surgery Group. Results of cancer and leukemia group B protocol 8935A mutiinstitutional phase II trimodality trial for Stage IIIa (N2) non-smallcell lung cancer. *J Thorac Cardiovasc Surg* 1995;109:473–85.
[23] Albain KS, Rusch VW, Crowley JJ, et al. Concurrent cisplatin/etoposide plus chest radiotherapy followed by surgery for Stages IIIA (N2) and IIIB non-smallcell lung cancer: mature results of Southwest Oncology Group phase II study 8805. *J Clin Oncol* 1995;13:1880–92.
[24] Rusch VW, Giroux DJ, Kraut MJ, et al. Induction chemoradiation and surgical resection for non-small cell lung carcinomas of the superior sulcus: initial results of Southwest Oncology Group Trial 9416 (Intergroup trial 0160). *J Thorac Cardiovasc Surg* 2001;121:472–83.
[25] Rusch VW, Giroux DJ, Kraut MJ, et al. Induction chemoradiation and surgical resection for superior sulcus non-small cell lung carcinomas: long-term results of Southwest Oncology Group Trial 9416 (Intergroup trial 0160). *J Clin Oncol* 2007;25:313–8.

[26] Albain KS, Swann RS, Rusch VW, et al. Radiotherapy plus chemotherapy with or without surgical resection for stage III non-small-cell lung cancer: a phase III randomised controlled trial. *Lancet* 2009; 374:379.
[27] Thomas M, Macha HN, Ukena D, et al. Cisplatin/etoposide (PE) followed by twice-daily chemoradiation (hfRT/CT) versus PE alone before surgery in stage III non-small cell lung cancer (NSCLC): a randomized phase III trial of the German Lung Cancer Cooperative Group (GLCCG). *J Clin Oncol* 2004;22:14S.
[28] Strauss GM, Herndon JE, Sherman DD, et al. Neoadjuvant chemotherapy and radiotherapy followed by surgery in stage IIIA non-small-cell carcinoma of the lung: report of a Cancer and Leukemia Group B phase II study. *J Clin Oncol* 1992;10:1237–44.
[29] Cerfolio RJ, Bryant AS, Spencer SA, et al. Pulmonary resection after high-dose and low-dose chest irradiation. *Ann Thorac Surg* 2005;80:1224–30.
[30] van Meerbeeck JP, Kramer GW, Van Schil PE, et al. Randomized controlled trial of resection versus radiotherapy after induction chemotherapy in stage IIIA-N2 non-small-cell lung cancer. *J Natl Cancer Inst* 2007; 99:442.
[31] Daly BD, Cerfolio RJ, Krasna MJ. Role of surgery following induction therapy for stage III non-small cell lung cancer. *Surg Oncol Clin N Am.* 2011; 20(4):721-32.
[32] Adelstein DJ, Rice TW, Rybicki LA, et al. Long-term follow-up after chemoradiotherapy (CRT) in patients (pts) with stage III non-small cell lung cancer (NSCLC): is bulky mediastinal nodal disease of prognostic importance? [abstract]. *J Clin Oncol* 2004;22:14S.
[33] Stamatis G, Eberhardt W, Stuben G, et al. Preoperative chemoradiotherapy and surgery for selected non-small cell lung cancer IIIB subgroups: long-term results. *Ann Thorac Surg* 1999;68:1144–9.
[34] Allen AM, Mentzer SJ, Yeap BY, et al. Pneumonectomy after chemoradiation: the Dana-Farber cancer Institute/Brigham and Women's Hospital Experience. *Cancer* 2008;112:1106–13.
[35] Weder W, Colland S, Eberhardt WE, et al. Pneumonectomy is a valuable treatment option after neoadjuvant therapy for stage III non-small-cell lung cancer. *J Thorac Cardiovasc Surg* 2010;139:1424–30.
[36] Barnett SA, Rusch VW, Zheng J, et al. Contemporary results of surgical resection of non-small cell lung cancer after induction therapy: a review of 549 consecutive cases. *J Thorac Oncol* 2011; 6:1530.
[37] Soresi E, Clerici M, Grilli R, Borghini R, Zucali R, Leoni M, et al. A randomized clinical trial comparing radiation therapy vs radiation therapy plus cis-dichlorodiammine platinum (II) in the treatment of locally advanced non-small cell lung cancer. *Semin Oncol* 1988; 15: 20-5.
[38] Chemotherapy in non-small cell lung cancer: a meta-analysis using updated data on individual patients from 52 randomised clinical trials. Non-small Cell Lung Cancer Collborative Group. *BMJ* 1995;311:899-909.
[39] Diillman RO, Herndon J, Seagren SL, et al. Improved survival in stage III non –small-cell lung cancer: seven-year follow-up of cancer and leucemia Group B (CALGB) 8433 trial. *J Natl cancer Inst* 1996;88:1210-5.
[40] Sause W, Kolesar P, Taylor S, et al. Final results of phase III trial in regionally advanced unresectable non-small cell lung cancer: Radiation Therapy Oncology Group,

Eastern Cooperative Oncology Group, And Southwest Oncology Group. *Chest* 2000;117:358-64.
[41] Le Chevaliar T, Arriagada R, Quoix E, et al. Radiotherapy alone versus combined chemotherapy and radiotherapy in nonresectable non-small-cell lung cancer: first analysis of a randomised trial in 353 patients. *J Natl cancer Inst* 1991;83:417-23.
[42] Okawara G, Mackay JA, Evans WK, et al. Management of unresected stage III non-small cell lung cancer: a systematic review. *J Thorac Oncol* 2006; 1:377.
[43] Jeremic B, Shibamoto T, Acimovic L, et al. Hyperfractionated radiation therapy with or without concurrent low-dose daily carboplatin/etoposide for stage III non-small-cell lung cancer: a randomized study. *J Clin Oncol* 1996;14:1065-70.
[44] Curran WJ Jr, Paulus R, Langer CJ, et al. Sequential vs. concurrent chemoradiation for stage III non-small cell lung cancer: randomized phase III trial RTOG 9410. *J Natl Cancer Inst* 2011; 103:1452.
[45] Furuse K, Fukuoka M, Kawahara M, et al. Phase III study of concurrent versus sequential thoracic radiotherapy in combination with mitomycin, vindesine, and cisplatin in unresectable stage III non-small-cell lung cancer. *J Clin Oncol* 1999; 17:2692.
[46] Zatloukal P, Petruzelka L, Zemanova M, et al. Concurrent versus sequential chemoradiotherapy with cisplatin and vinorelbine in locally advanced non-small cell lung cancer: a randomized study. *Lung Cancer* 2004;46:87-98.
[47] Fournel P, Robinet G, Thomas P, et al. Randomized phase III trial of sequential chemoradiotherapy compared with concurrent chemoradiotherapy in locally advanced non small- cell lung cancer: Groupe Lyon-Saint-Etienne d`Oncologie Thoracique Groupe Fancais de Pneumo-Cancérologic NPC 95-01 Study. *J Clin Oncol* 2005;23:5910-7.
[48] El-Sharouni SY, Kal HB, Battermann JJ, et al. Sequential versus concurrent chemoradiotherapy in inoperable stage III non-small cell lung cancer. Anticancer Res 2006;26:495-505.
[49] Aupérin A, Le Péchouw C, Pignon JP, et al. Concomitant radio-chemotherapy based on platin compounds in patients with locally advanced non-small cell lung cancer (NSCLC): a meta-analysis of individual data from 1764 patient. *Ann Oncol* 2006;17:473-83.
[50] Aupérin A, Le Péchouw C, Rolland E, et al. Meta-analysis of concomitant versus sequential radiochemotherapy in locally advanced non-small-cell lung cancer. *J Clin Oncol* 2010;28:2181-90.
[51] Phernambucq EC, Spoelstra FO, Verbakel WF, et al. Outcomes of concurrent chemoradiotherapy in patients with stage III non-small-cell lung cancer and significant comorbidity. *Ann Oncol* 2011;22:132-8.
[52] Vokes EE, Herndon JE, Kelley MJ et al. Induction chemotherapy followed by chemoradiotherapy compared with chemoradiotherapy alone for regionally advanced unresectable stage III Non-small-cell lung cancer: Cancer and Leukemia Group B. *J Clin Oncol* 2005;25:1698-704.
[53] Belani CP, Choy H, Bonomi P, et al. Combined chemoradiotherapy regimens of paclitaxel and carboplatin for locally advanced non-small-cell lung cancer: a randomized phase II locally advanced multi-modality protocol. *J Clin Oncol* 2005;23:5883-91.

[54] Mok TS, Wu YL, Thongprasert S, et al. Gefitinib or carboplatin-paclitaxel in pulmonary adenocarcinoma. *N Engl J Med* 2009; 361:947-957.

[55] Rosell R, Carcereny E, Gervais R, et al. Erlotinib versus standard chemotherapy as first-line treatment for European patients with advanced EGFR mutation-positive non-small-cell lung cancer (EURTAC): a multicentre, open-label, randomised phase 3 trial. *Lancet Oncol* 2012; 13:239-246.

[56] Kwak EL, Bang YJ, Camidge DR, et al. Anaplastic lymphoma kinase inhibition in non-small-cell lung cancer. *N Engl J Med* 2010; 363:1693-1703.

[57] Spiro SG, Rudd RM, Souhami RL, et al. Chemotherapy versus supportive care in advanced non-small cell lung cancer: improved survival without detriment to quality of life. *Thorax* 2004; 59:828-836.

[58] Chemotherapy in non-small cell lung cancer: a meta-analysis using updated data on individual patients from 52 randomised clinical trials. Non-small Cell Lung Cancer Collaborative Group. *BMJ* 1995; 311:899-909.

[59] Schiller JH, Harrington D, Belani CP, et al. Comparison of four chemotherapy regimens for advanced non-small-cell lung cancer. *N Engl J Med* 2002; 346:92-98.

[60] Scagliotti GV, De Marinis F, Rinaldi M, et al. Phase III randomized trial comparing three platinum-based doublets in advanced non-small-cell lung cancer. *J Clin Oncol* 2002; 20:4285-4291.

[61] Paccagnella A, Oniga F, Bearz A, et al. Adding gemcitabine to paclitaxel/carboplatin combination increases survival in advanced non-small-cell lung cancer: results of a phase II-III study. *J Clin Oncol* 2006; 24:681-687.

[62] Comella P, Filippelli G, De Cataldis G, et al. Efficacy of the combination of cisplatin with either gemcitabine and vinorelbine or gemcitabine and paclitaxel in the treatment of locally advanced or metastatic non-small-cell lung cancer: a phase III randomised trial of the Southern Italy Cooperative Oncology Group (SICOG 0101). *Ann Oncol* 2007; 18:324-330.

[63] Jiang J, Liang X, Zhou X, Huang R, Chu Z. A meta-analysis of randomized controlled trials comparing carboplatin-based to cisplatin-based chemotherapy in advanced non-small cell lung cancer. *Lung Cancer* 2007; 57:348-358.

[64] Azzoli GC, Kris MG, Pfister DG. Cisplatin versus carboplatin for patients with metastatic non-small cell lung cancer- an old rivalry renewed. *J Natl Cancer Inst* 2007; 99: 828-829.

[65] Ardizzoni A, Boni L, Tiseo M, et al. For the CISCA (CISplatin versus CArboplastin) Meta-analysis Group. Cisplatin-versus carboplatin-based chemotherapy in first-line treatment of advanced non-small cell lung cancer: an individual patient data metaanalysis. *J Natl Cancer Inst* 2007; 99: 847-857.

[66] Georgoulias V. Vinorelbine plus cisplatin versus docetaxel plus gemcitabine in advanced non-small cell lung cancer: a phase II randomized trial. *J Clin Oncol* 2005; 23: 2937-2945.

[67] D´Addario, Pintilie M, Leighl NB, Feld R, Cerny T, Shepherd FA. Platinum-based versus non-platinum based chemotherapy in advanced non-small cell lung cancer. *J Clin Oncol* 2005; 23:29-26-2936.

[68] Rajeswaran A, Trojan A, Burnand B, Giannelli M. Efficacy and side effects of cisplatin- and carboplatin-based doublet chemotherapeutic regimens versus non-platinum-based doublet chemotherapeutic regimens as first line treatment of metastatic

non-small cell lung carcinoma: a systematic review of randomized controlled trials. *Lung Cancer* 2008; 59:1-11.
[69] Scagliotti GV, Parikh P, von Pawel J, et al. Phase III study comparing cisplatin plus gemcitabine with cisplatin plus pemetrexed in chemotherapy-naive patients with advanced-stage non-small-cell lung cancer. *J Clin Oncol* 2008; 26:3543-3551.
[70] Johnson DH, Fehrenbacher L, Novotny WF, et al. Randomized phase II trial comparing bevacizumab plus carboplatin and paclitaxel with carboplatin and paclitaxel alone in previously untreated locally advanced or metastatic NSCLC. *J Clin Oncol* 2004; 22: 21-84-2191.
[71] Sandler A, Gray R, Perry MC, et al. Paclitaxel-carboplatin alone or with bevacizumab for non-small-cell lung cancer. *N Engl J Med* 2006; 355:2542-2550.
[72] Reck M, von Pawel J, Zatloukal P, et al. Phase III trial of cisplatin plus gemcitabine with either placebo or bevacizumab as first-line therapy for nonsquamous non-small-cell lung cancer: AVAiL. *J Clin Oncol* 2009; 27:1227-1234.
[73] Sandler AB, Schiller JH, Gray R, et al. Retrospective evaluation of the clinical and radiographic risk factors associated with severe pulmonary hemorrhage in first-line advanced, unresectable non-small-cell lung cancer treated with Carboplatin and Paclitaxel plus bevacizumab. *J Clin Oncol* 2009; 27:1405-1412.
[74] Dahlberg SE, Sandler AB, Brahmer JR, et al. Clinical course of advanced non-small-cell lung cancer patients experiencing hypertension during treatment with bevacizumab in combination with carboplatin and paclitaxel on ECOG 4599. *J Clin Oncol* 2010; 28:949-954.
[75] Sandler A, Yo J, Dahlbers S, et al. Treatment outcomes by tumor histology in Eastern Cooperative Group Study E4599 of bevacizumab with paclitaxel/carboplatin for advanced non-small cell lung cancer. *J Thorac Oncol* 2010; 5: 1416-1423.
[76] Ramalingam SS, Dahlberg SE, Langer CJ, et al. Outcomes for elderly, advanced-stage non small-cell lung cancer patients treated with bevacizumab in combination with carboplatin and paclitaxel: analysis of Eastern Cooperative Oncology Group Trial 4599. *J Clin Oncol* 2008; 26:60-65.
[77] Reck M, von Pawel J, Zatloukal P, et al. Overall survival with cisplatin-gemcitabine and bevacizumab or placebo as first-line therapy for nonsquamous non-small-cell lung cancer: results from a randomised phase III trial (AVAiL). *Ann Oncol* 2010; 21:1804-1809.
[78] Patel JD, Hensing TA, Rademaker A, et al. Phase II study of pemetrexed and carboplatin plus bevacizumab with maintenance pemetrexed and bevacizumab as first-line therapy for nonsquamous non-small-cell lung cancer. *J Clin Oncol* 2009; 27:3284-3289.
[79] Patel JD, Bonomi P, Socinski MA, et al. Treatment rationale and study design for the pointbreak study: a randomized, open-label phase III study of pemetrexed/carboplatin/bevacizumab followed by maintenance pemetrexed/bevacizumab versus paclitaxel/carboplatin/bevacizumab followed by maintenance bevacizumab in patients with stage IIIB or IV nonsquamous non-small-cell lung cancer. *Clin Lung Cancer* 2009; 10:252-256.
[80] Crinò L, Dansin E, Garrido P, et al. Safety and efficacy of first-line bevacizumab-based therapy in advanced non-squamous non-small-cell lung cancer (SAiL, MO19390): a phase 4 study. *Lancet Oncol* 2010; 11:733-740.

[81] Wozniak AJ, Garst J, Jahanzeb M, et al. Clinical outcomes (CO) for special populations of patients (pts) with advanced non-small cell lung cancer (NSCLC): Results from ARIES, a bevacizumab (BV) observational cohort study (OCS). *J Clin Oncol* 2010; 28:15s (Abstr 7618).

[82] Pirker R, Filipits M. Monoclonal antibodies against EGFR in non-small cell lung cancer. *Crit Rev Oncol Hematol* 2011;80:1-9.

[83] Pirker R, Pereira JR, Szczesna A, et al. Cetuximab plus chemotherapy in patients with advanced non-small-cell lung cancer (FLEX): an open-label randomised phase III trial. *Lancet* 2009;373:1525-31.

[84] Lynch TJ, Patel T, Dreisbach L, et al. Cetuximab and first-line taxane/ carboplatin chemotherapy in advanced non-small-cell lung cancer: results of the randomized multicenter phase III trial BMS099. *J Clin Oncol* 2010;28:911-7.

[85] Rosell R, Robinet G, Szczesna A, et al. Randomized phase II study of cetuximab plus cisplatin/vinorelbine compared with cisplatin/vinorelbine alone as first-line therapy in EGFR-expressing advanced non-small-cell lung cancer. *Ann Oncol* 2008;19:362-9.

[86] Butts CA, Bodkin D, Middleman EL, et al. Randomized phase II study of gemcitabine plus cisplatin or carboplatin [corrected], with or without cetuximab, as first-line therapy for patients with advanced or metastatic non-small-cell lung cancer. *J Clin Oncol* 2007;25:5777-84.

[87] Thatcher N, Linchy TJ. Cetuximab plus platinum-based chemotherapy as 1st-line treatment in patients with non-small cell lung cancer (NSCLC): A meta-analysis of randomized phase II/III trials. *WCLC* 2009 (Abstr A3.7).

[88] Gatzemeier U, von Pawel J, Vynnychenko I, et al. First-cycle rash and survival in patients with advanced non-small-cell lung cancer receiving cetuximab in combination with first-line chemotherapy: a subgroup analysis of data from the FLEX phase 3 study. *Lancet Oncol* 2011;12:30-7.

[89] Hirsch FR, Herbst RS, Olsen C, et al. Increased EGFR gene copy number detected by fluorescent in situ hybridization predicts outcome in non-small-cell lung cancer patients treated with cetuximab and chemotherapy. *J Clin Oncol* 2008; 26:3351-3357.

[90] Khambata-Ford S, Harbison CT, Hart LL, et al. Analysis of potential predictive markers of cetuximab benefit in BMS099, a phase III study of cetuximab and first-line taxane/carboplatin in advanced non-small-cell lung cancer. *J Clin Oncol* 2010; 28:918-927.

[91] O'Byrne KJ, Bondarenko I, Barrios C, et al. Molecular and clinical predictors of outcome for cetuximab in non-small cell lung cancer (NSCLC): Data from the FLEX study. *J Clin Oncol* 2009; 27:408s (Abstr 8007)

[92] Pirker R, Pereira JR, von Pawel J, et al. EGFR expression as a predictor of survival for first-line chemotherapy plus cetuximab in patients with advanced non-small-cell lung cancer: analysis of data from the phase 3 FLEX study. *Lancet Oncol* 2012; 13:33.

[93] Fidias PM, Dakhil SR, Lyss AP, et al. Phase III study of immediate compared with delayed docetaxel after front-line therapy with gemcitabine plus carboplatin in advanced non-small-cell lung cancer. *J Clin Oncol* 2009; 27:591-598.

[94] Ciuleanu T, Brodowicz T, Zielinski C, et al. Maintenance pemetrexed plus best supportive care versus placebo plus best supportive care for non-small-cell lung cancer: a randomised, double-blind, phase 3 study. *Lancet* 2009; 374:1432-1434.

[95] Smith IE, O'Brien ME, Talbot DC, et al. Duration of chemotherapy in advanced non-small cell lung cancer: a randomized trial of three versus six courses of mitomycin, vinblastine and cisplatin. *J Clin Oncol* 2001,19: 1336-1343.
[96] Park JO, Kim SW, Ahn JS,et al. Phase III trial of two versus four additional cycles in patients who are nonprogressive after two cycles of platinum-based chemotherapy in non-small cell lung cancer. *J Clin Oncol* 2007, 25:5233-5239.
[97] Pfister DG, Johnson DH, Azzoli CG, et al. American Society of clinical Oncology treatment of unresectable non-small cell lung cancer guideline. Update 2003. *J Clin Oncol* 2004; 22: 330-353.
[98] Azzoli CG, Baker S, Termin S, et al. American Society of clinical Oncology practice guideline update on chemotherapy for stage IV Non-small cell lung cancer. *J Clin Oncol* 2009; 36: 6251-6266.
[99] Perol M, Chouaid C, Milleron BJ, et al. Maintenance with either gemcitabine or erlotinib versus observation with predefined second-line treatment after cisplatin-gemcitabine induction chemotherapy in advanced NSCLC: IFCT-GFPC 0502 phase III study. *J Clin Oncol* 2010; 28:540s (Abstr 7507).
[100] Paz-Ares L, de Marinis F, Dediu M, et al. Maintenance therapy with pemetrexed plus best supportive care versus placebo plus best supportive care after induction therapy with pemetrexed plus cisplatin for advanced non-squamous non-small-cell lung cancer (PARAMOUNT): a double-blind, phase 3 randomised controlled trial. *Lancet Oncol* 2012; 13: 247-255.
[101] Barlesi F, de Castro J, Dvornichenko, V, et al. AVAPERL (MO22089): Final efficacy outcomes for patients with advanced nonsquamous non-small cell lung cancer randomized to continuation maintenance with bevacizumab or bevacizumab + pemetrexed after first-line bevacizumab-cisplatin + pemetrexed. *European Multidisciplinary Cancer Congress*, September, 2011.
[102] Goldie JH, Coldman AJ. A mathematic model for relating the drug sensitivity of tumours to their spontaneous mutation rate. Cancer Treat Rep 1979, 63:1727-17233.
[103] Cappuzzo F, Ciuleanu T, Stelmakh L, et al. Erlotinib as maintenance treatment in advanced non-small-cell lung cancer: a multicentre, randomised, placebo-controlled phase 3 study. *Lancet Oncol* 2010; 11:521-529.
[104] Gaafar RM, Surmont V, Scagliotti G, et al. A double-blind, randomized, placebo-controlled phase III intergroup study of gefitinib (G) in patients (pts) with advanced NSCLC, non-progressing after first-line platinum-based chemotherapy (EORTC 08021-ILCP 01/03). *J Clin Oncol* 2010; 28:15s (Abstr 7518).
[105] Miller V, O'Connor P, Soh C, et al. A randomized, double-blind, placebo-controlled, phase IIIb trial (ATLAS) comparing bevacizumab (B) therapy with or without erlotinib (E) after completion of chemotherapy with B for first-line treatment of locally advanced, recurrent, or metastatic non-small cell lung cancer (NSCLC). *J Clin Oncol* 2009; 27:799s (Abstr #LBA8002).
[106] Takeda K, Hida T, Sato T, et al. Randomized phase III trial of platinum-doublet chemotherapy followed by gefitinib compared with continued platinum-doublet chemotherapy in Japanese patients with advanced non-small-cell lung cancer: results of a west Japan thoracic oncology group trial (WJTOG0203). *J Clin Oncol* 2010; 28:753.
[107] Shepherd FA, Rodrigues Pereira J, Ciuleanu T, et al. Erlotinib in previously treated non-small-cell lung cancer. *N Engl J Med* 2005; 353:123-132.

[108] Thatcher N, Chang A, Parikh P, et al. Gefitinib plus best supportive care in previously treated patients with refractory advanced non-small-cell lung cancer: results from a randomised, placebo-controlled, multicentre study (Iressa Survival Evaluation in Lung Cancer). *Lancet* 2005; 366:1527-1537.

[109] Keedy VL, Temin S, Somerfield MR, et al. American Society of Clinical Oncology provisional clinical opinion: epidermal growth factor receptor (EGFR) Mutation testing for patients with advanced non-small-cell lung cancer considering first-line EGFR tyrosine kinase inhibitor therapy. *J Clin Oncol* 2011; 29:2121-2127.

[110] Mitsudomi T, Morita S, Yatabe Y, et al. Gefitinib versus cisplatin plus docetaxel in patients with non-small-cell lung cancer harbouring mutations of the epidermal growth factor receptor (WJTOG3405): an open label, randomised phase 3 trial. *Lancet Oncol* 2010; 11:121-128.

[111] Maemondo M, Inoue A, Kobayashi K, et al. Gefitinib or chemotherapy for non-small-cell lung cancer with mutated EGFR. *N Engl J Med* 2010; 362:2380-2388.

[112] Zhou C, Wu YL, Chen G, et al. Erlotinib versus chemotherapy as first-line treatment for patients with advanced EGFR mutation-positive non-small-cell lung cancer (OPTIMAL, CTONG-0802): a multicentre, open-label, randomised, phase 3 study. *Lancet Oncol* 2011; 12:735-742.

[113] Gridelli C, Ciardiello R, Feld R, et al. International multicenter randomized phase III study of first-line erlotinib (E) followed by second-line cisplatin plus gemcitabine (CG) versus first-line CG followed by second-line E in advanced non-small cell lung cancer (aNSCLC): The TORCH trial. *J Clin Oncol* 2010; 28:540s (Abst 7508).

[114] Herbst RS, Prager D, Hermann R, et al. TRIBUTE: a phase III trial of erlotinib hydrochloride (OSI-774) combined with carboplatin and paclitaxel chemotherapy in advanced non-small-cell lung cancer. *J Clin Oncol* 2005; 23:5892-5889.

[115] Gatzemeier U, Pluzanska A, Szczesna A, et al. Phase III study of erlotinib in combination with cisplatin and gemcitabine in advanced non-small-cell lung cancer: the Tarceva Lung Cancer Investigation *Trial. J Clin Oncol* 2007; 25:1545-1552.

[116] Giaccone G, Herbst RS, Manegold C, et al. Gefitinib in combination with gemcitabine and cisplatin in advanced non-small-cell lung cancer: a phase III trial--INTACT 1. *J Clin Oncol* 2004; 22:777-784.

[117] Herbst RS, Giaccone G, Schiller JH, et al. Gefitinib in combination with paclitaxel and carboplatin in advanced non-small-cell lung cancer: a phase III trial--INTACT 2. *J Clin Oncol* 2004; 22:785-774.

[118] Pao W, Miller V, Zakowski M, et al. EGF receptor gene mutations are common in lung cancers from "never smokers" and are associated with sensitivity of tumors to gefitinib and erlotinib. *Proc Natl Acad Sci U S A* 2004; 101:13306-11.

[119] Lynch TJ, Bell DW, Sordella R, et al. Activating mutations in the epidermal growth factor receptor underlying responsiveness of non-small-cell lung cancer to gefitinib. *N Engl J Med* 2004; 350:2129-2139.

[120] Rosell R, Moran T, Queralt C, et al. Screening for epidermal growth factor receptor mutations in lung cancer. *N Engl J Med* 2009; 361:958-967.

[121] D'Angelo SP, Pietanza MC, Johnson ML, et al. Incidence of EGFR exon 19 deletions and L858R in tumor specimens from men and cigarette smokers with lung adenocarcinomas. *J Clin Oncol* 2011; 29: 2066-2070.

[122] Linardou H, Dahabreh IJ, Kanaloupiti D, et al. Assessment of somatic k-RAS mutations as a mechanism associated with resistance to EGFR-targeted agents: a systematic review and meta-analysis of studies in advanced non-small-cell lung cancer and metastatic colorectal cancer. *Lancet Oncol* 2008; 9:962-972.

[123] Schneider CP, Heigener D, Schott-von-Römer K, et al. Epidermal growth factor receptor-related tumor markers and clinical outcomes with erlotinib in non-small cell lung cancer: an analysis of patients from german centers in the TRUST study. *J Thorac Oncol* 2008; 3:1446-1453.

[124] Shaw AT, Solomon B. Targeting anaplastic lymphoma kinase in lung cancer. *Clin Cancer Res* 2011; 17:2081-2086.

[125] Soda M, Choi YL, Enomoto M, et al. Identification of the transforming EML4-ALK fusion gene in non-small-cell lung cancer. *Nature* 2007; 448:561-566.

[126] Choi YL, Takeuchi K, Soda M, et al. Identification of novel isoforms of the EML4-ALK transforming gene in non-small cell lung cancer. *Cancer Res* 2008; 68:4971-4976.

[127] Soda M, Takada S, Takeuchi K, et al. A mouse model for EML4-ALK-positive lung cancer. *Proc Natl Acad Sci U S A* 2008; 105:19893-7.

[128] Takeuchi K, Choi YL, Togashi Y, et al. KIF5B-ALK, a novel fusion oncokinase identified by an immunohistochemistry-based diagnostic system for ALK-positive lung cancer. *Clin Cancer Res* 2009; 15:3143-3149.

[129] Wong DW, Leung EL, So KK, et al. The EML4-ALK fusion gene is involved in various histologic types of lung cancers from nonsmokers with wild-type EGFR and KRAS. *Cancer* 2009; 115:1723-1733.

[130] Shaw AT, Yeap BY, Mino-Kenudson M, et al. Clinical features and outcome of patients with non-small-cell lung cancer who harbor EML4-ALK. *J Clin Oncol* 2009; 27:4247-4253.

[131] Roding SJ, Mino-Kenudson M, Dacic S, et al. Unique clinicopathological features characterize ALK-rearranged lung adenocarcinoma in the western population. *Clin Cancer Res* 2009; 15:5216-5223.

[132] Wong DW, Leung EL, So KK, et al. The EML4-ALK fusion gene is involved in various histologic types of lung cancers from nonsmokers with wild-type EGFR and KRAS. *Cancer* 2009; 115:1723-1733.

[133] Boland JM, Erdogan S, Vasmatzis G, et al. Anaplastic lymphoma kinase immunoreactivity correlates with ALK gene rearrangement and transcriptional up-regulation in non-small cell lung carcinomas. *Hum Pathol* 2009; 40:1152-1158.

[134] Christensen JG, Zou HY, Arango ME, et al. Cytoreductive antitumor activity of PF-2341066, a novel inhibitor of anaplastic lymphoma kinase and c-Met, in experimental models of anaplastic large-cell lymphoma. *Mol Cancer Ther* 2007; 6:3314-3322.

[135] Shepherd FA, Dancey J, Ramlau R, et al. Prospective randomized trial of docetaxel versus best supportive care in patients with non-small-cell lung cancer previously treated with platinum-based chemotherapy. *J Clin Oncol* 2000; 18:2095-2103.

[136] Hanna N, Shepherd FA, Fossella FV, et al. Randomized phase III trial of pemetrexed versus docetaxel in patients with non-small-cell lung cancer previously treated with chemotherapy. *J Clin Oncol* 2004; 22:1589-1597.

[137] Dancey J, Shepherd FA, Gralla RJ, Kim YS. Quality of life assessment of second-line docetaxel versus best supportive care in patients with non-small-cell lung cancer

previously treated with platinum-based chemotherapy: results of a prospective, randomized phase III trial. *Lung Cancer* 2004; 43:183-194.

[138] Fossella FV, DeVore R, Kerr RN, et al. Randomized phase III trial of docetaxel versus vinorelbine or ifosfamide in patients with advanced non-small-cell lung cancer previously treated with platinum-containing chemotherapy regimens. The TAX 320 Non-Small Cell Lung Cancer Study Group. *J Clin Oncol* 2000; 18:2354-2362.

[139] Pujol JL, Paul S, Chouaki N, et al. Survival without common toxicity criteria grade 3/4 toxicity for pemetrexed compared with docetaxel in previously treated patients with advanced non-small cell lung cancer (NSCLC): a risk-benefit analysis. *J Thorac Oncol* 2007; 2:397-401.

[140] Scagliotti G, Hanna N, Fossella F, et al. The differential efficacy of pemetrexed according to NSCLC histology: a review of two Phase III studies. *Oncologist* 2009; 14:253-263.

[141] Douillard JY, Shepherd FA, Hirsh V, et al. Molecular predictors of outcome with gefitinib and docetaxel in previously treated non-small-cell lung cancer: data from the randomized phase III INTEREST trial. *J Clin Oncol* 2010; 28:744-752.

[142] Maruyama R, Nishiwaki Y, Tamura T, et al. Phase III study, V-15-32, of gefitinib versus docetaxel in previously treated Japanese patients with non-small-cell lung cancer. *J Clin Oncol* 2008; 26:4244-4252.

[143] Wheatley-Price P, Ding K, Seymour L, et al. Erlotinib for advanced non-small-cell lung cancer in the elderly: an analysis of the National Cancer Institute of Canada Clinical Trials Group Study BR.21. *J Clin Oncol* 2008; 26:2350-2357.

[144] Bezjak A, Tu D, Seymour L, et al. Symptom improvement in lung cancer patients treated with erlotinib: quality of life analysis of the National Cancer Institute of Canada Clinical Trials Group Study BR.21. *J Clin Oncol* 2006; 24:3831-3837.

[145] Ciuleanu T, Stelmakh L, Cicenas S, et al. Efficacy and safety of erlotinib versus chemotherapy in second-line treatment of patients with advanced, non-small-cell lung cancer with poor prognosis (TITAN): a randomised multicentre, open-label, phase 3 study. *Lancet Oncol* 2012; 13:300-308.

[146] Herbst RS, O'Neill VJ, Fehrenbacher L, et al. Phase II study of efficacy and safety of bevacizumab in combination with chemotherapy or erlotinib compared with chemotherapy alone for treatment of recurrent or refractory non-small-cell lung cancer. *J Clin Oncol* 2007; 25:4743-4750.

[147] Herbst RS, Ansari R, Bustin F, et al. Efficacy of bevacizumab plus erlotinib versus erlotinib alone in advanced non-small-cell lung cancer after failure of standard first-line chemotherapy (BeTa): a double-blind, placebo-controlled, phase 3 trial. *Lancet* 2011; 377:1846-1854.

[148] Pepe C, Hasan B, Winton TL, et al Adjuvant vinorelbine and cisplatin in elderly patients: National Cancer Institute of Canada and Intergroup Study JBR.10. *J Clin ONcol* 2007;25(12):1553.61

[149] Strauss GM, Herndon JE, Maddaus MA, et al. Adjuvant paclitaxel plus carboplatin compared with observation in stage IB non-small-cell lung cancer: CALGB 9633 with the Cancer and Leukemia Group B, Radiation Therapy Oncology Group, and North Central Cancer Treatment Group Study Groups. *J Clin Oncol* 2008; 26(31):5043-51

[150] Mathisen DJ, Wain JC, Wright C, et al. Assessment of preoperative accelerated radiotherapy and chemotherapy in stage IIIA (N2) non-small-cell lung cancer. *J Thorac Cardiovasc Surg* 1996;111:123–33

[151] Bueno R, Richards WC, Swanson SJ, et al. Nodal stage after induction therapy for stage IIIA lung cancer determines patient survival. *Ann Thorac Surg* 2000;70: 1826–31.

[152] Rice TW, Adelstein DJ, Ciezki JP, et al. Short-course induction chemoradiotherapy with paclitaxel for stage III non-small-cell lung cancer. *Ann Thorac Surg* 1998;66:1909–14.

[153] Granetzny A, Striehn E, Bosse U, et al. A phase II single-institution study of neoadjuvant stage IIIA/B chemotherapy and radiochemotherapy in non-small cell lung cancer. *Ann Thorac Surg* 2003;75:1107–12.

In: Lung Cancer: A Comprehensive Overview
Editor: Kathy Gately
ISBN: 978-1-62618-447-3


*Chapter VI*

# Management of Stage III N2 NSCLC

***Mark J. Krasna****
Meridian Cancer Care, Neptune, NJ, US

## Abstract

Stage III non-small cell lung cancer (NSCLC) represents approximately 30 to 40% of all newly diagnosed NSCLC patients. This heterogeneous group of patients requires careful preoperative assessment to determine the best management strategy. Stage IIIA and IIIB each contain very heterogeneous groups of patients. Very careful clinical evaluation is required in determining the best treatment strategy, starting with invasive mediastinal staging to accurately identify patients with N2 or N3 disease. When N2 disease is identified preoperatively, patients should be treated with either induction chemotherapy or chemoradiation, followed by surgery. For patients with resectable T4 disease, N0-N1 status, chemoradiation followed by resection in good risk candidates may be recommended. Stage IIIB patients by virtue of N3 status are unlikely to experience significant benefit from surgery and should generally be offered definitive chemoradiation.

## Introduction

Stage III non-small cell lung cancer (NSCLC) represents approximately 30 to 40% of all newly diagnosed NSCLC patients. It is a heterogeneous group of patients and therefore careful preoperative assessment is essential to determine the best management strategy. Using the 7th edition American Joint Committee on Cancer (AJCC) staging classification, survival rates at 5 years for clinical stage IIIA patients is 19%; 7% for IIIB; and for pathological stage IIIA and B, 24% and 9% respectively [1]. Preoperative identification of mediastinal lymph

* Mark J. Krasna, MD, Corporate Medical Director, Meridian Cancer Care, 1945 Hwy 33, Neptune, NJ 07753, US, mkrasna@meridianhealth.com, 732-776-2474.

node (LN) disease, and subsequent use of neoadjuvant therapy hold promise for improved survival even for patients with N2/N3 disease.

## Staging

Stage IIIA consists of T3N1, T1-3N2, and T4N0-1 non small cell lung cancer (NSCLC). Stage IIIB includes T4N2 and TanyN3 disease. T3 refers to local chest wall or pleural invasion and includes tumors larger than 7 cm and satellite nodules in the revised staging system. Tumors that are T3N1 based on the new T3 descriptors have not been studied in the context of treatment for stage IIIA disease. In addition, the vast majority of trials have involved N2 disease only, as it was difficult to establish T3N1 clinically reliably prior to resection. With the advent of endobronchial ultrasound and esophageal ultrasound (EBUS/EUS) it may be more likely that these patients too will be identified pretreatment. T4N0-1 tumors are now also considered IIIA; it is likewise unknown at this time if these patients should be treated in the same manner as other IIIA patients. Several phase II studies describe the treatment of T4N0-1 patients but the outcomes from randomized trials do not necessarily apply to this subset.

There is considerable heterogeneity in both clinical presentation and outcomes of stage III/ N2 NSCLC, ranging from radiographically (PET and CT) negative lymph nodes (LN); negative LN by invasive staging and microscopic disease discovered only at the time of final pathologic review of resected nodes. Clinically negative N2 nodes that are found to be positive on an intraoperative frozen section analysis during lung resection and N2 nodes that are enlarged or FDG-avid by PET, typically biopsy-proven by invasive staging techniques, but are still considered potentially resectable are the other end of this spectrum. Finally, there is bulky N2 disease typically defined as >2 cm nodes, or extranodal extension usually with multiple stations involved [2].

## Proving N2 Disease

A thorough preoperative assessment includes: pulmonary function testing (PFTs), bronchoscopy, CT chest/upper abdomen, PET/CT, invasive mediastinal staging, and occasionally brain MRI. The key is to follow up suspicious LN with cytologic or pathologic proof of stage. There are several methods to stage the mediastinum. The less invasive methods endobronchial ultrasound transbrachial needle aspiration (EBUS-TBNA), esophageal ultrasound fine needle aspiration (EUS-FNA), CT guided biopsy all have lower rates of accuracy than do cervical mediastinoscopy and thoracoscopic lymphadenectomy, but also lower rates of morbidity. Mediastinoscopy has a false positive rate of 0% and false negative rate of 9%, mostly because of nodes that are inaccessible such as levels 5, 6, posterior 7, 8 or 9. This remains the best test to confirm a negative mediastinum. For suspicious, enlarged mediastinal nodes, EBUS or EUS can be very helpful to establish N2 or N3 disease; it also leaves the option to perform mediastinoscopy after preoperative treatment to check for nodal clearance as a response to neoadjuvant therapy [3].

# Treatment

Surgery alone for stage III NSCLC is inadequate. When stage III NSCLC patients recur it is almost always systemically, thus a combined modality approach is necessary. For unsuspected N2 disease, there are data supporting adjuvant chemotherapy. Whether radiation therapy (XRT) should also be given postoperatively is debatable; microscopic N2 may have improved local control whereas macroscopic N2 disease may have less chance of recurring during adjuvant radiation. Prolongation of survival has not clearly been demonstrated using routine adjuvant XRT [4].

Following an R0 resection with an unsuspected N2 NSCLC, chemotherapy and radiation would typically be given sequentially. If margins are positive, then concurrent therapy is warranted. Treatment related toxicity may be higher with this aggressive regimen but several important steps can limit this: use of muscle flaps for bronchial stump coverage, judicious fluid administration intraoperatively, and low ventilatory pressures intraoperatively and early extubation to limit barotraumas [5].

Treatment of patients who have N2 disease documented preoperatively usually involves combination therapy. A recent German cooperative study [6] compared preoperative chemotherapy with preoperative chemoradiation for stage IIIA and IIIB. Patients received cisplatin and etoposide for 3 cycles followed by surgery and adjuvant radiation to 54 Gy, or cisplatin/etoposide for 3 cycles, then concurrent chemoradiation with hyperfractionated radiation to a dose of 45 Gy, followed by surgery. No difference in overall survival or progression free survival was demonstrated: median survival of 33 (induction chemotherapy) and 32.4 (induction chemotherapy + chemoradiation) months, 3 year survival of 45% and 48%, respectively, and 5 year survival of 31% and 39%, respectively. Although more patients in the chemoradiation group had mediastinal nodal sterilization, this did not translate to an increase in survival. It is unlikely that another attempt at a phase III trial will be undertaken in the wake of this and the North American Intergroup studies.

The remaining subset of IIIA patients are those with bulky mediastinal lymphadenopathy. The EORTC Lung Cancer Group reported a randomized trial of surgery vs. thoracic radiotherapy in patients with proven stage IIIA-N2 NSCLC that were considered unresectable at the time of presentation (predominantly because of extensive nodal disease) [7]. Those who responded to induction chemotherapy with 3 cycles of platinum-based therapy were randomized to either radiation (60 Gy) or surgery for local control. Median and disease-free survival were the same (17.5 and 16.4 months, respectively, p NS). Of note, the complete resection rate was only 50% and pneumonectomy rates were high (47%, although mortality was only 7%). The authors concluded that radiation therapy is the preferred method of locoregional control in unresectable/bulky nodal disease patients. Another study out of China from 2009 [8] studied a similar population in a phase II trial – 30 with bulky N2 disease and 18 with stage IIIB tumors. Patients were treated with induction chemotherapy followed by chemoradiation (45 Gy hyperfractionated) followed by resection in the absence of disease progression. Thirty-nine patients underwent thoractomy; 30 of whom had a complete resection (62.5% of the initial treatment group). Pneumonectomy was required in 6 of the 30 patients (20%). Median survival was 23 months for the entire group and 58 months (5 year survival 43.3%) for the 30 patients who were completely resected. A major limitation to this study is that no patient had histologic confirmation of N2 disease pre-treatment, it was simply defined by initial imaging and the pathologic findings at resection. The authors concluded that trimodality therapy is appropriate in select bulky N2 and IIIB patients that respond to induction therapy.

The treatment of Stage III NSCLC has evolved over the last thirty years. Prior to the advent of cisplatin, the overall survival of patients with Stage IIIA-N2 disease was dismal and a major focus of management was surgery used exclusively as a staging tool (9). Pearson et al., reported a 9% five year survival in 62 patients with a positive mediastinoscopy who underwent a complete surgical resection compared to a 24% five year survival in 79 patients who had a negative mediastinoscopy and who after a complete resection were found to have unsuspected mediastinal nodal disease [10]. Postoperative adjuvant chemotherapy and radiotherapy had little impact on the survival of these patients [11]. The early standard for these patients was definitive chemoradiation after the studies by Dillman et al., (CALGB 8834) followed by comparisons of concurrent or sequential chemoradiation [12]. Early phase II trials of neoadjuvant chemotherapy improved survivals of 20% in patients with preoperatively identified N2 disease [13]. Similar results were seen in early phase II studies carried out combining radiation (3000 to 4500cGy) with platinum containing chemotherapy. In the trial by Roth et al, patients underwent induction therapy with a combination of cyclophosphamide, etoposide, and cisplatin followed by surgery and then three additional cycles postoperatively [14]. Thirty-five percent of the patients had a major clinical response and their two and three year survivals were 60% and 50% compared to the surgery alone group that were 25% and 15%. In the trial by Rossel et al, patients were treated with induction mitomycin, ifosfamide, and cisplatin followed by surgery and postoperative radiation compared to surgery and radiation [15]. The two and five year survivals were 29% and 17% in the chemotherapy/surgery/radiation arm and 5% and 0% in the surgery/radiation arm. CALGB 8935 was a multi-institutional phase II trial of high-intensity trimodality therapy for patients with surgically staged IIIA-N2 non-small cell lung cancer [16].

This trial combined two cycles of neoadjuvant cisplatin and vinblastine with surgical resection and radical lymphadenectomy followed by two additional cycles of adjuvant chemotherapy followed by radiation therapy (5400cGy to 6000 cGy). The operative mortality was 3.2% and the morbidity 30%. R0 resections had a three year survival of 46% compared to 21% for those having an incomplete resection (R1), and 0% for unresectable patients. SWOG 8805 evaluated the impact of induction chemotherapy and concomitant radiotherapy on survival in 126 patients with Stage IIIA/B non-small cell lung cancer. All patients had biopsy proven N2 or N3 disease or T4 lesions. The induction regimen consisted of two cycles of cisplatin and etoposide with concurrent radiation to 4500 cGy. Seventy-five patients had stage IIIA-N2 and 51 patients had stage IIIB disease (including 27 patients with Stage IIIB / N3 disease. Unresectable patients or patients with positive nodes received additional chemotherapy and radiation postoperatively. 85% of patients with Stage IIIA-N2 and 80% of patients with Stage IIIB were resected with 10% treatment related deaths. With this aggressive induction approach 21% of patients had a complete pathologic response (path CR) and 37% had only residual microscopic disease. There was no difference in the survival of patients with Stage IIIA and Stage IIIB disease. The two year survivals were 37% and 39% and the three year survivals 27% and 24% respectively. This study demonstrated the importance of downstaging on survival as the strongest predictor of survival was an absence of tumor in the mediastinal lymph nodes at resection. The median five year survival for these patients was 30 months and 44% versus 10 months and 18% for patients with residual nodal disease. In 2001 Rusch et al., published the initial results of SWOG 9416 which adopted the protocol of 8805 and applied it to superior sulcus tumors [17]. Eighty T3 and 31 T4 patients were enrolled without N2 or N3 disease. The resection rate was 91% for T3 tumors and 87% for T4 tumors. 28 patients had a complete pathologic response (35%) and only 26 patients had microscopic residual disease. The long-term results of this study demonstrated a 54% survival for patients undergoing a complete resection. RTOG 9309, Intergroup trial 0139, was a randomized trial of definitive chemo-radiotherapy (194 patients) versus induction chemo-radiotherapy followed by surgical resection (202 patients) for patients with Stage III-N2 non-small cell lung cancer [18]. Patients received two cycles of chemotherapy with cisplatin and etoposide: The patients randomized to go onto surgical resection received a total dose of 4500 cGy and the patients randomized to definitive radiation received a total dose of 6100 cGy. Postoperative/ consolidation chemotherapy, was delivered in 55% of the surgical group and 74% of the non-surgical group. While there was a difference in the progression free survival between the two groups (12.8 months in the surgical group versus 10.5 months in the non-surgical group; $p = 0.017$), there was no difference in the overall survival (23.6 months versus 22.2 months; $p = 0.24$). The operative mortality for patients undergoing pneumonectomy, however, was 26%. In the lobectomy group there was a difference in survival (33.6. months versus 21.7 months in a matched chemotherapy-radiation group; $p =0.002$).

Several authors have reported single institution experiences utilizing neoadjuvant concurrent chemoradiotherapy with platinum based chemotherapy protocols and high dose radiation (approximately 6000 cGy) followed by surgical resection for patients with Stage III A/B NSCLC and for locally advanced T3N0 or T4N0 tumors or tumors of the superior sulcus. These studies highlight the importance of surgical resection for local control even after relatively high doses of radiation as approximately 50% of patients will have residual tumor at the time of resection. In addition, these regimens have relatively high success in effecting nodal downstaging. Operating after higher doses of radiation can be technically challenging and performing pneumonectomy in this setting carries significant risk that has to be weighed against the potential benefit [19-21].

## Goals of Neoadjuvant Therapy

Neoadjuvant therapy has several purposes: to increase the resectability of locally advanced disease, permit an R0 resection, downstage the mediastinal lymph nodes, and eliminate the presence of micro-metastatic disease. In some patients this may make a lobectomy rather than a pneumonectomy possible and thereby reduce the operative risk. While postoperative radiotherapy may improve local control and postoperative chemotherapy may reduce the risk of systemic metastases, these regimens are less likely to be effective in patients with gross disease and these patients may not tolerate or complete the planned postoperative therapy.

The resectability rate for patients with stage III NSCLC entered into several multi-institutional and single institution studies employing neoadjuvant chemotherapy or chemoradiotherapy is variable ranging from 50% to 80% on average. It is also clear that the percentage of patients undergoing an R0 resection is approximately 10% to 20% lower than the percentage of patients resected. These regimens, therefore, are only partially successful in fulfilling the goals of neoadjuvant therapy. Many of these trials include adjuvant therapy in their protocols but in virtually all of these studies patients undergoing an incomplete resection do significantly poorer. It is also unclear whether radiation added to the induction regimen improves the resectability rate. The study by the German Lung Cancer Cooperative Group demonstrated only a five percent difference in resectability between patients receiving induction chemotherapy versus induction chemotherapy followed by concurrent chemotherapy and radiation favoring the group that did not receive the radiation. While the resectability rates of patients receiving high dose radiation and chemotherapy have not always been published, in our experience it has been approximately 75 to 80%. It is possible; therefore, that the resectability in this group of patients may be higher but this awaits further study.

Achieving a complete pathologic response with induction therapy is met with variable success but overall appears to be higher in those patients receiving neoadjuvant chemotherapy and concurrent high dose radiation as opposed to chemotherapy alone or chemotherapy and lower doses of radiation. The significance of this ultimately remains to be determined although it has been suggested that patients who achieve a complete pathologic response have a survival advantage. A more important determinant of survival has been the downstaging of involved mediastinal lymph nodes from N3 or N2 to N0 or N1 (so called "mediastinal nodal clearance") and this finding has been consistently demonstrated in multiple studies. While the definition of absence of tumor in the mediastinal lymph nodes may be variously classified as no viable tumor or no tumor seen, and there may be inter-observer variability from institution to institution, there is no disagreement that nodal downstaging is an important determinant of survival in patients with Stage III disease. High dose radiation in a neoadjuvant protocol limited to patients with N2 disease was reported by Cerfolio et al. [22] This retrospective study demonstrated higher mediastinal nodal downstaging in patients receiving high dose radiation (83%) versus those receiving low dose radiation (median 4500 cGy; 74%). Consistent with other studies there was an increase in the disease free survival in the high dose radiation group versus the low dose radiation group (estimated 3 year survival 65% vs. 30%; $p = 0.047$). Overall, patients receiving high dose radiation have a higher rate of nodal downstaging than patients in studies utilizing either chemotherapy alone or chemotherapy and lower doses of radiation in the induction protocol and a significant survival benefit. In a study from Boston University BU, 32 patients with N2 disease treated with concurrent platinum based chemotherapy and high dose radiation, the median and estimated five year survivals for the 14 patients who had mediastinal nodal down staging were 58 months and 49% compared to the 18 patients with residual mediastinal nodal disease who had a median survival of 38 months and an estimated five year survival of 41% [23]. In RTOG 0229, patients with pathologically proven stage IIIA/B NSCLC underwent induction chemoradiation consisting of carboplatin andpaclitaxel every week for 6 weeks with 61.2 Gy to the mediastinum and primary tumor. Surgeons were required to demonstrate expertise in surgery after induction chemoradiation. 60 patients were accrued between 9/04 and 11/08. 57 patients were eligible from 22 institutions. 88% received radiation therapy (RT) and 91% received induction chemotherapy per protocol. 43 patients (75%) were evaluable for analysis of the primary endpoint of LN clearance. 37 patients underwent surgical resection (76% R0/24% R1). There were 34 lobectomies and 3 pneumonectomies (2 right sided). There was a 16% (6/37) incidence of grade 3 postoperative pulmonary complications but only one death (3%). 27/37(75%) had an intercostal muscle flap (and 1 serratus) at surgery. 36 of 37 had adequate

LN sampling. The authors concluded that Tri-modality therapy remains a viable option for carefully selected NSCLC patients presenting with stage III disease with the ability to sterilize known mediastinal LN disease [24] Currently a follow-up study (RTOG 0839) is evaluating patients with potentially operable N2 disease treated with induction chemotherapy, high dose radiation with or without panutumumab. This study will provide further insight into the impact of nodal staging on survival [25].

## Current Controversies

The first controversy is whether patients with N2 disease should be operated upon at all. This controversy is primarily based on the early results of the Intergroup 0139 study that showed no difference in the overall survival of patients undergoing neoadjuvant chemoradiotherapy followed by surgery versus definitive chemoradiotherapy. The more mature results of this study, however, do show a difference for patients undergoing lobectomy. The poor results in the pneumonectomy group are largely due to the high operative mortality of 26% in these patients.

When we look at the number of patients with residual disease in the primary tumor who have been resected after high dose radiation and concurrent chemotherapy, it is likely that 50% of patients will ultimately fail locally if they do not succumb to metastases. Thus, the rationale for surgery in NSCLC after treatment with concurrent chemotherapy and high dose radiation is local control and subsequent systemic metastases [26-31].

The second controversy is whether patients with gross mediastinal nodal disease, multi-station mediastinal nodal disease or even residual nodal disease after induction therapy should be offered resection. While it is intuitive that patients with gross or multi-station N2 disease are more likely to do poorly with any treatment algorithm, this is not universally accepted. It is clear, however, that in most studies of patients with Stage III-N2 disease, survival is significantly compromised when residual nodal disease is present after induction therapy and that they might do as well overall without surgery. However, a median survival of 41 months in patients with residual nodal disease with an induction regimen that includes high dose radiation has been noted and we should continue to offer these patients resection [32-33].

The most significant controversy is whether pneumonectomy should be offered to patients undergoing resection after induction therapy particularly when radiation is included in the induction regimen. Some surgeons omit radiation when pneumonectomy is contemplated. Unfortunately, many of these patients have advanced disease and the incidence of pneumonectomy in these patients is relatively high. The operative mortality rate in several recent series is significant and in several recent large series has varied from 6% to 12 % with 90 day mortalities significantly higher [34]. In fact, it has been suggested that for these patients 90 day mortality should be the gold standard for reporting. On the other hand the higher mortality is not a universal experience. In the recent study by Weder et al., 176 patients (21% of the resections) underwent pneumonectomy (49% right) for Stage III disease following neoadjuvant treatment and 141 of these received chemoradiotherapy [35]. The 90 day mortality rate was only 3%. Krasna et al., reported no mortality in a group of pneumonectomy patients even though they received high dose radiation [36]. While the operative risk is higher with pneumonectomy, the overall survival of this group of patients is probably higher than if they did not undergo resection. Even so, these patients tend to have a shorter survival than a comparable group of patients undergoing lobectomyThis is likely due both to their more advanced disease and the physiological consequences of the resection. Some authors express additional caution when considering right pneumonectomy although this has not been an issue in our series [37].

While the optimal dose of preoperative radiation as well as fractionation and sequence remain controversial, more groups are utilizing higher effective doses of radiation (6000 cGy and higher) since this provides definitive treatment for those patients who do not go on to surgery for a variety of reasons. In most series this approximates 20% or more of patients. Based on recent experience, there is the additional advantage of better nodal downstaging and potential survival advantage. In addition, the number of cycles of chemotherapy given preoperatively, the number of drug combinations in the protocol and whether chemotherapy postoperatively affords an additional benefit are other issues that have not been definitively determined. These will change as other drug and drug combinations become available, genetic profiling or *in vitro* testing for drug sensitivity become more widely used, and immunotherapy advances.

Another advantage of utilizing high or curative doses of radiation initially pre-operatively is that many patients are denied surgery after re-staging. If repeat EUS or EBUS or even repeat mediastinoscopy yield pathology that show recalcitrant N2 disease, surgery need not be offered. If this occurs and patients have received sub-curative doses of radiation (less than 6000 cGy) the several week hiatus that has occurred during the restaging process negatively affects the efficacy of the completion of the patient's radiation. If the patient is sent back for completion of their radiation the efficacy is less because of this several week hiatus that was caused by the surgeon. By utilizing a curative dose up front and then embarking on restaging this delay is avoided and the patient can still undergo pulmonary resection safely even after high doses of pre-operative radiation. Reevaluation and careful patient selection should not be seen by the surgeon as bias, but rather a judicious process of including those patients most likely to have a good outcome (no residual N2 disease) in whom the benefits outweigh the risks, as opposed to those patients with obvious residual disease or poor performance status who are likely not going to have a good outcome.

## Conclusion

Neoadjuvant treatment followed by surgical resection has significantly improved the overall results of treatment for patients with Stage III disease as well as patients with locally invasive tumors. Significant controversies still exist regarding treatment, especially with the new categories included in the revised staging system. Different chemotherapy regimens have been used although the majority of studies include combinations with a standard platinum. Radiation when given as part of the induction protocol appears to offer a higher rate of resection and complete resection, and higher doses of radiation (6000 cGy or higher) are associated with better nodal downstaging whereafter pulmonary resection can be safely performed. Pneumonectomy should be undertaken with caution and in patients with residual nodal disease risk assessment is important. In the final analysis, every patient is different and the overall risks and benefits of surgical resection have to be evaluated individually.

Randomized and multi-institutional trials will clarify the issues regarding treatment and new drugs or drug combinations especially targeted therapy will improve results further. Whether postoperative adjuvant chemotherapy adds to the benefit of neoadjuvant therapy followed surgery remains to be determined.

## References

[1] Goldstraw P, Crowley J, Chansky K et al. The IASLC Lung Cancer Staging Project: proposals for the revision of the TNM stage groupings in the forthcoming (seventh) edition of the TNM Classification of malignant tumours. *J Thorac Oncol*. 2007;2,706-714.

[2] Reed CE, Harpole DH, Posther KE et al. Results of the American College of Surgeons Oncology Group Z0050 trial: the utility of positron emission tomography in staging potentially operable non-small cell lung cancer. *J Thorac Cardiovasc Surg*. 2003;126, 1943.

[3] Ettinger DS, Akerley W, Bepler G et al. Non-small cell lung cancer. *J Natl Compr CancNetw*. 2010;8,740.

[4] Postoperative radiotherapy in non-small-cell lung cancer: systematic review and meta-analysis of individual patient data from nine randomized controlled trials. PORT Meta-analysis Trialists Group. *Lancet*. 1998;352,257.

[5] Sonett JR, Krasna MJ, Suntharalingam M, et al. Safe pulmonary resection after chemotherapy and high-dose thoracic radiation. *Ann Thorac Surg*. 1999;68,316.

[6] Thomas M, Rube C, Hoffknecht P et al. Effect of preoperative chemoradiation in addition to preoperative chemotherapy: a randomised trial in stage III non-small-cell lung cancer. *The Lancet Oncology*. 2008;9,636.

[7] Van Meerbeeck JP, Kramer GW, Van Schil PE et al. Randomized controlled trial of resection versus radiotherapy after induction chemotherapy in stage IIIA-N2 non-small-cell lung cancer. *J Natl Cancer Inst*. 2007;99,442.

[8] Li J, Dai CH, Yu LC et al. Results of trimodality therapy in patients with stage IIIA (N2-bulky) and stage IIIB non-small-cell lung cancer. *Clin Lung Cancer*. 2009;10, 353.

[9] Martini N, Flehinger BJ. The role of surgery in N2 lung cancer. *Surg Clin North Am*. 1987; 67,037.

[10] Pearson FG, DeLarue NC, Ilves R, et al. Significance of positive superior mediastinal nodes identified at mediastinoscopy in patients with resectable lung cancer. *J Thorac Cardiovasc Surg*. 1982;83,1.

[11] Sugarbaker DJ, Herndon J, Kohman LJ, Krasna MJ, Green MR , the Cancer and Leukemia Group B Thoracic Surgery Group. Results of cancer and leukemia group B protocol 8935A mutiinstitutional phase II trimodality trial for Stage IIIa (N2) non-small-cell lung cancer. *J Thoarac Cardiovasc Surg*. 1995;109, 473.

[12] Dillman RO, Herndon J, Seagren SL, et al. Improved survival in stage III non-small-cell *Cancer Inst*. 1996;88(17):1210-5.

[13] Martini N, Kris M, Flehinger BJ, et al. Preoperative chemotherapy for stage IIIa (N2) lung cancer:the Sloan-Kettering experience with 136 patients. *Ann Thorac Surg*. 1993;55,1365.

[14] Roth JA, Fosella F, Komaki R, et al. A randomized trial comparing perioperative chemotherapy and surgery with surgery alone in resectable Stage IIIA non-small cell lung cancer. *J Natl Cancer Inst.* 1994;86, 673.

[15] Rosell R, Gomez-Codina J, Camps C, et al. A randomized trial comparing preoperative chemotherapy plus sugery with surgery alone in patients with non-small cell lung cancer. *NEJM.* 1994;330,153.

[16] Albain KS, Rusch VW, Crowley JJ, et al. Concurrent cisplatin/etoposide plus chest radiotherapy followed by surgery for Stages IIIA (N2) and IIIB non-small-cell lung cancer: mature results of Southwest Oncology Group phase II study 8805. *J Clin Oncol.* 1995;13,1880.

[17] Rusch VW, Giroux DJ, Kraut MJ, et al. Induction chemoradiation and surgical resection for non-small cell lung carcinomas of the superior sulcus: initial results of Southwest Oncology Group Trial 9416 (Intergroup trial 0160). *J Thorac Cardiovasc Surg.* 2001;121, 472.

[18] Albain KS, Swann RS, Rusch VW, et al. Radiotherapy plus chemotherapy with or without surgical resection for stage III non-small-cell lung cancer: a phase III randomized controlled trial. *Lancet.* 2009;374,379.

[19] Daly BD, Ebright MI, Walkey AJ, et al. Impact of neoadjuvant chemoradiotherapy followed by surgical resection on node-negative T3 and T4 non-small cell lung cancer. *J Thorac Cardiovasc Surg.* 2011; Jun;141(6):1392-7.

[20] Sonett JR, Suntharalingam M, Edelman MJ, et al. Pulmonary resection after curative intent radiotherapy (>59Gy) and concurrent chemotherapy in non-small-cell lung cancer. *Ann Thorac Surg.* 2004;78, 1200.

[21] Kwong KF, Edelman MJ, Suntharalingam M, et al. High-dose radiotherapy in trimodality treatment of Pancoast tumors results in high pathologic complete response rates and excellent long-term survival. *J Thorac Cardiovasc Surg.* 2005;129,1250.

[22] Cerfolio RJ, Bryant AS, Spencer SA, Bartolucci AA. Pulmonary resection after high-dose and low-dose chest irradiation. *Ann Thorac Surg.* 2005;80,1224.

[23] Daly BD, Fernando HC, Ketchedjian A, et al. Pneumonectomy after high-dose radiation and concurrent chemotherapy for nonsmall cell lung cancer. *Ann Thorac Surg.* 2006;82, 227-231.

[24] Suntharalingam M, Paulus R, Edelman MJ, et al. Radiation Therapy Oncology Group Protocol 02-29: A Phase II Trial of Neoadjuvant Therapy With Concurrent Chemotherapy and Full-Dose Radiation Therapy Followed by Surgical Resection and Consolidative Therapy for Locally Advanced Non-small Cell Carcinoma of the Lung. *Int J Radiat Oncol Biol Phys.* 2012;84(2):456-63.

[25] ref.0839http:*//www.rtog.org/ClinicalTrials/ProtocolTable/StudyDetails.aspx?study=0839*

[26] Edelman MJ, Suntharalingam M, Burrows W, et al Phase I/IItrial of hyperfractionated radiation and chemotherapy followed by surgery in stage III lung cancer. *Ann Thorac Surg.* 2008;86,903.

[27] Junker K, Langner K, Klinke F, Bosse U, Thomas M. Grading of tumor regression in non-small cell lung cancer: morphology and prognosis. *Chest.* 2001;120,1584.

[28] Betticher DC, Schmitz SH, Totsch M, et al. Mediastinal lymph node clearance after docetaxel-cisplatin neoadjuvant chemotherapy is prognostic of survival in patients with

stage IIIA pN2 non-small-cell lung cancer: a multicenter phase II trial. *J Clin Oncol.* 2003;21(9):1752-9.

[29] Bueno R, Richards WC, Swanson SJ, et al. Nodal stage after induction therapy for stage IIIA lung cancer determines patient survival. *Ann Thorac Surg*. 2000;70,826.

[30] Stefani A, Alifano M, Bobbio A, et al. Which patients should be operated on after induction chemotherapy for non-small cell lung cancer? Analysis of a 7-year experience in 175 patients. *J Thorac Cardiovasc Surg*. 2010;140; 356.

[31] Paul S, Mirza F, Port JL, et al. Survial of patients with clinical stage IIIA non-small cell lung cancer after induction therapy: age, mediastinal downstaging, and extent of resection as independent predictors. *J Thoracic Cardiovasc Surg*. 2011;141,48.

[32] [Adelstein DJ, Rice TW, Rybicki LA, et al. Longterm follow-up after chemoradiotherapy (CRT) in patients (pts) with stage III non-small cell lung cancer (NSCLC): Is bulky mediastinal nodal disease of prognostic importance? *J Clinic Oncol*. 2004;22,14S.

[33] Okada M, Tsubota N, Yoshimura M, et al. Induction therapy for non-small cell lung cancer with involved mediastinal nodes in multiple stations. *Chest*. 2000;118,123.

[34] Doddoli CD, Barlesi F, Trousse D, et al. One hundred consecutive pneumonectomies after induction therapy for non-small cell lung cancer; an uncertain balance between risks and benefits. *J Thorac Cardiovasc Surg*. 2005;130,416.

[35] Weder W, Colland S, Eberhardt WE, et al. Pneumonectomy is a valuable treatment option after neoadjuvant for stage III non-small-cell lung cancer. *J Thoracic Cardiovasc Surg*. 2010;139(6):1424-30.

[36] Krasna MJ, Gamliel Z, Burrows WM, et al. Pneumonectomy for lung cancer after preoperative concurrent chemotheraphy and high-dose radiation. *Ann Thorac Surg*. 2010;89:200.

[37] Martin J, Ginsberg RJ, Abolhoda A, et al. Morbidity and mortality after neoadjuvant therapy for lung cancer: the risks of right pneumonectomy. *Ann Thorac Surg*. 2001;72,11494.

In: Lung Cancer: A Comprehensive Overview
Editor: Kathy Gately
ISBN: 978-1-62618-447-3


Chapter VII

# Targeted Therapies in Non-Small Cell Lung Cancer

***Susan Heavey, Ken O'Byrne and Kathy Gately*** *
Department of Clinical Medicine, Trinity College Dublin,
St. James's Hospital, Dublin, Ireland

## Abstract

The majority of non-small cell lung cancer (NSCLC) patients present with advanced disease and with a 5 year survival rate of <15% for these patients, treatment outcomes are considered extremely disappointing. Standard chemotherapy regimens provide some improvement to ~40% of patients. However, intrinsic and acquired chemoresistance are a significant problem and hinder sustained long term benefits of such treatments. Advances in proteomic and genomic profiling have increased our understanding of the aberrant molecular mechanisms that are driving an individual's tumour. The increased sensitivity of these technologies has enabled molecular profiling at the stage of initial biopsy thus paving the way for a more personalised approach to the treatment of cancer patients. Improvements in diagnostics together with a wave of new targeted small molecule inhibitors and monoclonal antibodies have revolutionised the treatment of cancer.

To date there are essentially three targeted agents approved for clinical use in NSCLC. The tyrosine kinase inhibitor (TKI) erlotinib, which targets the epidermal growth factor receptor (EGFR) TK domain, has proven to be an effective treatment strategy in patients who harbour activating mutations in the *EGFR* TK domain. Bevacizumab a monoclonal antibody targeting the vascular endothelial growth factor (VEGF) can improve survival, response rates, and progression-free survival when used in combination with chemotherapy. Crizotinib, a small-molecule drug, inhibits the tyrosine kinase activity of the echinoderm microtubule-associated protein-like 4 anaplastic lymphoma kinase (EML4-ALK) fusion protein, resulting in decreased tumour cell growth, migration, and invasiveness in patients with locally advanced or metastatic NSCLC. The clinical relevance of several other targeted agents are under investigation in distinct molecular subsets of patients with key "driver" mutations including: *KRAS,*

* Email: kgately@stjames.ie.

*HER2, BRAF, MET, PIK3CA, AKT1,* and *MAP2K1*.. Often several pathways are activated simultaneously and crosstalk between pathways allows tumour cells to escape the inhibition of a single targeted agent. This chapter will explore the clinical development of currently available targeted therapies for NSCLC as well as those in clinical trials and will examine the synergy between cytotoxic therapies.

## Introduction

Only approximately 20-30% of newly diagnosed NSCLC patients present with early stage disease and are suitable candidates for resection. Traditionally decisions on therapeutic options were based on the histology of the tumour. The standard treatment for advanced NSCLC patients with a good performance status (0-1) is platinum-based chemotherapy and partial responses are achieved in 30-40% of patients [1]. Complete responses are very rare in advanced NSCLC and those that do respond initially will develop acquired resistance to treatment. With a 5 year survival rate of <15% for patients with advanced disease, treatment outcomes are considered disappointing.

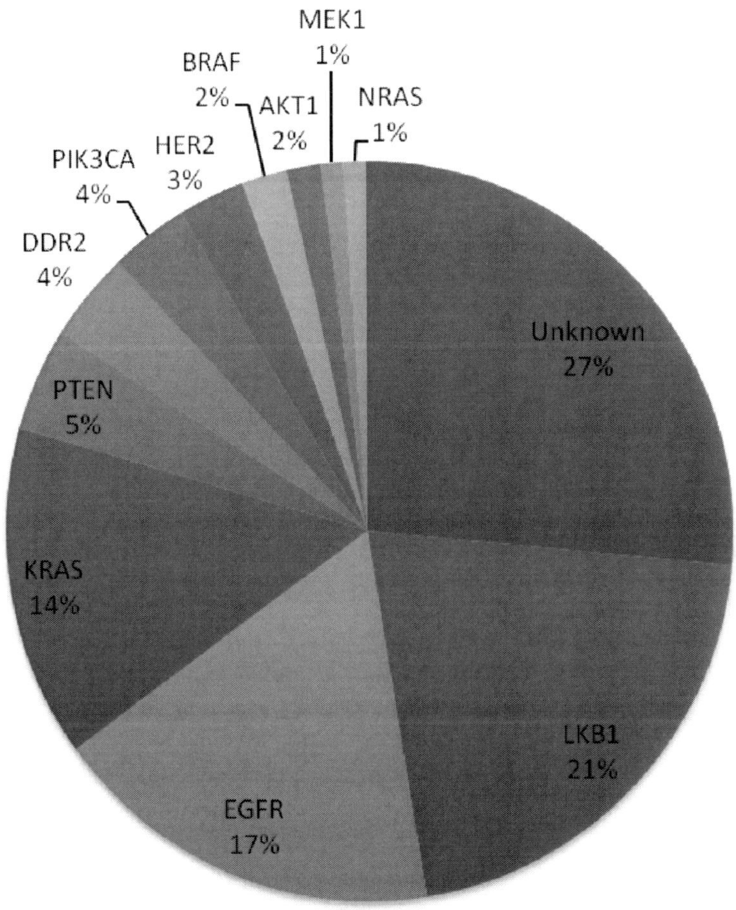


Figure 1. Mutation rates in Non-Small Cell Lung Cancer.

A randomised phase III trial demonstrated less toxicity and better overall survival (OS) in the cisplatin/pemetrexed arm than the cisplatin/gemcitabine arm in patients with non-squamous NSCLC [2]. However, conventional chemotherapy has reached a plateau of effectiveness in improving patient survival in all tumour histologies and a concerted effort to further classify tumours at the molecular level is critical. NSCLC is a heterogeneous disease and often several signalling pathways are driving the oncogenic behaviour of tumours. Several key "driver" genes are mutated in NSCLC including;*EGFR*, *ALK*, *KRAS*, *HER2*, *BRAF*, *MET*, PIK3CA, AKT1 and *MAP2K1* (*MEK1*) (Figure 1). In fact, these genes contribute to the pathogenesis of several cancer types. Other aberrations such as variation in gene copy numbers, translocations between genes and single nucleotide polymorphisms (SNPs) can occur in a proportion of cells within a tumour. These aberrant genes are obvious targets for inhibition and thus the design of drugs that will selectively block these oncogenic varieties while sparing their normal counterparts seems like the ideal strategy to destroy these rogue cells. A table summarising the frequency of mutations and availability of targeted therapies in NSCLC is shown below (Table 1). However, there is no guarantee that only the oncogenic variant is druggable, and like all targeted therapies the cancer cell will eventually activate alternative signalling pathways to evade these targeted inhibitors.

**Table 1. Frequency of mutations and availability of targeted therapies in NSCLC**

| Gene | Alteration | Frequency in NSCLC |
|---|---|---|
| AKT1 | Mutation | 1-2% |
| ALK | Rearrangement | 3–7% |
| BRAF | Mutation | 1–3% |
| DDR2 | Mutation | ~4% |
| EGFR | Mutation | 10–35% |
| FGFR1 | Amplification | 20% |
| HER2 | Mutation | 2–4% |
| KRAS | Mutation | 8-21% |
| LKB1 | Mutation | 9-33% |
| MEK1 | Mutation | 1% |
| MET | Amplification | 2–4% |
| NRAS | Mutation | 1% |
| PIK3CA | Mutation | 2-5% |
| PIK3CA | Amplification | 12-20% |
| PTEN | Mutation | 4–5% |
| PTEN | Loss | 24-44% |
| RET | Rearrangement | 1% |
| ROS1 | Rearrangement | 1% |

Key:

| |
|---|
| Drugs approved in NSCLC |
| Drugs approved in NSCLC for ALK subtype and effective here |
| Drugs approved in other cancers |
| Drugs in clinical development |

Intrinsic resistance or the development of acquired resistance to targeted therapies may be due to the multilevel complex cross-talk that occurs between the targets of the biological agent and several signal transduction pathways. Blocking only one of these pathways may not always be an effective treatment strategy as this approach may open the door for others to act as bypass mechanisms within tumour cells. The most promising approaches to the treatment of NSCLC, will be drugs with multiple targets or the use of a combination of targeted therapies.

# Targeted Therapy in Lung Cancer

A deeper understanding of the pathobiology of human malignancies has led to successful application of targeted therapeutic strategies in several cancers [3-6].

In NSCLC several targeted inhibitors are currently being evaluated in clinical trials and there are essentially three targeted agents approved for clinical use (Figure 2). The EGFR TKIs gefitinib and erlotinib which target the EGFR TK domain, have proven to be an effective treatment strategy in patients who harbour activating mutations in the *EGFR* TK domain. Bevacizumab a monoclonal antibody targeting VEGF can improve survival, response rates, and progression-free survival when used in combination with chemotherapy. Crizotinib, a small-molecule drug, inhibits the tyrosine kinase activity of the EML4-ALK fusion protein, resulting in decreased tumour cell growth, migration, and invasiveness in patients with locally advanced or metastatic NSCLC. With increasing studies showing the importance of matching the treatment to the mutation the Lung Cancer Mutation Consortium (LCMC) in collaboration with the National Lung Cancer Partnership was established in the United States (US) to promote molecular tumour mutation testing for lung cancer patients.

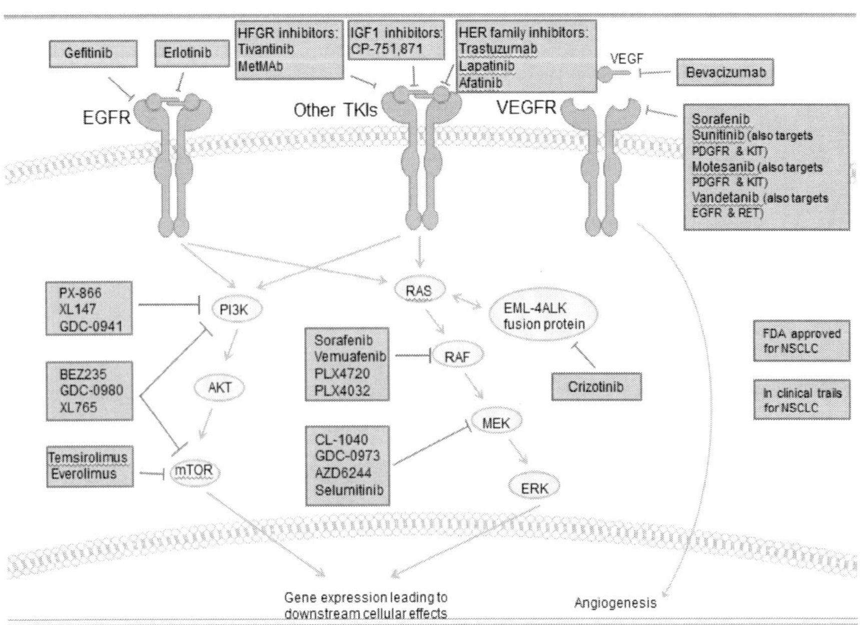


Figure 2. Targeted Therapies in NSCLC.

The LCMC aims to screen a large population of patients to create a unique national data set to determine the frequency of certain driver mutations and explore opportunities for clinical trial enrollment. Molecular profiling of 830 patients, indicated that 60% of tumors exhibit known driver mutations including 25% *KRAS*, 23% *EGFR*, and 6% ALK rearrangements [7].

These data remind us that in 40% of tumours there are as yet unknown lung cancer drivers. Interestingly 95% of molecular lesions are mutually exclusive and the presence of one mutation in lieu of another can influence response to targeted therapy. Companion diagnostics that enable the monitoring of changes in patients' tumour genotypes throughout the course of their disease together with a combination approach to targeted therapy can potentially reduce toxicities and improve patient outcomes.

## EGFR

The EGFR signalling pathway plays an essential role in the pathogenesis of NSCLC with EGFR protein expression seen in up to 85% of NSCLC patients. Initial studies failed to demonstrate the prognostic relevance of EGFR expression in NSCLC or to predict response to oral EGFR TKIs [8-12].

However, a recent study has shown that EGFR expression does predict response to EGFR-TKIs if an intracellular binding antibody is used for immunohistochemistry analysis [13]. Somatic mutations in the *EGFR* TK domain proved to be a better predictor of response to EGFR TKIs and were first described in 2004. Mutations are either in-frame deletions or amino acid substitutions clustered around the ATP-binding pocket of the TK domain (exons 18-21). The two most common mutations are in-frame deletions in exon 19 (del 19) or a substitution mutation in exon 21 (L858R) and these account for 85-90% of the drug-sensitive *EGFR* mutations seen in NSCLC. Two other sensitising mutations are substitutions in exons 18 (G719A/C) and 21 (L861Q) [14].

These mutations are more common in female, never smokers with adenocarcinomas, who are of Asian ethnicity [15, 16]. Cells harbouring these "driver" *EGFR* mutations are said to be in a state of "oncogenic addiction" and are highly dependent on the constitutively active EGFR signalling pathway [17]. A germline T790M *EGFR* mutation was reported in a family with multiple cases of NSCLC and was shown to confer a growth advantage to the cancer cells [18]. Both T790M positive cells and those having a "double mutant" (T790M and L858R mutations) have been shown to have enhanced kinase activity [19] and increased tyrosine phosphorylating activity, respectively [20].

The T790M mutation has also emerged as a secondary point mutation that is present in approximately half of lung cancer patients who develop resistance to EGFR TKIs. Pinter et al. have shown that there is little correlation between EGFR expression (IHC) and *EGFR*-activating mutations, increased *EGFR* gene copy number or response to EGFR TKI [9]. Although *EGFR* amplification can indicate response to EGFR TKIs, mutation status is the best predictor of response and is used routinely to identify NSCLC tumours that are most likely to benefit from treatment [15, 21-25].

## Targeting EGFR

Cetuximab (Erbitux) is a chimeric monoclonal G1 (IgG1) antibody that binds to EGFR with high affinity and blocks ligand binding, inducing receptor internalisation and degradation resulting in inhibition of EGFR expression. It is licensed to treat both metastatic colorectal cancer (mCRC) and squamous cell carcinoma of the head and neck (SCCHN). However, after initial positive results in Phase II trials in patients with advanced NSCLC, two Phase III trials evaluating cetuximab in addition to first-line chemotherapy showed only a small benefit in overall survival (OS). Interestingly, a subgroup analysis of patients with high EGFR expression by IHC from the FLEX Phase III trial demonstrated a greater survival benefit [26]. If this data can be validated prospectively than cetuximab may be approved as a standard treatment in the future.

The EGFR TKIs gefitinib (Iressa) and erlotinib (Tarceva) have been licensed to treat advanced or metastatic NSCLC. Activating mutations in the *EGFR* TK domain have been shown to demonstrate different sensitivities to EGFR TKIs, with exon 19 deletions being more likely to respond than those of exon 21 [27-31]. Conversely, some substitution mutations in exon 20 (T790M) and exon 21 (T854A) are known to confer resistance to some EGFR TKIs [32-34] Of the mutated tumours that initially respond to treatment with the EGFR TKIs erlotinib and gefitinib, almost all will eventually develop acquired resistance to these drugs [32, 35]. T790M confers resistance in 50% of cases [36-38] and it was initially thought that the substitution of the larger methionine residue may cause steric hindrance to the binding of the drugs [32, 39] however, a structurally similar reversible TKI is able to overcome resistance [40]. The T790M mutation may result in increased affinity of EGFR for ATP compared with erlotinib or gefitinib and this is the primary mechanism by which the mutation confers drug resistance [41] Thus, it should be possible to overcome the resistance by developing TKIs that have a higher affinity for the T790M kinase [33, 42, 43]. New-generation EGFR TKIs, that bind irreversibly to the EGFR-TK, forming covalent cross-links with EGFR, such as afatinib (BIBW 2992), have been shown to be active against tumours resistant to reversible EGFR TKIs [32, 42-46] and offer an alternative therapy strategy. New-generation TKIs may have a longer duration of action than reversible agents. In order to change the therapeutic agent at the optimal time to prevent tumour progression, it is crucial patients are screened regularly for the emergence of the T790M mutation. Interestingly, a study by Maheswaran et al. also found T790M in up to 38% of patients not previously treated with a TKI [47].

This existence of the T790M mutation in a few cancer cells at diagnosis confers a shorter time to tumour progression [48]. These mutant cells are subsequently 'cloned out' during the patient's treatment with EGFR TKIs indicating that these patients may benefit from treatment with new-generation EGFR TKIs from the beginning. In addition to these specific *EGFR* mutations, other factors such as amplification or activation of the insulin-like growth factor receptor [49] and *MET* amplification [50] have also been shown to confer resistance to EGFR TKIs. These nuances of the EGFR discussed above demonstrate that both preselection of patients most likely to respond to EGFR-targeted therapy and screening during therapy are crucial to determine the appropriate treatment regimen.

## VEGF and VEGFR

The vascular endothelial growth factor (VEGF) ligand is released from endothelial cells in response to tissue injury or hypoxia, and leads to the formation of new blood vessels. It has been implicated in tumorigenesis and metastasis and is an important pro-angiogenic mediator. There are five members of the VEGF family (VEGF-A, VEGF-B, VEGF-C, VEGF-D and PIGF) with VEGF-A the most clinically active. There are 3 VEGF receptor (VEGFR) tyrosine kinases (VEGFR-1, VEGFR-2 and VEGFR-3) with VEGFR-2 involved in most angiogenic responses. Overexpression of VEGF promotes vascular permeability, which enhances tumor nutrient exchange, extravasation of macromolecular proteins and the influx of tumor cells [51]. Several studies have identified VEGF overexpression as a poor prognostic indicator in NSCLC and SCLC [52, 53].

## Targeting VEGFR with Bevacizumab

The anti-tumor effects of VEGF pathway inhibition have been validated in preclinical models [54, 55], and subsequently led to the development of VEGF antagonists such as the monoclonal antibody, bevacizumab (Avastin). The Phase III ECOG 4599 trial established the efficacy of bevacizumab by randomizing metastatic, non-squamous lung cancer patients to carboplatin, paclitaxel and bevacizumab versus chemotherapy alone [56]. The addition of bevacizumab to chemotherapy resulted in better median survival (12.3 vs 10.3 months, hazard ratio (HR) 0.79) and a higher response rate (RR; 35 vs 15%, $p < 0.001$) when compared with chemotherapy alone. Based on this study, bevacizumab gained FDA and EMEA approval in 2006 as first-line therapy in combination with carboplatin and paclitaxel for advanced nonsquamous NSCLC.

## Targeting VEGFR with TKIs

After the success of bevacizumab a number of compounds targeting angiogenesis have since gone into preclinical and clinical testing. Several of these newer agents are multitarget tyrosine kinase inhibitors (MTKIs) which target several pathways concomitantly. Sorafenib inhibits the kinase activity of C-RAF, B-RAF and targets platelet-derived growth factor receptor family (PDGFR-β and stem cell factor receptor (KIT)) as well as VEGFR2/3. Sorafenib inhibits MEK and ERK phosphorylation in various cancer cell lines and tumor xenografts [57]. Sunitinib is a multitargeted inhibitor of VEGFR, PDGFR, KIT and FLT3 (FMS-like tyrosine kinase 3). Both MTKIs were approved by the FDA to treat metastatic renal cell carcinoma and sunitinib has been approved for gastrointestinal stromal tumours. However these drugs have not produced as promising results as in the non-specific biomarker setting. These drugs are also associated with having higher toxicities.

In a large Phase III placebo-controlled study investigating the efficacy of sorafenib with carboplatin and pacliltaxel (CP), the addition of sorafenib to chemotherapy-naïve patients with advanced NSCLC failed to show clinical benefit [58]. In a setting where the biomarker status of a patient is known, such as in the case of the BATTLE trial, sorafenib has shown varying results [59]. Sorafenib was found to have activity against tumors in patients with wild-type *KRAS,* whereas patients who had *EGFR* mutations fared worse on sorafenib. Such results illustrate the importance of biomarkers in predicting the sensitivity or resistance of patients to targeted therapy. BATTLE-2 is a follow-up trial seeking to pursue the interesting data found in BATTLE-1 regarding *KRAS* mutations and the positive results of sorafenib. Thus, only two arms from the original BATTLE-1 trial (erlotinib and sorafenib) were continued in BATTLE-2.

Another MTKI that has been investigated in NSCLC is Motesanib which targets VEGFR 1 - 3, PDGFR and KIT. A Phase II three arm study comparing motesanib and CP with single agent motesanib and single agent bevacizumab showed comparable results between the motesanib and bevacizumab arms in advanced NSCLC patients but with higher toxicity in the motesanib arms [60]. A larger Phase III placebo-controlled study with motesanib and CP was temporarily halted due to a high incidence of hemoptysis in patients with squamous cell histology, but reopened later for non-squamous NSCLC patients with results available in 2013 [61].

Other therapies that target and antagonize circulating VEGF are currently undergoing investigations [62]. VEGF and EGFR have interconnected downstream pathways, potentiating the effectiveness of their dual inhibition in cancer therapy. Vandetanib is a small molecule that inhibits VEGFR, EGFR as well as RET and additional kinases, and may be beneficial in treating patients with solid tumors [63]. The effectiveness of dual EGFR/VEGF inhibition compared to single EGFR blockade was evaluated in a two-part crossover, randomized Phase II trial [64]. Vandetanib (300 mg) was tested against gefitinib (250 mg) and following progression on the randomized primary treatment, patients were crossed over to the opposing treatment arm. Median PFS was 11.0 weeks for vandetanib and 8.1 weeks for gefitinib (HR = 0.69) with no difference found in OS. Disease control (DC) for more than 8 weeks was observed in 45% of patients in the vandetanib arm compared with only 34% patients taking gefitinib.

The efficacy of vandetanib was evaluated in four randomized phase III clinical trials in NSCLC in combination with docetaxel (ZODIAC) [65], pemetrexed (ZEAL) [66] or as a single agent (ZEST and ZEPHYR) [67, 68]. Both combination trials with vandetanib resulted in the improvement of lung cancer symptom control. However, ZODIAC was the only trial to meet its primary endpoint of progression free survival (PFS) while no study showed advantage in overall survival (OS). As of October 2009, there are no longer planned developments for the use of vandetanib in treating advanced NSCLC in the US or the EU. The decision was made based on the lack of benefit to OS and the insufficiency of using PFS as the primary end point for approval.

## EML4-ALK

*EML4-ALK* is an aberrant fusion gene that is the result of a chromosomal rearrangement between the N-terminal half of the echinoderm microtubule-associated protein-like 4 (*EML4*) gene and intracellular kinase domain of the anaplastic lymphoma kinase (*ALK*) gene. This leads to constitutive, ligand-independent activation of the ALK kinase, resulting in aberrant activation of downstream oncogenic signalling pathways including PI3K and MAPK, as well as STAT3 dependent pathways that promote cell proliferation, stromal invasion, and apoptotic inhibition. Other reported ALK fusions in NSCLC including TFG [69] and kinesin family member 5B (KIF5B) [70, 71] are less frequently observed. EML4-ALK was initially discovered in anaplastic large-cell lymphoma [72] however, in 2007, Soda et al. described *ALK* activation in a subset of NSCLC that exhibited this fusion between *EML4* and *ALK* in the short arm of chromosome 2p [73]. This study detected the EML4–ALK fusion transcript in 5 of 75 Japanese (6.7%) NSCLC patients however further studies revealed that it occurs in approximately in 2-7% of patients with NSCLC adenocarcinomas. *ALK* rearrangements are more common in never smokers or light smokers and in those with adenocarcinoma especially the acinar histology in East Asia or the signet-ring or cribriform morphology in the West. This variant is always positive for thyroid transcription factor 1 (TTF-1) [74, 75]. In general, EML4–ALK and *EGFR* and *KRAS* mutations are mutual exclusive [76] however counterexamples have also been reported [77]. Patients with *ALK* rearrangements are not thought to benefit from EGFR TKIs.

## Targeting EML4-ALK

Although the incidence of EML4–ALK is low in NSCLC its importance is significant due to its relatively specific and well-tolerated ALK inhibitor, crizotinib (Xalkori) [78, 79]. Crizotinib is a small molecule TKI originally developed as a mesenchymal epithelial transition growth factor (c-Met) inhibitor [80] but was discovered to be a potent ALK inhibitor. It binds to ALK blocking the driver kinase activity and inhibiting tumour growth. This inhibitor was first described in 2007 and in less than 3 years an early-phase clinical trial yielded impressive responses in patients with advanced lung cancer containing *ALK* rearrangements. Eighty-two patients, most of whom were previously treated, were enrolled in the study and received crizotinib (250 mg) twice daily in 28-day cycles [81]. At a mean treatment duration of 6.4 months, the overall response rate was 57% (47 of 82 patients, with 46 confirmed partial responses and 1 confirmed complete response); 27 patients (33%) had stable disease. A total of 63 of 82 patients (77%) were continuing to receive crizotinib at the time of data cut-off, and the estimated probability of 6-month progression-free survival was 72%, with no median for the study reached. The drug resulted in grade 1 or 2 (mild) gastrointestinal side effects. The benefit of testing for *ALK* rearrangements was demonstrated in phase I and phase II trials of crizotinib. Patients with the EML4-ALK fusion, nearly all of whom had progressed despite at least 1 prior line of therapy, showed response rates of approximately 50% to 60% crizotinib. Response duration was 42-48 weeks [78, 79].

Data obtained from clinical trials has shown that in patients who had received prior treatments that either failed or worked only for a brief period of time, crizotinib offered a 72% chance that the tumour would shrink or remain stable for at least six months. In August 2011,the FDA granted accelerated approval for crizotinib along with a companion diagnostic to evaluate *ALK* rearrangements by FISH (Vysis ALK Break-Apart FISH Probe Kit (Abbott Molecular, Inc.)), for advanced stage non-small cell lung cancer which has been determined to be ALK positive. Immunohistochemistry, may become a standard-of-care, as high concordance with FISH has been established for IHC 3+ or IHC 0 scores [82]. As with HER2 in breast cancer intermediate IHC scores may, however, still require FISH. Several different antibodies are in development [76].

As with the EGFR TKIs, tumours eventually develop mechanisms of resistance to crizotinib including secondary mutations in the *ALK* TK domain or gene amplification [83].

Treatment strategies to overcome resistance mechanisms are currently under investigation including a potent, selective, and orally available ALK inhibitor (CH5424802) which has a unique chemical scaffold that has been shown to inhibit the "gatekeeper" mutation L1196M [84-86].

Interestingly the *ROS* gene is also an "off-target" of crizotinib. Activation of *ROS* can be found in about 1.7% of NSCLC and crizotinib appears to have marked activity in these cases [87]. There is also a case report of a patient with NSCLC harboring *MET* amplification who responded to crizotinib [88].

Pemetrexed has been shown to have exceptional activity in *ALK*-rearranged NSCLC [89], with a response (in monotherapy or in platinum-based combinations) of 42% and a PFS of 9 months. Other publications have appeared to support this [90, 91] but more recently, these findings have been questioned. The ongoing profile studies should be informative.

## KRAS

*RAS* oncogenes were first identified as the transforming factor in the Harvey and Kirsten strains of a mouse sarcoma virus [92]. KRAS is a member of a family of intracellular GTP-binding switch proteins called the GTPase superfamily. KRAS alternates between an active "on" state with a bound GTP and an inactive "off" state with a bound GDP. It plays a key role in signal transduction downstream of transmembrane receptor tyrosine kinases, e.g. EGFR. After binding of growth factors such as the epidermal growth factor (EGF) and transforming growth factor α (TGFα) to the EGFR, GDP bound KRAS is then recruited by adaptor molecules. KRAS activation is accelerated by a protein called guanine nucleotide–exchange factor (GEF), which binds to the KRAS-GDP complex, causing dissociation of the bound GDP. GTP binds spontaneously to "empty" KRAS molecules, with release of GEF, activating downstream signalling predominantly via the RAF/MEK/ERK downstream signal transduction pathway (the classical MAPK pathway). Several other pathways may be stimulated by KRAS, including PI3K/AKT [93, 94]. Deactivation of KRAS, requires the assistance of a GTPase-activating protein (GAP), which binds to KRAS-GTP and accelerates its intrinsic GTPase activity by a hundredfold.

Homologous *KRAS* mutations have been identified in several human cancers. These missense mutations impair GTP hydrolysis and thus promote formation of constitutively activated GTP-bound KRAS. In NSCLC, 97% of *KRAS* mutations occur in exon 2, codon 12 or 13 [95] and are more common in "smoking adenocarcinoma" patients (30%–40%) hence the hypothesis that there is a direct relationship to tobacco exposure. The mutations are G-to-T or G-to-C transversions (pyrimidine swapped for purine); however, in never-smokers with adenocarcinoma, "transition" mutations (G to A (purine for purine)) have occasionally been found (approximately 15%) [96]. Mutation subtype may alter downstream signal activation, with potential implications [97] for prognosis. *KRAS* mutations are rarer in never smokers and less common in East Asian vs. US/European patients [98]. In general, *KRAS* mutations are found in tumors wild type for *EGFR* or *ALK* defining a distinct molecular subset of the disease. *KRAS* mutations are prognostic for poor survival, independent of therapy and patients fail to benefit from adjuvant chemotherapy and seem to be resistant to EGFR-TKIs [99, 100].

# Targeting KRAS

Unlike inactivating mutations which "switch off" signalling, *KRAS* mutations results in its persistent signal activation. For this reason KRAS has been difficult to target directly; as it requires reactivation, not inactivation, to switch the signalling off.

Potentially KRAS itself could be targeted by; inhibition of protein expressionor membrane localization through posttranslational modification or trafficking, blocking its interaction with GEFs, or enhancing KRAS/GAP interactions [101]. Although extensive studies have been undertaken to block prenylation of the KRAS C-terminal membrane anchoring by farnesyltransferase inhibiton, unfortunately to date, no agent has been developed that can modulate any of the above processes with success. Efforts to target downstream effector pathways including BRAF, MEK, and PI3K either singularly or in combination have been more successful and are described below.

Targeted inhibition of the molecular chaperone Hsp90 by investigational drug ganetespib, a synthetic second-generation Hsp90 inhibitor, slowed the growth of NSCLC cells which were *KRAS* mutation positive. The drug was even more active when combined with traditional lung cancer treatments and other investigational targeted therapies, according to preclinical study data [102].

The indirect value of KRAS in determining sensitivity to other targeted agents or to pemetrexed remains controversial. Recent data in NSCLC has shown that *KRAS* mutations may sensitize tumours to antifolates such as pemetrexed [105], possibly by upregulation of mir-181c, a micro RNA that can downregulate *KRAS*. As clinical evidence emerges, it is apparent that both *KRAS* mutation and amplification status should be considered for patient stratification prior to antifolate treatment.

# HER2

HER2 is a member of the EGFR family of tyrosine kinase receptors that drive and regulate cell proliferation [103]. HER2 is overexpressed in 20% of NSCLC patients resulting in poor patient prognosis and survival [104]. Increased gene amplification has been documented in 2% to 23% of cases depending on the study [105, 106] and is more frequent (30%) in tumors with bronchioloalveolar carcinoma histology [107]. Mutations in the tyrosine kinase domain of *HER2* were first identified by the Cancer Genome Project [108]. Occurring in 2 to 4% of cases somatic mutations are predominantly insertion/duplications between amino acids 774 and 779, or a missense mutation at 755 and result in the continuous activation of the HER2 receptor pathway [109]. *EGFR* and *HER2* mutations are located in the C-helix region of the kinase domain and interestingly, *HER2* in-frame insertions are found in a similar position to the deletion mutations observed in *EGFR* in NSCLC. Similar to *EGFR* and *ALK*, mutations occur more frequently in women, never-smokers and those with an adenocarcinoma sub-type. Studies have shown *HER2* mutations, in exon 20 of the tyrosine kinase domain, are found in 3 to 10% of lung adenocarcinomas [110, 111]. *HER2, EGFR*, and *KRAS* mutations seem to be mutually exclusive although a small proportion of patients may have coexisting *HER2* and *EGFR* mutations [112]. At present, due to the relatively low mutation rate in the *HER2* tyrosine kinase domain, routine patient screening and the availability of clinical trials has been limited.

## Targeting HER2

Early trials with the anti-HER2 monoclonal antibody (Trastuzumab) combined with chemotherapy in lung cancer patients with HER2 overexpression did not show a benefit for patients like the exceptional results seen in breast cancer [113]. Patients with amplified *HER2* do not seem to benefit from anti- HER2 monoclonal antibodies (trastuzumab) or HER2 TKIs (lapatinib) [105-107, 114, 115].

Although patients with *HER2* mutations are resistant to EGFR TKIs irrespective of their EGFR mutation status, they do benefit from HER2 targeted therapy. Patients who have previously shown resistance to chemotherapy and/or EGFR inhibitors benefit from trastuzumab plus chemotherapy [116]. The dual tyrosine kinase inhibitors lapatinib and afatanib, which target both EGFR and HER2, have shown evidence of activity in lung cancer patients with *HER2* mutations [117]. Similarly, the pan-HER TKI (PF00299804) inhibited cell growth in *HER2*- amplified and *HER2*-mutated NSCLC cell lines resistant to gefitinib [118].

At present, patients who are identified as *HER2*-mutant are treated with first-line chemotherapy, with HER2 specific trials designated as second-line or greater therapy. The Lung Cancer Mutation Consortium is offering tumor testing for *HER2* mutations with the aim of promoting, within all participating medical institutions, clinical trials for this uncommon mutation.

## B-RAF

B-RAF is a serine/threonine-protein kinase that plays a role in linking RAS GTPases with proteins of the MAPK family which are involved in cell division and differentiation [119]. Three members of RAF kinase family have been identified and include: A-RAF, B-RAF and c-RAF. *BRAF* mutations are among the most common in cancer in general, and were first described in melanomas [120].

They are present in only 1% to 3% of lung cancers and are most commonly found in adenocarcinomas and in former or current smokers. In melanoma, where the most promising results with B-RAF inhibitors have been seen, about 80% of mutations affect the Val600 residue (exon 15) within the kinase domain.

Lung tumours also harbour non-Val600Glu mutations including the Leu596Val mutation in the kinase domain and the Gly468Ala mutation in the G loop of the activation domain, making testing more complicated [57, 120, 121]. The Lung Cancer Mutation Consortium is testing for multiple *BRAF* mutations, with direction to clinical trials being offered through the consortium.

## Targeting B-RAF

Sorafenib (BAY43-9006, Nexavar) was the first RAF kinase inhibitor to enter clinical testing. This compound was initially developed as a selective inhibitor of RAF, however studies revealed other targets included VEGF receptor 2 and 3, PDGFR, FLT-3, c-KIT, and FGFR-1 [122]. The anti-tumor activity of sorafenib is actually thought to be anti-angiogenic rather than through RAF inhibition in patients with advanced cancer. Second-generation RAF inhibitors with greater selectivity for B-RAF are in development and include PLX4032 (vemurafenib) and its close analogue PLX4720 (Plexxikon, Berkeley, CA, USA). Both are small molecule inhibitors selective for B-RAF and have shown excellent results in the treatment of melanoma patients with the Val600Glu mutation [123]. PLX4032 potently inhibits MAPK pathway activity in cells expressing $^{V600E}$BRAF, however paradoxically it induces activation of ERK in *BRAF* wild-type tumor and normal cells [132, 133]. In *BRAF* wild-type tumor and normal cells, low concentrations of PLX4032 induces ERK signaling by transactivating non-drug bound RAF protomers in a process that is RAS-dependent. At higher concentrations, PLX4032 binds to both protomers within a dimer and inhibits all RAF activation [124]. Novel RAF inhibitors that potently suppress ERK activation in *BRAF* mutant cells but lack the paradoxical activation of ERK noted with PLX4032 in normal cells are also in development on the basis of the presumption that such agents would exhibit a broader therapeutic index [125].

## C-Met

The *MET* gene is located on chromosome 7q21-q31 and encodes hepatocyte growth factor receptor (HGFR) [126]. Its paracrine ligand, hepatocyte growth factor (HGF), is produced by stromal cells. Met signals via RAS, PI3K/AKT, and STAT, affecting mitosis, survival, angiogenesis, migration, invasion as well as mesenchymal–epithelial transversion. Upregulation in cancer cells results in "invasive growth" [127]. In NSCLC, *MET* amplification occurs in squamous-cell carcinoma and adenocarcinoma but HGFR overexpression maybe more common. Mutations in *MET* are rare with one study identifying only 3 mutations in a cohort of 188 lung adenocarcinomas; two in exon 13 encoding the juxtamembrane domain (Arg988del and Tyr1021Asn) and one in exon 18 encoding the kinase domain (Gly1260Cys) [128]. Two Japanese studies also identified an intronic splice variant leading to exon 14 deletions in 2–3% of NSCLC [129, 130]. Upregulation of MET may depend on prior exposure to therapy and may mediate resistance to it. Several studies indicate that *MET* amplification is responsible for ±20% of resistance to EGFR TKIs through a mechanism termed kinase switch [131–133], prompting the development of Met-inhibitory strategies.

## Targeting C-Met

Interestingly, crizotinib (PF-02341066 (Pfizer) described above as an approved targeted therapy for *ALK*-rearranged metastatic NSCLC, was originally developed as a c-MET inhibitor. A recent report [88] of a *MET*-amplified NSCLC patient with normal *ALK* treated with crizotinib showed the patient had a rapid, durable response to the dual inhibitor. As seen with other cancers crizotinib has a role in treating NSCLC patients with *ALK* rearrangements or *MET* amplification [134, 135].

Tivantinib (ARQ 197) is a small molecule inhibitor of c-Met with potential antineoplastic activity. A randomized, double-blind study (MARQUEE) evaluating erlotinib plus tivantinib versus erlotinib plus placebo, in previously treated patients with locally advanced or metastatic, non-squamous NSCLC, was recently halted after interim analysis showed it was not expected to reach its primary endpoint of improvement in OS. This trial was based on a randomized phase II study (erlotinib ± tivantinib) in which non-squamous and *KRAS* M+ patients had benefited most with PFS (4.4 vs 2.3 months, $P = 0.12$) and OS (10.1 vs 6.9 months, $P = 0.18$) [136]. Tivantinib continues to be studied as a monotherapy and as a part of combinations to treat many cancers including NSCLC.

MetMAb (Hoffmann–La Roche), an anti-Met monoclonal antibody, achieved significant PFS and OS benefit in a randomized phase II trial (OAM4558g), comparing MetMAb plus erlotinib (ME) to placebo plus erlotinib (PE) in 2nd/3rd line NSCLC. Benefit was not restricted to *EGFR* M+ or *MET* FISH + but was also seen in *MET* FISH-/IHC + [137]). Therefore MET expression may be more reliable than amplification in predicting MetMAb benefit. The effect in low expressors of Met appeared actually harmful, highlighting the importance of a companion diagnostic as MetMAb proceeds into phase III. Several phase I trials are in progress with inhibitors targeted towards specific and multiple kinases that are also active against c-Met. Multikinase inhibitor of c-Met and VEGFR-2 foretinib (GSK1363089 or XL880), and cabozantinib XL184 (Exelixis) demonstrate strong affinity for the hepatocyte growth factor receptor (Met) and vascular endothelial growth factor receptor 2 (VEGFR2).

Rilotumumab (AMG 102) (Amgen) is a fully humanised IgG2 monoclonal antibody that binds to and neutralises HGF, which prevents its binding to c-MET. A phase II trial of this drug in combination with chemotherapy is underway. MET appears to be the next major biomarker in metastatic NSCLC, with several inhibitors fast approaching the clinic.

## PI3K

Phosphatidylinositol 3-kinases (PI3Ks) were discovered by Lewis Cantley and colleagues, who first published on their association with the polyoma middle T protein in 1985 [138]. PI3Ks have since been shown to be signal transducer enzymes that have the ability to phosphorylate the 3 position hydroxyl group of the inositol ring of phosphatidylinositol and phosphoinositides. The signals that PI3K family members help to potentiate induce the cell to grow, differentiate, proliferate, and increase survival, motility and intracellular trafficking. As such, these enzymes are strongly implicated in the development of the malignant phenotype. The PI3K/AKT/mTOR pathway has been implicated in lung tumourigenesis, with mutations, amplifications and epigenetic alterations observed at various points in the cascade [139]. The catalytic subunit of PI3K, p110, occurs in multiple isoforms, with the p110α isoform being encoded by *PIK3CA*. *PIK3CA* is frequently amplified or mutated in NSCLC, and is associated with increased AKT activity. *PIK3CA* aberrations are more frequently observed in squamous cell carcinomas (mutations: 2-7%; amplifications: 33-70%) than adenocarcinomas (mutations: 2%; amplifications: 6-19%) [140]. *PIK3CA* promoter methylation has also been observed in NSCLC, implying an alternative mechanism underlying inactivation of tumor-associated genes in lung carcinogenesis [139]. Further alterations in PI3K pathway genes such as *PTEN* (mutation: 4-5%, loss 24-44%), *LKB1* (mutation: 9-33%) and *AKT1* (mutation: 1-2%) are all found in NSCLC. Alterations in these genes lead the PI3K pathway to become constitutively activated. Activated mTOR (p-mTOR) has been shown to be present in up to 90% of adenocarcinomas, 60% of large cell carcinomas and 40% of squamous cell carcinomas cases. We and others have shown that activation of this pathway in NSCLC leads to a more aggressive, drug-resistant disease which correlates to poor prognosis for patients [141].

## Targeting PI3K

The PI3K pathway represents an attractive target for therapeutic intervention and recently we have seen the development of several inhibitors targeting strategic points in the signalling cascade. Analogues of mTOR inhibitor rapamycin (or 'rapalogues') were first investigated as a method of inhibiting PI3K pathway signalling. The mTOR protein kinase nucleates two distinct multiprotein complexes, mTOR complex1 and 2 (mTORC1 and mTORC2), and these rapalogues (including Everolimus and Temsirolimus) only inhibit mTORC1. Disappointing results from clinical trials indicated that this treatment strategy was not ideal, and as such 'second generation inhibitors' of mTOR, which inhibit the adenosine triphosphate site of the mTOR kinase domain, and crucially are able to block both mTORC1 and mTORC2 complexes, were developed [142].

Several second generation mTOR inhibitors also exert effects on PI3K, and as such several of these 'dual PI3K/mTOR inhibitors' such as BEZ235, GDC-0980 and XL765 are currently in clinical trials, with promising *in vitro* and *in vivo* data indicating that this dual inhibition strategy may be superior to targeting mTORC1 or PI3K alone. Pan PI3K inhibitors such as GDC-0941, XL147 and PX-866, and isoform-specific PI3K inhibitors such as p110α inhibitor BYL719, p110β inhibitor GSK2636771 and p110δ inhibitor GS1101 have also been developed and are currently under investigation.

AKT, NFκB and other PI3K pathway protein inhibitors have also been investigated in the laboratory and clinical setting for effectiveness in NSCLC, with more recent strategies involving a combined treatment approach, as discussed later in this chapter. NSCLC represents a cancer which could benefit greatly from use of PI3K pathway targeted inhibitors such as these, due to the limited effectiveness of current standard treatments as well as the crucial role that the PI3K pathway has been shown to play in the progress, maintenance and inherent/acquired chemoresistance of NSCLC tumours.

# MEK

The most common oncogene in human cancer is RAS, with 20% of all tumours harbouring an activating mutation in one of the *RAS* genes. As discussed earlier in this chapter, this gene plays a particularly important role in NSCLC, with 35% of NSCLC tumours having undergone a *RAS* activating mutation [143]. It is generally accepted that the RAS protein superfamily plays an important role in lung carcinogenesis and the maintenance of the malignant phenotype, with *KRAS* and *BRAF* being frequently mutated in NSCLC. It has been reported that one or other of *KRAS* and *BRAF* is mutated in 50% of NSCLC cases [144]. While strategies for targeting KRAS and BRAF have already been discussed here, the relevance of KRAS downstream signalling effectors to NSCLC treatment will be examined.

Once activated through the binding of an extracellular mitogen to a membrane-bound ligand, RAS exchanges its GDP for a GTP, allowing it to activate signalling proteins which ultimately exert effects on cell proliferation, cell survival and other pro-carcinogenic phenotypes. The first identified and most extensively investigated effector of RAS is RAF, a serine/threonine kinase which phosphorylates MEK1 and MEK2, which in turn activate ERK1 and ERK2 by phosphorylation. Once activated, ERK can translocate to the nucleus and activate transcription factors such as ETS family members that can transcribe genes involved in the promotion of cell cycle progression.

Glu56Pro, Lys57Asn and GLN56Pro mutations occur in the non-kinase portion of MEK1. Somatic mutations including these have been identified in approximately 1% of NSCLC, predominantly adenocarcinoma [145].

# Targeting MEK

With the RAS-RAF-MEK signalling cascade offering a cancer cell ample opportunity to grow, divide and survive, there has been significant interest in developing methods of 'switching off' the pathway in cancers including NSCLC. A number of inhibitors of RAF have been investigated in both the laboratory and clinical settings, and are discussed earlier in this chapter.

The only known substrate for MEK is ERK, and since activation of MEK and ERK can be independent of RAS activation, inhibition of MEK has become a major focus of research over the last number of years. Marks et al. demonstrated in 2008 that cells harbouring *MEK1* Lys57Asn and Gln56Pro mutations (which are both gain-of-function mutations) can be sensitive to MEK inhibitor AZD6244 [145]. Results from a Phase II, open-label, randomized study to assess the efficacy and safety of AZD6244 versus pemetrexed in patients with NSCLC who had failed prior chemotherapeutic regimens indicated that while AZD6244 showed clinical activity as a second- or third- line treatment for patients with advanced NSCLC, it did not offer any advantage over standard treatment with pemetrexed [146]. A phase II study of the oral MEK inhibitor, CI-1040, in patients with cancers including advanced NSCLC concluded that it demonstrated insufficient antitumor activity to warrant further development [147]. Other inhibitors of MEK currently under investigation include PD0325901 [148], selumitinib [149] and GDC-0973 [150].

With numerous points of cross-talk between the RAS-RAF-MEK pathway and other pathways including the PI3K/AKT/mTOR pathway, cancer cells have the ability to overcome MEK targeted inhibition by utilising alternative signalling routes, which could explain the disappointing results that have been observed thus far with clinical MEK inhibition. As such recent thinking suggests a more promising role for these inhibitors in combination with other pathway inhibitors, as discussed below.

## PI3K and MEK Co-Targeted Inhibition

RAS has the ability to activate both the PI3K and MEK pathways, resulting in pro-carcinogenic phenotypes being expressed by a cell in response to an extracellular stimulus such as the binding of a growth factor to a receptor. Once one of these two pathways is blocked by a targeted therapy, it is both possible and plausible that the cell can overcome the treatment by signalling through the other pathway at any of a number of points of convergence, i.e. by using a 'bypass track'. This is one increasingly discussed explanation for the high frequency of resistance observed when patients are treated with cell signalling protein targeted inhibitors. As such, a promising strategy going forward is to utilize a combination approach to therapy for NSCLC patients, where both the PI3K and MEK pathways are inhibited. Research published in 2009 identified a robust increase in apoptosis and tumour shrinkage upon combined blockade of both of these pathways [151], with further *in vitro* and *in vivo* work showing promise for this strategy [152-154].

Recent *in vitro* data demonstrates that PI3K/mTOR inhibitor GDC-0941 synergizes with the MEK inhibitor U0126 in NSCLC cells [155]. A phase I trial is currently recruiting patients with solid tumours for combination treatment with PI3K pathway inhibitor BKM120 and MAPK pathway inhibitor MEK162. Another Phase I trial is currently recruiting patients with locally advanced or metastatic solid tumours for co-targeted inhibition treatment with MEK inhibitor GDC-0973 and PI3K inhibitor GDC-0941. This approach may become more common in lung cancer treatment, as an estimated 70% of lung tumours display RAS-RAF-MEK pathway activation [144].

## IGF1-R

The insulin-like growth factor receptor-1 (IGF-1R) is a transmembrane tyrosine kinase and is structurally homologous to the Insulin Receptor (IR). IGF-1R overexpression has been identified in several tumour types and protects cells from apoptosis-inducing agents, including hypoxia and anti-cancer drugs. The IGF-1R suppresses apoptosis primarily through the phosphoinositide 3-kinase (PI3K) pathway [156] and has been shown to activate other receptors involved in cancer including EGFR, VEGFR, ERα and AR [157]. Although several studies have shown that IGF-1R is not a prognostic marker in NSCLC [158-160]. Merrick et al showed that high IGF-1R expression is associated with ADC histology and a poorer survival in 191 resected NSCLC patients [161]. We have shown that high levels of both IGF-1R and EGFR correlates to poor survival in NSCLC patients (unpublished data) and high levels of IGF-1R correlates to a poor prognosis in SCLC [162]. Activation of the IGF-1R signalling pathway is also involved in the development of resistance to EGFR TKIs [163].

## Targeting IGF-1R

Several different approaches are being investigated for targeting the IGF-1R, including small-molecule kinase inhibitors and IGF-1R antibodies. Initial results of a randomized phase II study showed that combining an anti-IGF-1R monoclonal antibody (figitumumab) with a platinum doublet (paclitaxel–carboplatin) in NSCLC patients resulted in a higher response rate and trends for superior progression-free survival and overall survival. The best results were observed in squamous cell patients [164]. However, a subsequent phase III study failed to validate these results although in a subset of patients with high IGF serum levels, the addition of figitumumab appeared to offer benefit over carboplatin–paclitaxel [165]. Studies have shown mTOR inhibition can activate AKT through IGF-1R resulting in a synergistic interaction with IGF-1R inhibitors [166]. To this end, a phase I trial with cixutumumab in combination with temsirolimus was undertaken and resulted in stable disease in 47% of patients, although only 1 patient in this trial had NSCLC [167]. These clinical trials have indicated that high circulating levels of IGF-1 may be a potential biomarker that could identify patients who may benefit from IGF-1R inhibitors. Currently, the monoclonal antibody IMC-A12 is being tested in combination with a platinum doublet in stage IV NSCLC and in extensive stage SCLC. Several trials are ongoing that are testing the inhibition of both the EGFR and IGF-1R pathways. In one study, cetuximab is combined with cixutumumab and patients are randomized to gemcitabine–cisplatin or carboplatin–cetuximab with or without cixutumumab. Two randomized trials with the IGF-1R tyrosine kinase inhibitor (OSI-906) combined with erlotinib are ongoing. The first study, chemotherapy naïve patients with EGFR mutations are randomized to erlotinib combined with OSI-906 or to erlotinib and placebo. In the second study, patients who are eligible for erlotinib maintenance are assigned to the EGFR TKI plus OSI-906 *versus* placebo. Importantly the collection of of blood and tumor specimens for molecular marker testing is mandatory in these trials, which is crucial in determining markers of response to treatment.

## The Future of Targeted Therapy

The implementation of treatment protocols tailored to the molecular profile of an individual's tumour represents an important paradigm shift in how we treat cancer patients. This personalised approach will hopefully lead to substantial therapeutic improvements and increased patient survival. The success of EGFR and ALK targeted therapies have taught us that a greater emphasis should be placed on the collection of tumor specimens in "real-time" during clinical trials as in the case of the BATTLE trial. Further analyses of these tumor and blood specimens may identify unique patient subgroups that are sensitive to targeted treatments. A recently published study by Tsimberidou and colleagues describes a personalised medicine program undertaken, at the MD Anderson cancer center, in the context of early clinical trials, which involved using targeted agents matched with tumor molecular aberrations [168]. Of 1,144 patients analyzed, 460 (40.2%) had 1 or more aberration. Patients with one aberration treated with a matched therapy (n =175), compared with treatment without matching (n = 116) were associated with a higher overall response rate (27% vs. 5%; P < 0.0001), longer time-to-treatment failure (TTF; median, 5.2 vs. 2.2 months; P < 0.0001), and longer survival (median, 13.4 vs. 9.0 months; P = 0.017). These data, although not randomized and patients had diverse tumor types and a median of 5 prior therapies, are extremely encouraging and represent a promising future for targeted therapies.

## Conclusion

A deeper understanding of the aberrant molecular mechanisms involved in the pathogenesis and progression of NSCLChas led to a shift from a "one size fits all" therapeutic approach to a more personalised targeted approach defined by each tumour's molecular characteristics. Patient screening using companion diagnostics is key to ensuring those with a compatible molecular profile receive an appropriate targeted agent thus improving overall survival and decreasing toxicity. However, in NSCLC, the acquisition of sufficient biopsy material remains a stubborn obstacle to the identification of a patient's molecular signature. Therefore the development of more sensitive technologies, that can generate a comprehensive genetic profile of tumour specimens in a time- and cost-effective manner, is crucial to the success of targeted therapies in NSCLC.

## References

[1] Pfister DG, Johnson DH, Azzoli CG, Sause W, Smith TJ, Baker S et al. American Society of Clinical Oncology treatment of unresectable non-small-cell lung cancer guideline: Update 2003. *Journal of Clinical Oncology* 2004; 22(2): 330-53.

[2] Scagliotti GV, Parikh P, von Pawel J, et al. Phase III study comparing cisplatin plus gemcitabine with cisplatin plus pemetrexed in chemotherapy-naive patients with advanced-stage non-small-cell lung cancer. *J Clin Oncol* 2008; 26**:** 3543–551.

[3] Druker BJ, Talpaz M, Resta DJ, et al. Efficacy and safety of a specific inhibitor of the BCR-ABL tyrosine kinase in chronic myeloid leukemia. *N Engl J Med* 2001;344:1031–1037.

[4] Demetri GD, von Mehren M, Blanke CD, et al. Efficacy and safety of imatinib mesylate in advanced gastrointestinal stromal tumors. *N Engl J Med* 2002;347:472–480.

[5] Flaherty KT, Puzanov I, Kim KB, et al. Inhibition of mutated, activated BRAF in metastatic melanoma. *N Engl J Med* 2010;363:809–819.

[6] Janku F, Tsimberidou AM, Garrido-Laguna I, et al. PIK3CA mutations in patients with advanced cancers treated with PI3K/AKT/mTOR axis inhibitors. *Mol Cancer Ther* 2011;10:558 –565.

[7] Kris MG, Johnson BE, Kwiatkowski DJ, Iafrate AJ et al., Identification of driver mutations in tumor specimens from 1,000 patients with lung adenocarcinoma: The

NCI's Lung Cancer Mutation Consortium (LCMC) *J Clin Oncol.* 2011;29(Suppl):CRA7506.
[8] Nicholson RI, Gee JM, Harper ME. EGFR and cancer prognosis. *Eur J Cancer* 2001;37(Suppl 4):S9e15.
[9] Pinter F, Papay J, Almasi A, et al. Epidermal growth factor receptor (EGFR) high gene copy number and activating mutations in lung adenocarcinomas are not consistently accompanied by positivity for EGFR protein by standard immunohistochemistry. *J Mol Diagn* 2008;10:160e8.
[10] Cappuzzo F, Gregorc V, Rossi E, et al. Gefitinib in pretreated non-small-cell lung cancer (NSCLC): analysis of efficacy and correlation with HER2 and epidermal growth factor receptor expression in locally advanced or metastatic NSCLC. *J Clin Oncol* 2003;21:2658e63.
[11] Bailey R, Kris M, Wolf M, et al. Gefitinib ('Iressa,' ZD1839) monotherapy for pretreated advanced non-small-cell lung cancer in IDEAL 1 and 2: tumor response is not clinically relevantly predictable from tumor EGFR membrane staining alone. *Lung Canc* 2003;41(Suppl 2):S71.
[12] Parra HS, Cavina R, Latteri F, et al. Analysis of epidermal growth factor receptor expression as a predictive factor for response to gefitinib ('Iressa', ZD1839) in nonsmall-cell lung cancer. *Br J Cancer* 2004;91:208e12.
[13] Mascaux C, Wynes MW, Kato Y, et al. EGFR Protein Expression in Non–Small Cell Lung Cancer Predicts Response to an EGFR Tyrosine Kinase Inhibitor—A Novel Antibody for Immunohistochemistry or AQUA Technology. *Clin Cancer Res* December 15, 2011 17:7796-7807.
[14] Cappuzzo F. EGFR FISH versus mutation: different tests, different end-points. *Lung Canc* 2008;60:160e5.
[15] Lynch TJ, Bell DW, Sordella R, et al. Activating mutations in the epidermal growth factor receptor underlying responsiveness of non-small-cell lung cancer to gefitinib. *N Engl J Med* 2004;350:2129e39.
[16] Paez JG, Ja¨nne PA, Lee JC, et al. EGFR mutations in lung cancer: correlation with clinical response to gefitinib therapy. *Science* 2004;304:1497e500.
[17] Gazdar AF, Shigematsu H, Herz J, et al. Mutations and addiction to EGFR: the Achilles 'heal' of lung cancers? *Trends Mol Med* 2004;10:481e6.
[18] Li X, Hemminki K. Inherited predisposition to early onset lung cancer according to histological type. *Int J Cancer* 2004;112:451e7.
[19] Vikis H, Sato M, James M, et al. EGFR-T790M is a rare lung cancer susceptibility allele with enhanced kinase activity. *Cancer Res* 2007;67:4665e70.
[20] Mulloy R, Ferrand A, Kim Y, et al. Epidermal growth factor receptor mutants from human lung cancers exhibit enhanced catalytic activity and increased sensitivity to gefitinib. *Cancer Res* 2007;67:2325e30.
[21] Pao W, Miller V, Zakowski M, et al. EGF receptor gene mutations are common in lung cancers from 'never smokers' and are associated with sensitivity of tumors to gefitinib and erlotinib. *Proc Natl Acad Sci U S A* 2004;101:13306e11.
[22] Inoue A, Kobayashi K, Usui K, et al. First-line gefitinib for patients with advanced non-small-cell lung cancer harboring epidermal growth factor receptor mutations without indication for chemotherapy. *J Clin Oncol* 2009;27:1394e400.

[23] Mitsudomi T, Morita S, Yatabe Y, et al. Gefitinib versus cisplatin plus docetaxel in patients with non-small-cell lung cancer harbouring mutations of the epidermal growth factor receptor (WJTOG3405): an open label, randomised phase 3 trial. *Lancet Oncol* 2010;11:121e8.

[24] Inoue A, Kobayashi K, Maemondo M, et al. A randomized phase III study comparing gefitinib with carboplatin (CBDCA) plus paclitaxel (TXL) for the first-line treatment of non-small cell lung cancer (NSCLC) with sensitive EGFR mutations:NEJ002 study. *Eur J Cancer Suppl* 2009;7:Abstract 9 LBA.

[25] Lee J, Park K, Kim SW. A randomized phase III study of gefinitib (IRESSATM) versus standard chemotherapy (gemcitabane plus cisplatin) as a first-line treatment for never smokers with advanced or metastatic adenocarcinoma of the lung. 13th World Conference on Lung Cancer. San Francisco, *J Thorac Oncol* 2009;4(Suppl 1):S283e4.

[26] Pirker R, Pereira JR, von Pawel J, et al. EGFR expression as a predictor of survival for first-line chemotherapy plus cetuximab in patients with advanced non-small-cell lung cancer: analysis of data from the phase 3 FLEX study. *Lung Cancer*. 2012;77(2):376-82.

[27] Porta R, Queralt C, Cardenal F, et al. Erlotinib customization based on epidermal growth factor receptor (EGFR) mutations in stage IV non-small-cell lung cancer (NSCLC) patients (p). *J Clin Oncol* 2008;26:Abstract 8038.

[28] Mok TS, Wu YL, Thongprasert S, et al. Gefitinib or carboplatin-paclitaxel in pulmonary adenocarcinoma. *N Engl J Med* 2009;361:947e57.

[29] Rosell R, Perez-Roca L, Sanchez JJ, et al. Customized treatment in non-small-cell lung cancer based on EGFR mutations and BRCA1 mRNA expression. *PLoS One* 2009;4:e5133.

[30] Han SW, Kim TY, Hwang PG, et al. Predictive and prognostic impact of epidermal growth factor receptor mutation in non-small-cell lung cancer patients treated with gefitinib. *J Clin Oncol* 2005;23:2493e501.

[31] Takano T, Ohe Y, Sakamoto H, et al. Epidermal growth factor receptor gene mutations and increased copy numbers predict gefitinib sensitivity in patients with recurrent non-small-cell lung cancer. *J Clin Oncol* 2005;23:6829e37.

[32] Kobayashi S, Boggon TJ, Dayaram T, et al. EGFR mutation and resistance of nonsmall-cell lung cancer to gefitinib. *N Engl J Med* 2005;352:786e92.

[33] Pao W, Miller VA. Epidermal growth factor receptor mutations, small- molecule kinase inhibitors, and non-small-cell lung cancer: current knowledge and future directions. *J Clin Oncol* 2005;23:2556e68.

[34] Bean J, Riely G, Balak M, et al. Acquired resistance to epidermal growth factor receptor (EGFR) kinase inhibitors associated with a novel T854A mutation in a patient with EGFR-mutant lung adenocarcinoma. *American Society of Clinical Oncology*. Chicago, IL, 2008.

[35] Li D, Shimamura T, Ji H, et al. Bronchial and peripheral murine lung carcinomas induced by T790M-L858R mutant EGFR respond to HKI-272 and rapamycin combination therapy. *Cancer Cell* 2007;12:81e93.

[36] Balak MN, Gong Y, Riely GJ, et al. Novel D761Y and common secondary T790M mutations in epidermal growth factor receptor-mutant lung adenocarcinomas with acquired resistance to kinase inhibitors. *Clin Cancer Res* 2006;12:6494e501.

[37] Johnson BE, Jackman D, Janne PA. Impact of EGFR mutations on treatment of non-small cell lung cancer. *Canc Chemother Pharmacol* 2006;58(Suppl 7):5e9.
[38] Gazdar AF. Activating and resistance mutations of EGFR in non-small-cell lung cancer: role in clinical response to EGFR tyrosine kinase inhibitors. *Oncogene* 2009;28(Suppl 1):S24e31.
[39] Pao W, Miller VA, Politi KA, et al. Acquired resistance of lung adenocarcinomas to gefitinib or erlotinib is associated with a second mutation in the EGFR kinase domain. *PLoS Med* 2005;2:e73.
[40] Gendreau SB, Ventura R, Keast P, et al. Inhibition of the T790M gatekeeper mutant of the epidermal growth factor receptor by EXEL-7647. *Clin Cancer Res* 2007;13:3713e23.
[41] Yun CH, Mengwasser KE, Toms AV, et al. The T790M mutation in EGFR kinase causes drug resistance by increasing the affinity for ATP. *Proc Natl Acad Sci U S A* 2008;105:2070e5.
[42] Kobayashi S, Ji H, Yuza Y, et al. An alternative inhibitor overcomes resistance caused by a mutation of the epidermal growth factor receptor. *Cancer Res* 2005;65:7096e101.
[43] Kwak EL, Sordella R, Bell DW, et al. Irreversible inhibitors of the EGF receptor may circumvent acquired resistance to gefitinib. *Proc Natl Acad Sci U S A* 2005;102:7665e70.
[44] Li D, Ambrogio L, Shimamura T, et al. BIBW2992, an irreversible EGFR/HER2 inhibitor highly effective in preclinical lung cancer models. *Oncogene* 2008;27:4702e11.
[45] Carter TA, Wodicka LM, Shah NP, et al. Inhibition of drug-resistant mutants of ABL, KIT, and EGF receptor kinases. *Proc Natl Acad Sci U S A* 2005;102:11011e16.
[46] Regales L, Gong Y, Shen R, et al. Dual targeting of EGFR can overcome a major drug resistance mutation in mouse models of EGFR mutant lung cancer. *J Clin Invest* 2009;119:3000e10.
[47] Maheswaran S, Sequist LV, Nagrath S, et al. Detection of mutations in EGFR in circulating lung-cancer cells. *N Engl J Med* 2008;359:366e77.
[48] Inukai M, Toyooka S, Ito S, et al. Presence of epidermal growth factor receptor gene T790M mutation as a minor clone in non-small cell lung cancer. *Cancer Res* 2006;66:7854e8.
[49] Guix M, Faber AC, Wang SE, et al. Acquired resistance to EGFR tyrosine kinase inhibitors in cancer cells is mediated by loss of IGF-binding proteins. *J Clin Invest* 2008;118:2609e19.
[50] Engelman JA, Zejnullahu K, Mitsudomi T, et al. MET amplification leads to gefitinib resistance in lung cancer by activating ERBB3 signaling. *Science* 2007;316:1039e43.
[51] Dvorak HF, Detmar M, Claffey KP, et al. Vascular permeability factor/vascular endothelial growth factor: an important mediator of angiogenesis in malignancy and inflammation. *Int Arch Allergy Immunol* 1995;107(1-3):233-5.
[52] Shimanuki Y, Takahashi K, Cui R, et al. Role of serum vascular endothelial growth factor in the prediction of angiogenesis and prognosis for non-small cell lung cancer. *Lung* 2005;183(1):29-42.
[53] Zhan P, Wang J, Lv XJ, et al., Prognostic value of vascular endothelial growth factor expression in patients with lung cancer: a systematic review with meta-analysis. *J Thorac Oncol.* 2009 Sep;4(9):1094-103.

[54] Savai R, Langheinrich AC, Schermuly RT, et al. Evaluation of angiogenesis using micro-computed tomography in a xenograft mouse model of lung cancer. *Neoplasia* 2009;11(1):48-56.

[55] Takayama K, Ueno H, Nakanishi Y, et al. Suppression of tumor angiogenesis and growth by gene transfer of a soluble form of vascular endothelial growth factor receptor into a remote organ. *Cancer Res* 2000;60(8):2169-77.

[56] Sandler A, Gray R, Perry MC, et al. Paclitaxel-carboplatin alone or with bevacizumab for non-small-cell lung cancer. *N Engl J Med* 2006;355(24):2542-50.

[57] Wilhelm SM, Carter C, Tang LY et al. BAY 43-9006 exhibits broad spectrum oral antitumor activity and targets the RAF/MEK/ERK pathway and receptor tyrosine kinases involved in tumor progression and angiogenesis. *Cancer Res* 2005;64:7099–7109.

[58] Scagliotti G, Novello S, von Pawel J, et al. Phase III study of carboplatin and paclitaxel alone or with sorafenib in advanced non-small-cell lung cancer. *J Clin Oncol* 2010;28(11):1835-42.

[59] Kim ES, Herbst RS, Wistuba II, et al. The BATTLE Trial: personalizing therapy for lung cancer. *Cancer Discov* 2011;1:44-53.

[60] Blumenschein GR Jr, Kabbinavar F, Menon H, et al. A phase II, multicenter, open-label randomized study of motesanib or bevacizumab in combination with paclitaxel and carboplatin for advanced nonsquamous non-small-cell lung cancer. *Ann Oncol* 2011;22(9):2057-67.

[61] Amgen. A *Phase III, multicenter, randomized, placebo-controlled, double blind trial of AMG 706 in combination with paclitaxel and carboplatin for advanced non-small cell lung cancer.*

[62] Tew WP, Gordon M, Murren J, et al. Phase 1 study of aflibercept administeredsubcutaneously to patients with advanced solid tumors. *Clin Cancer Res*2010;16(1):358-66.

[63] Wedge SR, Ogilvie DJ, Dukes M, et al. ZD6474 inhibits vascular endothelial growth factor signaling, angiogenesis, and tumor growth following oral administration. *Cancer Res* 2002;62(16):4645-55

[64] Natale RB, Bodkin D, Govindan R. et al. Vandetanib versus gefitinib in patients with advanced non-small-cell lung cancer: results from a two-part, double-blind, randomized phase ii study. *J Clin Oncol.* 2009 May 20;27(15):2523-9.

[65] Herbst RS, Sun Y, Eberhardt WE, Germonpré P, Saijo N, Zhou C, et al. Vandetanib plus docetaxel versus docetaxel as second line treatment for patients with advanced non-small-cell lung cancer (ZODIAC): a double-blind, randomised, phase 3 trial. *Lancet Oncol* 2010;11:619-26

[66] De Boer R, Arrieta O, Gottfried M, Blackhall FH, Raats J, Yang CH, et al. Vandetanib plus pemetrexed versus pemetrexed as second-line therapy in patients with advanced non-small cell lung cancer (NSCLC): A randomized, double blind phase III trial (ZEAL) [abstract]. *J Clin Oncol* 2009;s27:8010.

[67] Natale RB, Thongprasert S, Greco FA, Thomas M, Tsai CM, Sunpaweravong P, et al. Vandetanib versus erlotinib in patients with advanced non-small cell lung cancer (NSCLC) after failure of at least one prior cytotoxic chemotherapy: A randomized, double-blind phase III trial (ZEST) [abstract]. *J Clin Oncol* 2009;s27:8009.

[68] Lee J, Hirsch V, Park K, Qin S, Blajman CR, Perng R, et al. Vandetanib versus placebo in patients with advanced non-small cell lung cancer (NSCLC) after prior therapy with an EGFR tyrosine kinase inhibitor (TKI): A randomized, double-blind phase III trial (ZEPHYR) [abstract]. *J Clin Oncol* 2010;s28:7525.

[69] Shiota M, Fujimoto J, Semba T, Satoh H, Yamamoto T, Mori S: Hyperphosphorylation of a novel 80 kDa protein-tyrosine kinase similar to Ltk in a human Ki-1 lymphoma cell line, AMS3. *Oncogene* 1994, 9:1567-74.

[70] Takeuchi, K, Choi YL, Togashi Y, Soda M, Hatano S, Inamura K, Takada S, Ueno T, Yamashita Y, Satoh Y, Okumura S, Nakagawa K, Ishikawa Y, Mano H: KIF5B-ALK, a novel fusion oncokinase identified by an immunohistochemistry-based diagnostic system for ALK-positive lung cancer. *Clin Cancer Res* 2009;15:3143-9.

[71] Wong DW, Leung EL, Wong SK, Tin VP, Sihoe AD, Cheng LC, Au JS, Chung LP, Wong MP: A novel KIF5B-ALK variant in nonsmall cell lung cancer. *Cancer* 2011, 117:2709-18.

[72] Morris SW, Kirstein MN, Valentine MB, et al. Fusion of a kinase gene, ALK, to a nucleolar protein gene, NPM, in non-Hodgkin's lymphoma. *Science* 1994;263:1281–4.

[73] Soda M, Choi YL, Enomoto M, et al. Identification of the transforming EML4–ALK fusion gene in non-small-cell lung cancer. *Nature* 2007;448:561–6.

[74] Inamura K, Takeuchi K, Togashi Y, et al. EML4–ALK lung cancers are characterized by rare other mutations, a ttf-1 cell lineage, an acinar histology, and young onset. *Mod Pathol* 2009;22:508–15.

[75] Shaw AT, Yeap BY, Mino–Kenudson M, et al. Clinical features and outcome of patients with non-small-cell lung cancer who harbour EML4–ALK. *J Clin Oncol* 2009;27:4247–53.

[76] Subramanian J, Corrales L, Soulieres D, Morgensztern D, Govindan R. Summary of presentations from the 46th Annual Meeting of the American Society of Clinical Oncology (2010) focus on tumor biology and biomarkers related to lung cancer. *J Thorac Oncol* 2011;6:399–403.

[77] Tiseo M, Gelsomino F, Boggiani D, et al. EGFR and *EML4-ALK* mutations in NSCLC: a case report of erlotinib-resistant patient with both concomitant mutations. *Lung Cancer.* 2011;71:241-3.

[78] Kwak EL, Bang YJ, Camidge DR, et al. Anaplastic lymphoma kinase inhibition in non-small-cell lung cancer. *N Engl J Med* 2010;363(18):1693-703.

[79] Crinò L, Kim D, Riely GJ, et al. Initial phase II results with crizotinib in advanced ALK-positive non-small cell lung cancer (NSCLC): PROFILE 1005. *J Clin Oncol.* 2011;29 (suppl 15):Abstract 7514.

[80] Ou SH. Crizotinib: a novel and first-in-class multitargeted tyrosine kinase inhibitor for the treatment of anaplastic lymphoma kinase rearranged non-small cell lung cancer and beyond. *Drug Des Devel Ther* 2011;5:471–85.

[81] Kwak EL, Camidge DR, Clark J, et al. Clinical activity observed in a phase i dose escalation trial of an oral c-Met and Alk inhibitor, PF-02341066 [abstract 3509]. *J Clin Oncol* 2009;27.

[82] Yang P, Kulig K, Boland JM, et al. Worse disease-free survival in never-smokers with ALK+ lung adenocarcinoma. *J Thorac Oncol* 2012;7:90–7.

[83] Katayama R, Shaw AT, Khan TM, et al. Mechanisms of acquired crizotinib resistance in ALK-rearranged lung Cancers. *Sci Transl Med* 2012;Feb 8;4(120):120ra17. Choi

YL, Soda M, Yamashita Y, et al. EML4–ALK mutations in lung cancer that confer resistance to Alk inhibitors. *N Engl J Med* 2010;363:1734–9.

[84] Katayama R, Khan TM, Benes C, et al. Therapeutic strategies to overcome crizotinib resistance in non-small cell lung cancers harboring the fusion oncogene EML4–ALK. *Proc Natl Acad Sci U S A* 2011;108:7535–40.

[85] Sakamoto H, Tsukaguchi T, Hiroshima S, et al. CH5424802, a selective Alk inhibitor capable of blocking the resistant gatekeeper mutant. *Cancer Cell* 2011;19:679–90.

[86] Bergethon K, Shaw AT, Ou SH, et al. ROS1 rearrangements define a unique molecular class of lung cancers. *J Clin Oncol* 2012;30:863–70.

[87] Ou SH, Kwak EL, Siwak-Tapp C, et al. 16. Activity of crizotinib (PF02341066), a dual mesenchymal-epithelial transition (MET) and anaplastic lymphoma kinase (ALK) inhibitor, in a non-small cell lung cancer patient with de novo MET amplification. *J Thorac Oncol*. 2011 May;6(5):942-6.

[88] Camidge DR, Kono SA, Lu X, et al. Anaplastic lymphoma kinase gene rearrangements in non-small cell lung cancer are associated with prolonged progression-free survival on pemetrexed. *J Thorac Oncol* 2011;6:774–80.

[89] Takeda M, Okamoto I, Sakai K, et al. Successful long-term treatment with pemetrexed of NSCLC associated with EML4– ALK and low thymidylate synthase expression. *Clin Lung Cancer* 2012;13:157–9.

[90] Lee JO, Kim TM, Lee SH, et al. Anaplastic lymphoma kinase translocation: a predictive biomarker of pemetrexed in patients with non-small cell lung cancer. *J Thorac Oncol* 2011;6:1474–80.

[91] Chang EH, Gonda MA, Ellis RW, Scolnick EM, Lowy DR. Human genome contains four genes homologous to transforming genes of Harvey and Kirsten murine sarcoma viruses. *Proc Natl Acad Sci U S A* 1982;79:4848–52.

[92] Vakiani E, Solit DB. KRAS and BRAF: drug targets and predictive biomarkers. *J Pathol* 2011;223:219–29.

[93] Xu N, Lao Y, Zhang Y, Gillespie DA. Akt: a double-edged sword in cell proliferation and genome stability. *J Oncol* 2012;2012:951724.

[94] Forbes S, Clements J, Dawson E, et al. COSMIC 2005. *Br J Cancer* 2006;94:318–22.

[95] Riely GJ, Kris MG, Rosenbaum D, et al. Frequency and distinctive spectrum of KRAS mutations in never smokers with lung adenocarcinoma. *Clin Cancer Res* 2008;14:5731–4.

[96] Ihle NT, Byers LA, Kim ES, et al. Effect of KRAS oncogene substitutions on protein behavior: implications for signalling and clinical outcome. *J Natl Cancer Inst* 2012;104:228–39.

[97] Sun Y, Ren Y, Fang Z, et al. Lung adenocarcinoma from East Asian never-smokers is a disease largely defined by targetable oncogenic mutant kinases. *J Clin Oncol.* 2010 Oct 20;28(30):4616-20.

[98] Eberhard DA, Johnson BE, Amler LC, et al. Mutations in the epidermal growth factor receptor and in *KRAS* are predictive and prognostic indicators in patients with non-small–cell lung cancer treated with chemotherapy alone and in combination with erlotinib. *J Clin Oncol.* 2005;23:5900-5909.

[99] Massarelli E, Varella-Garcia M, Tang X, et al. *KRAS* mutation is an important predictor of resistance to therapy with epidermal growth factor receptor tyrosine kinase inhibitors in non-small cell lung cancer. *Clin Cancer Res.* 2007;13:2890-2896.

[100] Adjei AA. K-ras as a target for Lung Cancer Therapy. *Journal of Thoracic Oncology* 2008; 3:6,S160-163.

[101] Acquaviva J, Smith DL, Sang J et al. Targeting KRAS-Mutant Non-Small Cell Lung Cancer with the Hsp90 Inhibitor Ganetespib. Mol Cancer Ther. 2012; Nov30.

[102] Bacus S. *KRAS* mutation and amplification status predicts sensitivity to antifolate therapies in non-small cell lung cancer [abstract PR-2*]. Mol Cancer Ther* 2011;10 (suppl 1).

[103] Yarden Y, Sliwkowski MX. Untangling the ErbB signalling network. *Nat Rev Mol Cell Biol.* 2001;2:127–137.

[104] Tan D, Deeb G,Wang J, et al. HER-2/neu protein expression and gene alteration in stage I-IIIA non-small-cell lung cancer: a study of140 cases using a combination of high throughput tissue microarray, immunohistochemistry, and fluorescent in situ hybridization. *Diagn Mol Pathol.* 2003;12:201-11.

[105] Cappuzzo F, Varella-Garcia M, Shigematsu H, et al. Increased HER2 gene copy number is associated with response to gefitinib therapy in epidermal growth factor receptor-positive non-small-cell lung cancer patients. *J Clin Onco*l. 2005;23:5007-18.

[106] Pellegrini C, Falleni M, Marchetti A, et al. HER-2/Neu alterations in non-small cell lung cancer: a comprehensive evaluation by real time reverse transcription-PCR, fluorescence in situ hybridization, and immunohistochemistry. *Clin Cancer Re*s 2003;9:3645-52.

[107] Hirsch FR, Varella-Garcia M, McCoy J, et al. Increased epidermal growth factor receptor gene copy number detected by fluorescence in situ hybridization associates with increased sensitivity to gefitinib in patients with bronchioloalveolar carcinoma subtypes: a Southwest Oncology Group Study. *J Clin Oncol.* 2005;23:6838-45.

[108] Stephens P, Hunter C, Bignell G, et al. Intragenic ERBB2 kinase mutations in tumours. *Nature*. 2004;431:525-6.

[109] Wang SE, Narasanna A, Perez-Torres M, et al. HER2 kinase domain mutation results in constitutive phosphorylation and activation of HER2 and EGFR and resistance to EGFR tyrosine kinase inhibitors. *Cancer Cell.* 2006;10:25–38.

[110] Shigematsu H, Takahashi T, Nomura M, et al. Somatic mutations of the HER2 kinase domain in lung adenocarcinomas. *Cancer Res.* 2005;65: 1642–1646.

[111] Pao W, Girard N. New driver mutations in non-small-cell lung cancer. *Lancet Oncol.* 2011;12(2):175-80.

[112] Gatzemeier U, Groth G, Butts C, et al. Randomized phase II trial of gemcitabine-cisplatin with or withour trastuzumab in HER2-positive non-small cell lung cancer. *Ann Oncology*. 2004; 15(1):19-27.

[113] Hirsch FR, Langer CJ. The role of HER2/neu expression and trastuzumab in non-small cell lung cancer. *Semin Oncol.* 2004; 31:75-82.

[114] Ross HJ, Blumenschein GR Jr, Aisner J, et al. Randomized phase II multicenter trial of two schedules of lapatinib as first- or second-line monotherapy in patients with advanced or metastatic non-small cell lung cancer. *Clin Cancer Res*. 2010;16:1938 – 1949.

[115] Cappuzzo F, Bemis L, Varella-Garcia M. HER2 mutation and response to trastuzumab therapy in non-small cell lung cancer. *N Engl J Med*. 2006; 354: 2619-2621.

[116] De Greve J, Teugels E, De Mey J, et al. Clinical activity of BIBW2992, an irreversible inhibitor of EGFR and HER2 in adenocarcinoma of the lung with mutations in the kinase domain of HER2neu. *J Thorac Oncol*. 2009; 4:S307 (abstr).
[117] Engelman JA, Zejnullahu K, Gale CM, et al. PF00299804, an irreversiblepan-ERBB inhibitor, is effective in lung cancer models with EGFR and ERBB2 mutations that are resistant to gefitinib. *Cancer Res*. 2007;67:11924 –11932.
[118] Davies H, Bignell GR, Cox C, et al. Mutations of the *BRAF* gene in human cancer. *Nature*. 2002;417:949–54.
[119] Naoki K, Chen TH, Richards WG, et al. Missense mutations of the *BRAF* gene in human lung Adenocarcinoma. *Cancer Res*. 2002;62:7001–03.
[120] Sasaki H, Kawano O, Endo K, et al. Uncommon V599E *BRAF* mutations in Japanese patients with lung cancer. *J Surg Res*. 2006;133:203–06.
[121] Tsai J, Lee JT, Wang W, et al. Discovery of a selective inhibitor of oncogenic B-Raf kinase with potent antimelanoma activity. *Proc Natl Acad Sci USA*. 2008;105:3041–46.
[122] Poulikakos PI, Zhang C, Bollag G, et al. RAF inhibitors transactivate RAF dimers and ERK signalling in cells with wild-type BRAF. *Nature*. 2010;464:427–30.
[123] Heidorn SJ, Milagre C, Whittaker S, et al. Kinase-Dead BRAF and Oncogenic RAS Cooperate to Drive Tumor Progression through CRAF. *Cell*. 2010;140:209–221.
[124] Bollag G. *Overcoming the paradoxical pathway activation of first-generation RAF kinase inhibitors AACR annual meeting;* Orlando, FL. 2011.
[125] Seki T, Hagiya M, Shimonishi M, et al. Organization of the human hepatocyte growth factor-encoding gene. *Gene*. 1991;102:213–19.
[126] Feng Y, Thiagarajan PS, Ma PC. Met signaling: novel targeted inhibition and its clinical development in lung cancer. J Thorac Oncol. 2012;7:459–67.
[127] Ding L, Getz G, Wheeler DA, et al. Somatic mutations affect key pathways in lung adenocarcinoma. *Nature*. 2008;455:1069–75.
[128] Onozato R, Kosaka T, Kuwano H, et al. Activation of MET by gene amplifi cation or by splice mutations deleting the juxtamembrane domain in primary resected lung cancers. *J Thorac Oncol*. 2009;4:5–11.
[129] Kong-Beltran M, Seshagiri S, Zha J, et al. Somatic mutations lead to an oncogenic deletion of met in lung cancer. *Cancer Res*. 2006;66:283–89.
[130] Ma PC, Tretiakova MS, MacKinnon AC, et al. Expression and mutational analysis of MET in human solid cancers. *Genes Chromosomes Cancer*. 2008;47:1025–37.
[131] Cappuzzo F, Jänne PA, Skokan M, et al. MET increased gene copy number and primary resistance to gefitinib therapy in non-small-cell lung cancer patients. *Ann Oncol*. 2009;20:298–304.
[132] Bean J, Brennan C, Shih JY, et al. MET amplification occurs with or without T790M mutations in EGFR mutant lung tumors with acquired resistance to gefitinib or erlotinib. *Proc Natl Acad Sci USA*. 2007;104:20932–7.
[133] Lennerz JK, Kwak EL, Ackerman A, et al. MET amplification identifies a small and aggressive subgroup of esophagogastric adenocarcinoma with evidence of responsiveness to crizotinib. *J Clin Oncol*. 2011;29:4803–10.
[134] Chi A, Kwak EL, Clark JW, et al. Clinical improvement and rapid radiographic regression induced by a Met inhibitor in a patient with MET-amplified glioblastoma. *Clin Oncol*. 2011; 29:(suppl; abstr 2072).

[135] Sequist LV, von Pawel J, Garmey EG, et al. Randomized phase II study of erlotinib plus tivantinib versus erlotinib plus placebo in previously treated non-small-cell lung cancer. *J Clin Oncol*. 2011;29:3307-15.

[136] Spigel DR, Ervin TJ, Ramlau R, et al. Final efficacy results from OAM4558g, a randomized phase II study evaluating MetMAb or placebo in combination with erlotinib in advanced NSCLC. *J Clin Oncol.* 2011;29(suppl; abstr 7505).

[137] Whitman M, Kaplan DR, Schaffhausen B, et al. Association of phosphatidylinositol kinase activity with polyoma middle-T competent for transformation. *Nature*. 1985; 315(6016):239-42.

[138] Ji M, Guan H, Gao C, et al. Highly frequent promoter methylation and PIK3CA amplification in non-small cell lung cancer (NSCLC). *BMC Cancer.* 11:147.

[139] Papadimitrakopoulou, V. Development of PI3K/AKT/mTOR pathway inhibitors and their application in personalized therapy for non-small-cell lung cancer. *J Thorac Oncol*. 2012;7(8):1315-26.

[140] Gately K, Al-Alao B, T Dhillon, et al. Overexpression of the mammalian target of rapamycin (mTOR) and angioinvasion are poor prognostic factors in early stage NSCLC: a verification study. *Lung Cancer*. 2012;75(2):217-22.

[141] Courtney K, Corcoran RB, Engelman JA. The PI3K pathway as drug target in human cancer. *J Clin Oncol*. 2010;28(6):1075-83.

[142] Downward J. Targeting RAS signalling pathways in cancer therapy. *Nat Rev Cancer*. 2003; 3(1):11-22.

[143] Adjei AA. The role of mitogen-activated ERK-kinase inhibitors in lung cancer therapy. *Clin Lung Cancer*. 2005;**7**(3):221-3.

[144] Marks JL, Gong Y, Chitale D, et al. Novel MEK1 mutation identified by mutational analysis of epidermal growth factor receptor signaling pathway genes in lung adenocarcinoma. *Cancer Res*. 2008;68(14):5524-8.

[145] Hainsworth JD, Cebotaru CL, Kanarev V, et al. A phase II, open-label, randomized study to assess the efficacy and safety of AZD6244 (ARRY-142886) versus pemetrexed in patients with non-small cell lung cancer who have failed one or two prior chemotherapeutic regimens. *J Thorac Oncol.* 2010;5(10):1630-6.

[146] Rinehart J, Adjei AA, Lorusso PM, et al. Multicenter phase II study of the oral MEK inhibitor, CI-1040, in patients with advanced non-small-cell lung, breast, colon, and pancreatic cancer. *J Clin Oncol*. 2004;22(22):4456-62.

[147] Hersey P, Bastholt L, Chiarion-Sileni V, et al. Small molecules and targeted therapies in distant metastatic disease. Ann Oncol. 2009,20 Suppl 6:vi35-40.

[148] Staehler M, Rohrmann K, Haseke N, et al. Targeted agents for the treatment of advanced renal cell carcinoma. *Curr Drug Targets*. 2005;6(7):835-46.

[149] Wong H, Vernillet L, Peterson A, et al. Bridging the gap between preclinical and clinical studies using pharmacokinetic-pharmacodynamic modeling: an analysis of GDC-0973, a MEK inhibitor. *Clin Cancer Res.* 2012;18:3090-9.

[150] Sos ML, Fischer S, Ullrich R, et al. Identifying genotype-dependent efficacy of single and combined PI3K- and MAPK-pathway inhibition in cancer. *Proc Natl Acad Sci USA*. 2009;106:18351-6.

[151] Engelman JA, Chen L, Tan X, et al. Effective use of PI3K and MEK inhibitors to treat mutant Kras G12D and PIK3CA H1047R murine lung cancers. *Nat Med.* 2008;14:1351-6.

[152] Mirzoeva OK, Das D, Heiser LM, et al. Basal subtype and MAPK/ERK kinase (MEK)-phosphoinositide 3-kinase feedback signaling determine susceptibility of breast cancer cells to MEK inhibition. *Cancer Res.* 2009;69:565-72.
[153] Hoeflich KP, O'Brien C, Boyd Z, et al. In vivo antitumor activity of MEK and phosphatidylinositol 3-kinase inhibitors in basal-like breast cancer models. *Clin Cancer Res.* 2009;15:4649-64.
[154] Zou ZQ, Zhang LN, Wang F, et al. The novel dual PI3K/mTOR inhibitor GDC-0941 synergizes with the MEK inhibitor U0126 in non-small cell lung cancer cells. *Mol Med Report.* 2012;5:503-8.
[155] LeRoith D, Roberts CT Jr. The insulin-like growth factor receptor system and cancer. *Cancer Lett.* 2003;195:127-137.
[156] Riedemann J, Takiguchi M, Sohail M, Macaulay VM. The EGF receptor interacts with the type 1 IGF receptor and regulates its stability. *Biochemical and Biophysical Research Communications.* 2007;355:707–714.
[157] Ludovini V, Bellezza G, Pistola L, et al. High coexpression of both insulin-like growth factor receptor-1 (IGFR-1) and epidermal growth factor receptor (EGFR) is associated with shorter disease-free survival in resected non-small-cell lung cancer patients. *Annals of Oncology.* 2009;20(5):842-9.
[158] Lee YC, Jeon HJ, Kim JH et al. Clinical significance of insulin-like growth factor-1 receptor expression in stage I non-small-cell lung cancer: immunohistochemical analysis. *Korean J Intern Med.* 2008;23(3):116–120.
[159] Cappuzzo F, Tallini G, Finocchiaro G, et al. Insulin-like growth factor receptor 1 (IGF1R) expression and survival in surgically resected non-small-cell lung cancer (NSCLC) patients. *Annals of Oncology.* 2010;21(3):562-7.
[160] Merrick DT, Dziadziuszko R, Szostakiewicz B, et al. High insulin-like growth factor1 receptor (IGF1R) expression is associated with poor survival in surgically treated non-small cell lung cancer (NSCLC) patients (pts*). J Clin Oncol* 2007; 25:18s (Abstr 7550).
[161] Gately K, Collins I, Forde L, et al. A role for IGF-1R-targeted therapies in small-cell lung cancer? *Clin Lung Cancer.* 2011;12(1):38-42.
[162] Morgillo F, Woo JK, Kim ES, et al. Heterodimerization of Insulin-like Growth Factor Receptor/Epidermal Growth Factor Receptor and Induction of Survivin Expression Counteract the Antitumor Action of Erlotinib. *Cancer Res.* 2006;66(20):10100-11.
[163] Karp DD, Paz-Ares LG, Novello S, et al. Phase II study of the anti-insulin-like growth factor type 1 receptor antibody CP-751,871 in combination with paclitaxel and carboplatin in previously untreated, locally advanced, or metastatic non-small-cell lung cancer. *J Clin On*col. 2009;27(15):2516–2522.
[164] Jassem J, Langer CM, Karp DD, et al. Randomized, open label, phase III trial of figitumumab in combination with paclitaxel and carboplatin *versus* paclitaxel and carboplatin in patients with non-small cell lung cancer. *J Clin Oncol.* 2010;28(15s):abstract 7500.
[165] Wan X, Harkavy B, Shen N, et al. Rapamycin induces feedback activation of Akt signaling through an IGF-1R dependent mechanism. *Oncogene.* 2007;26:1392–1340.
[166] Naing A, Kurzrok R, Burger A, et al. Phase I trial of cixutumumab combined with temsirolimus in patients with advanced cancer. *Clin Cancer Res.* 2011;17(18):6052-60.

[167] Tsimberidou AM, Iskander NG, Hong DS, et al. Personalized medicine in a phase I clinical trials program: the MD anderson cancer center initiative. *Clin Cancer Res.* 2012;18(22):6373-83

In: Lung Cancer: A Comprehensive Overview
Editor: Kathy Gately
ISBN: 978-1-62618-447-3


*Chapter VIII*

# Molecular Mechanisms of Cisplatin Resistance in Lung Cancer

***Martin P. Barr*** [*] ***and Ken O'Byrne***
Thoracic Oncology Research Group, Institute of Molecular Medicine,
Trinity Centre for Health Sciences, St. James's Hospital
and Trinity College Dublin, Ireland

## Abstract

Cisplatin is one of the most potent anticancer agents, displaying significant clinical activity against a variety of solid tumours. To date, cisplatin-based combination treatment remains the most effective systemic chemotherapy for non-small cell lung cancer (NSCLC) patients. Unfortunately, the outcome of cisplatin therapy in NSCLC has reached a plateau due to the development of both intrinsic and acquired resistance that have become a major obstacle in the use of cisplatin in the clinical setting. The molecular mechanisms that underlie chemoresistance are largely unknown. Mechanisms of acquired resistance to cisplatin include reduced intracellular accumulation of the drug, enhanced drug inactivation by metallothionine and glutathione, increased repair activity of DNA damage, and altered expression of oncogenes and regulatory proteins. Cisplatin-induced cytotoxicity is mediated through the induction of apoptosis and cell cycle arrest as a result of cisplatin-DNA adduct formation, which in turn, activates multiple signaling pathways and mediators. These include p53, Bcl-2 family, caspases, cyclins, CDKs, MAPK and PI3K/Akt. Increased expression of anti-apoptotic genes and mutations in the intrinsic apoptotic pathway may also contribute to the inability of cells to detect DNA damage or to induce apoptosis. This chapter will provide an insight into the mechanisms involved in cisplatin resistance and a better understanding of the molecular basis of the cellular response to cisplatin-based chemotherapy in lung cancer.

[*] Email: mbarr@stjames.ie.

# Introduction

Since its approval by the FDA (Food and Drug Administration) in 1978, cisplatin (cis-diamminedichloroplatinum(II) or CDDP), has been largely employed as a platinum agent in the treatment of a wide spectrum of solid malignancies including testicular, bladder, ovarian, colorectal, lung and head and neck cancers [1-4]. Cisplatin works by binding to DNA leading to different types of DNA lesions. The most frequently observed of these lesions include intra-strand DNA adducts between two guanines and adenines which account for approximately 25% of lesions (Figure 1). Inter-strand crosslinks on the other hand which occur between two guanines on opposite DNA strands account for less than 5% of all cisplatin-induced lesions. Although there is still some controversy surrounding which cross-links are responsible for cisplatin-induced toxicity, it has been proposed that cisplatin damage induces an arrest in the G2 phase of the cell cycle and subsequent apoptosis [5]. In reviewing mechanisms of platinum resistance, data strongly suggest similar mechanisms for both cisplatin and carboplatin. However, these are not always identical. The latter is a second generation platinum compound with a broad spectrum of anti-neoplastic properties. While carboplatin possesses anti-tumour activity similar to that of its parent compound, cisplatin, it is more stable and less toxic. Oxaliplatin, an organoplatinum complex, exhibits distinct pharmacological and immunological properties from cisplatin and carboplatin. However, despite the fact that cisplatin-refractory cancers are generally considered to be sensitive to oxaliplatin, clinical data suggest that there may be some degree of cross-resistance [6]. The efficacy of cisplatin in the treatment of cancer is limited due to resistance which may be either intrinsic (as observed in patients with colorectal, prostate and lung cancer) or acquired following cisplatin chemotherapy (often seen in patients with ovarian cancer). Mechanisms of cisplatin resistance have been studied in several preclinical studies and have been shown to be multifactorial. Some of the most critical molecular mechanisms that appear to account for the cisplatin-resistant phenotype include reduced intracellular accumulation of cisplatin, enhanced detoxification, aberrant DNA repair mechanisms and reduced apoptotic response, amongst others.

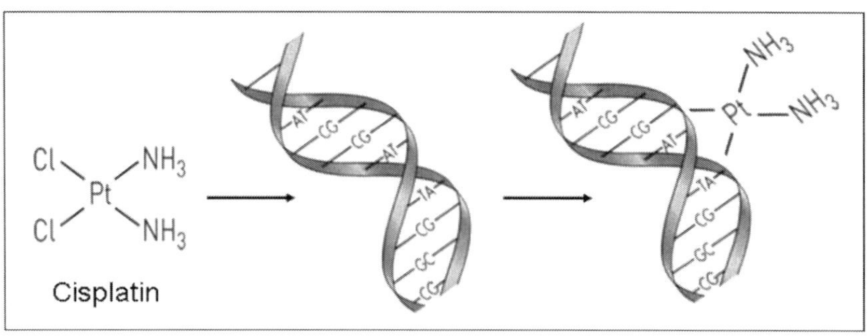


Figure 1. Structure and interaction of cisplatin with DNA. Cisplatin, an inorganic square planar complex reacts with DNA to induce its characteristic biological effects, which culminate in either repair of the DNA damage and cell survival, or activation of the irreversible apoptotic programme and subsequent cell death. It is generally accepted that the primary cytotoxic mode of action of cisplatin is the production of DNA adducts, the most prevalent adduct being the intra-strand linkage of two adjacent guanine bases.

Circumventing cisplatin resistance remains a critical goal for future anti-cancer therapy. While findings obtained to date have provided valuable information about the various factors implicated in cisplatin resistance, strategies to overcome this resistant phenotype may be exploited to reverse cisplatin resistance in the clinical setting.

# Resistance Mechanisms

## Intracellular Drug Accumulation

### *Drug Uptake*

Many resistant cell lines with acquired resistance to cisplatin have reduced cisplatin accumulation, in comparison to their parent counterparts [7]. Such findings suggest changes in the cisplatin transport system resulting in a decreased uptake and/or increased efflux of the drug as a mechanism of resistance. Cellular cisplatin uptake is not saturable with dose, but is altered by metabolic inhibitors which do not affect efflux [8]. Several studies found that cell membrane fluidity (which may potentially effect passive diffusion of a drug, or the activity of membrane transport systems) does not correlate with cisplatin uptake [9], while others suggested that resistant cell lines with reduced drug uptake have rigid cell membranes with high sphingomyelin and cholesterol content [10]]. Ganglioside expression has also been associated with cisplatin resistance [11]. More recently however, copper transporter 1 (CTR1), a transmembrane protein involved in copper homeostasis, has been shown to be involved in the uptake of cisplatin [12]. Copper transporters undergo rapid cytoplasmic internalisation following exposure to cisplatin, reducing transporter surface expression and limiting further cisplatin uptake. In studies using mouse $Ctr1^{-/-}$ embryonic fibroblasts, less cisplatin was shown to accumulate compared to their wild-type counterparts and were two- to three-fold more resistant to its cytotoxic effects [13]. Accordingly, cells pre-treated with the main CTR1 substrate, copper, are protected from cisplatin-induced cytotoxicity. On the contrary, copper chelators reverse this effect resulting in cisplatin accumulation and increased cytotoxicity [14].

### *Drug Efflux*

Copper competes with cisplatin for uptake into cells but also reduces cisplatin efflux and may therefore increase cisplatin net accumulation and cytotoxicity. Following the discovery of the role of CTR1 in cisplatin uptake, the copper-transporting P-type adenosine triphosphatases ATP7A and ATP7B were subsequently implicated in platinum efflux and resistance [15, 16]. Both proteins are up-regulated in cisplatin-resistant cancer cell lines and their transfection-enforced over-expression has been shown to drive the acquisition of the cisplatin-resistant phenotype. Over-expression of ATP7B is associated with poor outcome in oesophageal patients and squamous cell cancers of the head and neck treated with cisplatin [17], suggesting that the efflux of platinum drugs associated with ATP7B could potentially contribute to the clinical resistance of these drugs. Early reports suggested that alternative pumps may also play a role in cisplatin resistance by increasing cisplatin export, namely the multidrug resistance proteins MRP1, MRP2, MRP3 and MRP5 [18], P-glycoprotein [19] and major vault/lung resistance-related protein (MVP/LRP) [20]. Over-expression and RNAi studies point to MRP2 as the major ATPase responsible for an increased efflux of cisplatin in resistant cells [21] while more recent reports reinforce the notion that MRP2 expression levels may indeed predict tumour response to platinum-based therapies [22, 23].

### *Drug Detoxification*

Cisplatin resistance can arise as a result of increased inactivation of the drug by intracellular thiol-containing molecules such as glutathione (GSH) and metallothionein. Glutathione is a protective tri-peptide which scavanges free radicals thereby protecting cells from xenobiotic substances. Cisplatin can be conjugated with glutathione in a reaction catalysed by glutathione-S-transferase (GST), resulting in the prevention of its binding to DNA. The role of these inactivating thiol-containing proteins in cisplatin resistance has been extensively studied in cell lines and cancer tissues [24]. Increased GSH may cause resistance by binding/inactivating cisplatin, enhancing DNA repair or reducing cisplatin-induced oxidative stress [25]. Gene amplification [26], immunostaining [27], gene polymorphisms [29] and plasma levels [29] of GST-π (a member of the GSH superfamily of isoenzymes) correlate with clinical resistance to cisplatin, suggesting that platinum detoxification by GSH and GST may be of clinical importance. An increased concentration of glutathione or GST was correlated with cisplatin resistance in a number of different cancer cell lines such as ovarian, cervical, lung, embryonal and bladder [30-32]. In some studies, glutathione or GST expression was found to be associated with resistance to cisplatin in addition to poor clinical outcome in head and neck and NSCLC patients [26]. Other studies however, have reported no significant relationship of GST expression with either response rate or survival was observed in cervical, ovarian or NSCLC patients following treatment with cisplatin-based chemotherapy [33, 34]. It is of interest that glutathione S-conjugates are readily extruded by cells via MRP1 and MRP2 [35]. This may explain why the latter may more often be associated with cisplatin resistance than other ABC ATPases [36]. Other GSH-related enzymes have been linked to cisplatin resistance, such as gamma-glutamylcysteine synthetase [37], gamma-glutamyltransferase [38], glutamate cysteine ligase [39], GSH peroxidise [40], GSH reductase [41] and catalase [42]. The antioxidants superoxide dismutase and dihydrodiol dehydrogenase [43] have also been associated with cisplatin resistance in a number of preclinical systems. Sulphur-containing proteins involved in zinc homeostasis, know as the metallothioneins, have been associated with cisplatin resistance in a number of studies and correlate with clinical cisplatin resistance in hepatocellular carcinoma [8] and NSCLC [44].

## DNA Repair Mechanisms

The relevance of DNA repair in cisplatin resistance has been an area of interest for many years. The recognition of inter- and intra-strand DNA adducts and the consequent generation of apoptotic cell death is often impaired in cisplatin resistant cancer cells due to a variety of intracellular defects. Alternatively, many tumour cell lines with acquired resistance show an increased capacity for removal of cisplatin-induced DNA lesions in comparison with their cisplatin sensitive counterparts. In the human small cell lung cancer cell line, $GLC_{4}$-CDDP, increased removal of cisplatin-induced DNA adducts was found to be associated with increased resistance relative to the corresponding parental cells [45]. Similar observations have been reported in ovarian cancer cells [46] and colon carcinoma cells [47]. The latter study showed a higher extent of removal of DNA platination relative to the parental cells. While no enhanced removal of cisplatin-damaged DNA has been observed in other model systems of acquired resistance to cisplatin, such findings would suggest that cells may become resistant to cisplatin, in part, by increasing their DNA repair capacity [48]. On the contrary, a correlation between DNA repair capacity and cisplatin response has been reported in tumour cells exhibiting intrinsic sensitivity to cisplatin [49].

### *Nucleotide Excision Repair (NER)*

The majority of cisplatin-induced lesions are removed from DNA by nucleotide excision repair (NER) system. It is one of the main DNA repair pathways implicated in eradicating DNA lesions induced by many chemotherapeutic drugs, in particular cisplatin [50]. In this process, damaged nucleotides are excised from the DNA upon incision on both sides of the lesion, followed by DNA synthesis to replace the excised fragment [51]. Several protein factors participate in NER, where the core incision reaction requires the protein factors RPA (replication protein A), XPA (xeroderma pigmentosum complementation group A), XPC, XPG, TFIIH (containing XPB and XPD) and the ERCC1/XPF complex (excision repair cross-complementation group 1) [52]. Early reports pointed to a correlation between NER proficiency and cisplatin resistance in multiple preclinical models [53, 54], while subsequent studies reported this notion in the clinical setting of NSCLC [55]. ERCC1 expression (mRNA and protein) has been negatively correlated with survival and/or response to cisplatin-based chemotherapeutic regimens in a number of tumour types including bladder [56], colorectal [57], gastric [54], oesophageal [58], head and neck [59], ovarian [60] and NSCLC [61]. Inconclusive evidence for functionally increased NER in cisplatin resistant cancers may be due to a lack of methods that can easily and reliably measure NER activity in tissues in addition to mRNA and protein levels in correlating expression levels with cellular resistance to cisplatin or response to chemotherapy.

ERCC1 was one of the first DNA repair genes cloned [62] and whose over-expression is associated with reduced platinum-based therapy efficacy in NSCLC [63]. It is associated with its partner, XPF (xeroderma pigmentosum protein F) to form a specific endonuclease that acts by making a 5' incision [64]. In preclinical studies, a cisplatin resistant phenotype was postulated to correlate with ERCC1 expression. Conversely, downregulation of ERCC1-XPF using siRNA sensitised prostate cancer cells and testis tumour cells to cisplatin [10, 65]. A similar effect has been observed in cells derived from NSCLC [66]. Polymorphisms of the *XPD* gene, involved in the NER transcription-coupled repair pathway, confer reduced repair capacity and are associated with increased sensitivity to cisplatin [67] and are associated with an increasing trend towards improved outcome in some NSCLC patients [68] but not others [69]. Low levels of *BRCA1* mRNA, a related gene in the NER pathway, predicts for better survival in NSCLC patients treated with neoadjuvant cisplatin/gemcitabine [70].

While damage induced by cisplatin is removed by NER, some lesions may remain. The mechanism by which cells can tolerate these unrepaired DNA lesions is known as translesion synthesis (TLS) and is carried out by specialised DNA polymerases. Such polymerases can bypass unrepaired DNA lesions and have been implicated in tolerance of different types of DNA damage [71]. Depending on the type of damage, different TLS polymerases may act in concert to bypass lesions in mammalian cells [72]. The base excision repair enzyme DNA polymerase-β is over-expressed in several cisplatin resistant cell lines demonstrating translesion synthesis across platinated crosslinks [73]. Other polymerases such as DNA polymerase-zeta may enable the mutagenic bypass of replication-blocking DNA adducts [74], as may DNA polymerase-eta [75]. This bypass replication by DNA polymerase-eta may be more efficient and less error prone that with DNA polymerase-β [76]. Platinum DNA damage repair may also be increased by topoisomerase-II and homologous recombination repair while non-homologous end-joining repair may enhance the efficiency of platinum drugs [77]. Proteins that recognise DNA damage are over-expressed in many cisplatin resistance cancer cells such as HMG1 which functions by shielding DNA adducts from cell repair mechanisms [78].

### *DNA Mismatch Repair (MMR)*

Cisplatin-induced DNA lesions can be detected, but not repaired, by the mismatch repair (MMR) system, the major pathway that corrects erroneous insertions, deletions and mis-incorporations which arise during DNA replication, or as a result of DNA damage [79]. The MMR process consists of a number of steps consisting of the recognition of the mismatch, identification and excision of the mispairs or looped intermediates and re-synthesis of the excised strand. MMR-related proteins that participate in the recognition of GpG inter-strand adducts include MSH2 and MLH1. The first observation of the involvement of the MMR process in cisplatin-induced damage and cell death was proposed on the basis of the finding that the mismatch repair complex MutSα (a heterodimer consisting of MSH2 and MSH6) binds *in vitro* to cisplatin DNA adducts [80]. It has been reported that MMR proteins attempt to repair cisplatin adducts, fail and subsequently transmit an apoptotic signal to the cell. In agreement with this model, MSH2 and MLH1 are often mutated or under-expressed in the context of acquired resistance to cisplatin [81]. NSCLC patients however with high expression of MSH2 who do not receive cisplatin treatment upon tumour resection have a better prognosis than patients with low MSH2 levels [82]. This may reflect an intrinsic difference between naïve patients and those treated with chemotherapy, where previously untreated tumours with high MSH2 levels are a good prognostic indicator. Tumours that have acquired resistance following exposure to cisplatin are often associated with reduced levels of MSH2. Hence, in the clinical setting, while a high DNA repair capacity may protect against tumour relapse, it may on the contrary prevent patients from the benefits derived from treatments involving DNA-damaging agents. The clinical relevance of loss of MMR for chemotherapy regimens incorporating cisplatin has been investigated in a number of clinical studies involving other tumour types such as ovarian cancer and testicular germ cell tumours. Taken together the various studies on MMR in different tumour types and its impact on cisplatin-induced cell death, it is most likely only a small contributing factor in the development of cisplatin resistance in the clinic.

## DNA Damage Response and Apoptosis

Cisplatin exerts its effect on cancer cells via the induction of cell death, or apoptosis [83]. Cisplatin-induced DNA damage that is not repairable may lead to the activation of a number of signaling cascades with a pro-apoptotic outcome. Such pathways are a subject of considerable interest in the study of chemoresistance in cancer, albeit not fully understood.

While cisplatin-induced apoptosis may be mediated via the extrinsic death receptor pathway or the intrinsic mitochondrial pathway, the resistance phenotype associated with this chemotherapeutic drug may occur through decreased expression or loss of a number of pro-apoptotic factors, or increased expression of anti-apoptotic proteins [84].

### *Loss of p53 Function*

The p53 tumour suppressor protein plays a critical role in the apoptotic pathway in cancer cells in response to chemotherapeutic drugs. Several studies have been conducted *in vitro* in a large panel of cell lines with different p53 status [85] and also *in vivo* in the clinical setting [86]. In one study comparing the response to cisplatin in breast, lung, colon, kidney, ovarian, leukaemia, melanoma and prostate cancer cell lines, it was shown that cell lines harbouring a p53 mutation were more resistant to cisplatin compared to p53 wild-type cells [87]. Defective apoptosis may contribute to resistance to both p53-dependent and independent cisplatin cytotoxicity [88]. Alternatively, downregulation of p53 may confer resistance by possible over-expression of its negative feedback regulator, Mdm2, with or without downregulation of $p14^{ARF}$ [25] or reduced p53-binding protein-2 expression (53BP2) [89]. In a panel of lung cancer cell lines (H460, A549, SBC3, SBC5 and Lu99), although no gross genomic alteration or mutation of *53BP2* gene was observed, 53BP2 mRNA levels were highly variable [85]. There was no association between the 53BP2 mRNA level and the p53 status. However, when the sensitivities of these cell lines to DNA-damaging agents were examined, including UV irradiation, X-ray irradiation and cisplatin, higher 53BP2 mRNA expression was found to be correlated with their sensitivity to these agents. Mutations in p53 are generally associated with protein over-expression, but the mutant protein lacks normal tumour suppressor function. In some studies over-expression of p53 is associated with poor outcome in platinum-treated NSCLC patients [90] while this is not seen in other studies [91]. It was also shown that cisplatin resistant cancer cells lacking a functional p53 protein had reduced levels of Apaf-1, an important protein involved in the formation of the apoptosome complex [92]. Knockdown of Apaf-1 in A549 lung adenocarcinoma resulted in decreased cisplatin-induced apoptosis [93]. In contrast, there was no correlation between cisplatin resistance and p53 status in some cancer cell types, such as human testis tumour cells [94] and ovarian cancer cells [95]. Such observations would indicate that susceptibility of these cells to apoptosis is induced by cisplatin in a p53-independent manner.

### *Alterations in Apoptosis Family Members and Response to Cisplatin*

Alterations in any of the factors that regulate and execute the apoptotic process, whether it is triggered by DNA damage, oxidative stress or otherwise, have the potential to influence cisplatin sensitivity (Figure 2). Many proteins identified to date, including death receptors, cytoplasmic adaptors, pro- and anti-apoptotic members of the Bcl-2 family, caspases, calpains and mitochondrial proteins, participate in this tightly regulated process and have been shown to modulate the response of cells to cisplatin and other chemotherapeutic agents [96-98]. However, only some of these predict sensitivity to cisplatin in the clinical setting. In NSCLC cell lines A549 and Calu1, gene expression profiles of BAD, Bid and caspases 4 and 6 were examined and found to be significantly decreased in cisplatin resistant sublines, where the differential phosphorylation status of BAD played a roll in the development of cisplatin resistance in these cell lines [99]. In a study of SCLC cell lines H1339 and H187, the expression of Bad, Bim and Bid was comparable in naive and resistant cells while the expression of Bax was reduced in the resistant cells. Reducing Bax expression in naive cells did not alter cisplatin sensitivity in H1339 or H187 SCLC cells, suggesting that the reduced Bax expression observed following exposure to cisplatin is not sufficient to induce cisplatin-resistance in SCLC cells [100]. The inhibitor of apoptosis (IAP) gene family encodes proteins which have been shown to inhibit the endogenous expression of caspases, thereby resulting in cell death inhibition. Among the various IAP proteins identified, the X-linked inhibitor of apoptosis (XIAP) is probably the most potent regulator of apoptosis and has been shown to be implicated in the development of cisplatin resistance in a number of *in vitro* models [101, 102]. XIAP siRNA was shown to inhibit NSCLC cell growth specifically, down-regulate *XIAP* gene expression, promote apoptosis and increase sensitivity to chemotherapy. The effect of XIAP silencing on resistance to cisplatin, paclitaxel and gemcitabine was also studied in the NSCLC cell lines, A549 and H460. Transfection of these cells with small interfering RNA (siRNA) for XIAP blocked over-expression of the gene, suppressed cell proliferation, increased apoptosis and increased the cells sensitivity to cisplatin and paclitaxel by preventing the binding of XIAP to caspase 3 and increasing the activity of this enzyme. There was no significant difference in resistance to gemcitabine between XIAP-silenced cells and non-transfected cells and changes in chemoresistance were independent of the activity of caspase-9 [103].

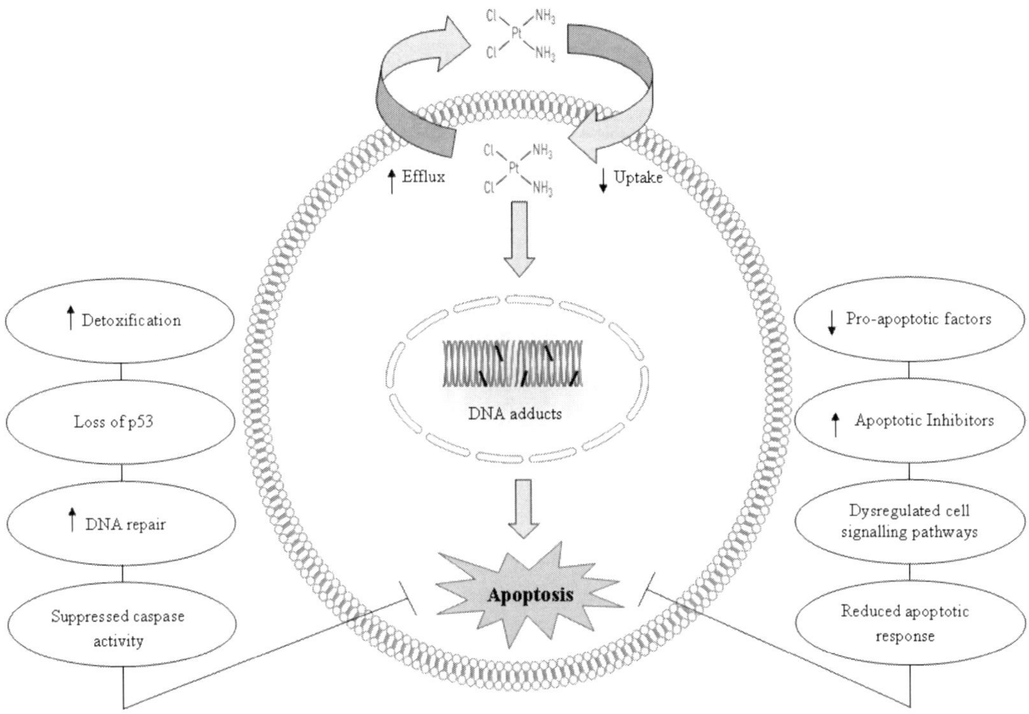


Figure 2. Mechanisms of apoptosis inhibition in cisplatin resistant tumour cells. The onset of cisplatin resistance and subsequent inhibition of apoptotic signalling is multifactorial, with multiple mechanisms and pathways contributing to the resistant phenotype in tumour cells.

Survivin, another member of the IAP family, is abundantly expressed in a variety of cancer cells in particular lung cancer cells and exerts its anti-apoptotic function by inhibition of caspase activation. High levels of survivin expression have been reported in SCLC [104] and NSCLC [105] in which the role of the phosphatidylinositol 3-kinase (PI3K)/Akt pathway has been implicated [106]. Moreover, the cytoprotective function of survivin in response to cisplatin was investigated and identified survivin as an anti-apoptotic protein in SCLC cells. Treatment with the DNA damaging agent activated the PI3K/Akt/survivin pathway which, in part, protected cells from drug-induced apoptosis. An investigation of survivin expression in cancer patient tissues following treatment with cisplatin chemotherapy revealed a negative correlation between survivin gene expression and response to cisplatin therapy in NSCLC [107].

## Aberrant Cell Signalling Pathways

While the exact mechanisms of the effects of cisplatin on cell signaling remains poorly understood, several signaling pathways and transcription factors have been identified that may enhance cisplatin resistance and promote cell survival.

### *MAPK Signal Transduction*

The activation of the MAP kinases SAPK/JNK (stress-activated protein kinases/c-Jun-N-terminal kinases) and p38 kinases are known to be involved in the cellular response to cisplatin. C-Myc, c-Fos and c-Jun are also activated by the MAPK pathway and may be over-expressed in cisplatin resistance (108). MAP kinases can be inactivated through dephosphorylation by members of the MAPK phosphatase (MKP) family, where MKP-1 is an important determinant of cisplatin resistance. It has been shown that cisplatin induces MKP-1, which correlates with inactivation of JNK and over-expression of MKP-1, and protects human lung cancer cells from cisplatin-induced death (109). Importantly, knockdown of MKP-1 by small interfering RNA (siRNA) sensitized human lung cancer cells to cisplatin-induced death. Moreover, blocking JNK, but not ERK and p38 activities, protected MKP-1 knockout cells from cisplatin-induced death, suggesting that the JNK-mediated apoptotic pathway may be critical for cisplatin-induced cell killing.

### *Epidermal Growth Factor (EGF)*

Inhibition of the epidermal growth factor receptor (EGFR) increases cisplatin sensitivity in NSCLC cell lines [110]. Induction of tumour cell migration as a result of EGF-induced chemotaxis upregulates a number of anti-apoptotic genes and downregulates various pro-apoptotic genes resulting in reduced cisplatin-induced apoptosis. Despite the observed increase in the sensitivity of cancer cell lines to cisplatin in response to EGFR inhibitors, the administration of EGFR inhibitors concurrently with platinum-based regimens has not proven clinically useful in NSCLC [111]. Epidermal growth factor receptor (EGFR) tyrosine kinase inhibitors (TKIs) given concurrently with chemotherapy do not improve patient outcomes compared with chemotherapy alone in advanced-stage NSCLC. One potential explanation for this lack of benefit is a negative interaction or antagonism between chemotherapy and EGFR TKIs when delivered concomitantly. Support for this line of reasoning is provided by preclinical data demonstrating that EGFR TKIs induce primarily a cytostatic effect resulting from a G1 cell cycle arrest in cell lines with wild-type EGFR. This results in reduced cell cycle phase-dependent activity of chemotherapy, whereas apoptotic cell death is induced in tumours with EGFR-activating mutations. As the great majority of NSCLC tumours consist of wild-type EGFR, sequence-specific interactions of EGFR TKI/chemotherapy combinations might negatively influence the efficacy of these regimens in patients with NSCLC. It is postulated that inhibition of cell growth by EGFR inhibitors may render tumour cells resistant to chemotherapy and as such, trials are ongoing where such therapies are administered sequentially rather than concurrently [112].

### *Phosphatidylinisotol-3-Kinase (PI3K)/AKT Pathway*

While there is little evidence to date of the role of PI3K inhibitors in sensitising cisplatin resistance in lung cancer cells, enhanced efficacy of cisplatin in response to inhibitors of the PI3K pathway has been reported in resistant cell lines [113] and in xenograft models of ovarian cancer [114], while knockdown of PTEN and p110α using siRNA blocked cisplatin-induced apoptosis and increased resistance. Lung cancer cells expressing Akt protein kinases display a cisplatin resistant phenotype with modulation of various apoptotic pathways, increased Bcl-$X_L$ expression and delayed activation of p53 [115]. There remains little knowledge of the importance and implications of this signaling pathway in cisplatin resistance in the clinical setting. However, clinical trials are ongoing combining chemotherapy with mammalian target of rapamycin inhibitors (mTOR inhibitors). In both SCLC and NSCLC cell lines, inhibition of mTOR restored sensitivity to cisplatin via the downregulation of the anti-apoptotic proteins, Bcl-2 and Bcl-$X_L$ [116].

Insulin-like growth factor-binding protein-3 (IGFBP-3) is a member of the insulin-like growth factor-binding protein family that binds IGF-1, blocking its mitogenic and anti-apoptotic functions. In the absence of IGFBP-3, IGF-1 binds and activates insulin-like growth factor-1 receptor (IGF-1R) and EGFR, commonly over-expressed in NSCLC which signal through the PI3K/Akt pathway, and therefore play a crucial role in cell growth, proliferation and survival. In addition, genetic and epigenetic alterations account for multiple genes in the pathway. The IGFBP-3/IGF-I/IGFIR axis exemplifies redundant routes to induce resistance to many drugs, where many proteins belonging to this pathway mediate chemotherapy resistance in NSCLC through the activation of Akt/mTOR (mammalian target of rapamycin) signaling [117].

## Epigenetic Regulation and Cisplatin Resistance

It is now clear that epigenetics and the cellular machinery involved in regulating the epigenetic regulation of gene expression play important roles in NSCLC tumorigenesis and cisplatin resistance in lung cancer. Epigenetics may be simply defined as stable and heritable changes in gene expression which are not due to changes in the primary DNA sequence. Some of the main epigenetic mechanisms currently known involve DNA CpG methylation, histone post-translational modifications (PTMs), gene imprinting and non-coding RNA (ncRNA).

Significant evidence is emerging linking loss of gene expression in NSCLC by DNA CpG methylation with cisplatin resistance. Indeed, pulsed exposure to cisplatin has been shown to result in drug-induced DNA hypermethylation both *in vitro* and *in vivo* [118, 119]. Checkpoint kinase 2 (*CHK2*) was one of the first examples of a gene whose downregulation by DNA CpG methylation in NSCLC was associated with resistance to standard chemotherapies including cisplatin [35]. EMX2, a human homologue of the Drosophila empty spiracles gene (ems), is a homeodomain-containing transcription factor with important functions during early development. It has been shown to be dramatically downregulated in lung cancer tissue samples by methylation of its promoter, while restoration of *EMX2* gene expression sensitised lung cancer cells to cisplatin [120]. The serine protease HtrA3 has also been shown to be reduced or completely lost in over 50% of lung cancer cell lines and primary lung tumours from heavy smokers. The loss of HtrA3 expression is due to DNA methylation and results in resistance to both etoposide and cisplatin [121]. Expression of transglutaminase 2 (TGM2) has been linked to cisplatin resistance in NSCLC where good responders could be identified by the promoter methylation of TGM2 and that TGase 2 inhibition was an effective cisplatin-sensitizing modality in NSCLC [122]. Other studies have shown that the *TGM2* gene is silenced by promoter CpG methylation in approximately one-third of all NSCLC cell lines examined. Cell lines which had loss of TGM2 were more sensitive to cisplatin, and targeting TGM2 using siRNA resulted in increased sensitivity to this drug [122]. Using microarray technology comparing isogenic parent and resistant cell lines, loss of expression of insulin-like binding protein-3 (IGFBP-3) was identified by DNA CpG methylation in cisplatin resistant cells. A strong correlation between IGFBP-3 methylation status and cisplatin response was found in patients, where methylated promoters were mostly found in patients with cisplatin resistant tumours [123].

## Novel Strategies for Overcoming Cisplatin Resistance

Cisplatin has remained a valuable therapeutic agent against several cancer types including head and neck, ovarian, testicular and lung cancers. Unfortunately, cancer cells eventually become resistant to cisplatin, resulting in relapse or treatment failure. The multifactorial nature of the cisplatin resistant phenotype, where more than one mechanism is normally activated, is a significant problem in overcoming this clinically important issue in lung cancer patients. Combination approaches using cisplatin or other platinum agents with human monoclonal antibodies may prove beneficial in improving the efficacy of cisplatin treatment in cancer patients. The combination of cisplatin and trastuzumab, an antibody raised against the EGF receptor subtype HER2, has shown promising clinical activity in patients with advanced breast cancer that over-express HER2 [124, 125]. In lung cancer patients, the addition of bevacizumab, a humanised monoclonal antibody against vascular endothelial growth factor (VEGF), to platinum-based chemotherapy resulted in an improved response and survival in NSCLC patients. Bevacizumab in combination with platinum-based therapy may therefore offer a significant clinical benefit for NSCLC patients [126, 1278].

While the platinum agents, mainly cisplatin, carboplatin and oxaliplatin have had a significant effect in the treatment of patients with malignancies such as testicular, ovarian, colorectal, and lung cancer patients, much studies are warranted to increase the therapeutic benefit of this important class of drug. In preclinical studies, new generation cisplatin analogues have been shown to overcome acquired resistance to cisplatin in certain tumour types. Two such analogues include satraplatin and picoplatin and have recently shown promising clinical activity in hormone-refractory prostate cancer and NSCLC [128]. Both analogues are in clinical trials and are thought to work by introducing bulkier DNA lesions than cisplatin, thereby making it more difficult for cells to remove or tolerate by translesion synthesis [129]. When satraplatin was used in the first-line treatment of SCLC, a response rate of 38% was reported [130]. Furthermore, there was a lack of satraplatin-induced nephrotoxicity during the course of the Phase I trial [131]. Picoplatin has been shown to circumvent acquired cisplatin resistance in ovarian cancer cell lines while similar findings of non-cross-resistance have also been demonstrated in pairs of cisplatin-sensitive and resistant human lung cancer cell lines [132]. In a more recent phase II study, the clinical efficacy of picoplatin was shown in SCLC patients who were refractory to other platinum compounds [133].

## Conclusion

Cisplatin continues to play a critical role in the treatment of a number of solid tumours such as head and neck, testicular, ovarian, bladder, breast and in particular, lung cancer. While the success of cisplatin in the treatment of lung cancer is often limited due to intrinsic or acquired tumour cell resistance, elucidation of the mechanisms by which tumours become refractory to cisplatin is essential. A better understanding of these fundamental mechanisms may lead to improved therapeutic strategies and will allow for better patient stratification in the clinical setting.

## References

[1] D'Aoust JC, Prestayko AW, Einhorn LH et al. Cisplatin, bleomycin, and vinblastine combination therapy of testicular tumors: an analysis. *Med Pediatr Oncol.* 1979;6(3):195-205.

[2] Garcia JA, Dreicer R. Systemic chemotherapy for advanced bladder cancer: update and controversies. *J Clin Oncol.* 2006 Dec 10;24(35):5545-51.

[3] Thigpen T, Vance RB, Khansur T. The platinum compounds and paclitaxel in the management of carcinomas of the endometrium and uterine cervix. *Semin Oncol.* 1995 Oct;22(5 Suppl 12):67-75.

[4] Lebwohl D, Canetta R. Clinical development of platinum complexes in cancer therapy: an historical perspective and an update. *Eur J Cancer.* 1998 Sep;34(10):1522-34.

[5] Kartalou M, Essigmann JM. Recognition of cisplatin adducts by cellular proteins. *Mutat Res.* 2001 Jul 1;478(1-2):1-21.

[6] Stordal B, Pavlakis N, Davey R. Oxaliplatin for the treatment of cisplatin-resistant cancer: a systematic review. *Cancer Treat Rev.* 2007 Jun;33(4):347-57.

[7] Loh SY, Mistry P, Kelland LR et al. Reduced drug accumulation as a major mechanism of acquired resistance to cisplatin in a human ovarian carcinoma cell line: circumvention studies using novel platinum (II) and (IV) ammine/amine complexes. *Br J Cancer.* 1992 Dec;66(6):1109-15.

[8] Shirazi FH, Molepo JM, Stewart DJ et al. Cytotoxicity, accumulation, and efflux of cisplatin and its metabolites in human ovarian carcinoma cells. *Toxicol Appl Pharmacol.* 1996 Oct;140(2):211-8.

[9] Mann SC, Andrews PA, Howell SB. Comparison of lipid content, surface membrane fluidity, and temperature dependence of cis-diamminedichloroplatinum(II) accumulation in sensitive and resistant human ovarian carcinoma cells. *Anticancer Res.* 1988 Nov-Dec;8(6):1211-5.

[10] Iwamori M, Iwamori Y, Kubushiro K et al. Characteristic expression of Lewis-antigenic glycolipids in human ovarian carcinoma-derived cells with anticancer drug-resistance. *J Biochem.* 2007 Mar;141(3):309-17.

[11] Kiura K, Watarai S, Ueoka H et al. An alteration of ganglioside composition in cisplatin-resistant lung cancer cell line. *Anticancer Res.* 1998 Jul-Aug;18(4C):2957-60.

[12] Safaei R, Howell SB. Copper transporters regulate the cellular pharmacology and sensitivity to Pt drugs. *Crit Rev Oncol Hematol.* 2005 Jan;53(1):13-23.

[13] Katano K, Kondo A, Safaei R et al. Acquisition of resistance to cisplatin is accompanied by changes in the cellular pharmacology of copper. *Cancer Res.* 2002 Nov 15;62(22):6559-65.

[14] Ishida S, McCormick F, Smith-McCune K, Hanahan D. Enhancing tumor-specific uptake of the anticancer drug cisplatin with a copper chelator. *Cancer Cell.* 2010 Jun 15;17(6):574-83.

[15] Samimi G, Safaei R, Katano K et al. Increased expression of the copper efflux transporter ATP7A mediates resistance to cisplatin, carboplatin, and oxaliplatin in ovarian cancer cells. *Clin Cancer Res.* 2004 Jul 15;10(14):4661-9.

[16] Nakayama K, Miyazaki K, Kanzaki A et al. Expression and cisplatin sensitivity of copper-transporting P-type adenosine triphosphatase (ATP7B) in human solid carcinoma cell lines. *Oncol Rep.* 2001 Nov-Dec;8(6):1285-7.

[17] Miyashita H, Nitta Y, Mori S et al. Expression of copper-transporting P-type adenosine triphosphatase (ATP7B) as a chemoresistance marker in human oral squamous cell carcinoma treated with cisplatin. *Oral Oncol.* 2003 Feb;39(2):157-62.

[18] transporters: the multidrug resistance-associated proteins. *J Natl Cancer Inst.* 2000 Aug 16;92(16):1295-302.

[19] Yeh JJ, Hsu NY, Hsu WH et al. Comparison of chemotherapy response with P-glycoprotein, multidrug resistance-related protein-1, and lung resistance-related protein expression in untreated small cell lung cancer. *Lung.* 2005 May-Jun;183(3):177-83.

[20] Berger W, Elbling L, Micksche M. Expression of the major vault protein LRP in human non-small-cell lung cancer cells: activation by short-term exposure to antineoplastic drugs. *Int J Cancer.* 2000 Oct 15;88(2):293-300.

[21] Liedert B, Materna V, Schadendorf D et al. Overexpression of cMOAT (MRP2/ABCC2) is associated with decreased formation of platinum-DNA adducts and decreased G2-arrest in melanoma cells resistant to cisplatin. *J Invest Dermatol.* 2003 Jul;121(1):172-6.

[22] Korita PV, Wakai T, Shirai Y et al. Multidrug resistance-associated protein 2 determines the efficacy of cisplatin in patients with hepatocellular carcinoma. *Oncol Rep.* 2010 Apr;23(4):965-72.

[23] Yamasaki M, Makino T, Masuzawa T et al. Role of multidrug resistance protein 2 (MRP2) in chemoresistance and clinical outcome in oesophageal squamous cell carcinoma. *Br J Cancer.* 2011 Feb 15;104(4):707-13.

[24] Lewis AD, Hayes JD, Wolf CR. Glutathione and glutathione-dependent enzymes in ovarian adenocarcinoma cell lines derived from a patient before and after the onset of drug resistance: intrinsic differences and cell cycle effects. *Carcinogenesis.* 1988 Jul;9(7):1283-7.

[25] Siddik ZH. Cisplatin: mode of cytotoxic action and molecular basis of resistance. *Oncogene.* 2003 Oct 20;22(47):7265-79.

[26] Cullen KJ, Newkirk KA, Schumaker LM et al. Glutathione S-transferase pi amplification is associated with cisplatin resistance in head and neck squamous cell carcinoma cell lines and primary tumors. *Cancer Res.* 2003 Dec 1;63(23):8097-102.

[27] Kase H, Kodama S, Nagai E, Tanaka K. Glutathione S-transferase pi immunostaining of cisplatin-resistant ovarian cancer cells in ascites. *Acta Cytol.* 1998 Nov-Dec;42(6):1397-402.

[28] Medeiros R, Pereira D, Afonso N et al. Platinum/paclitaxel-based chemotherapy in advanced ovarian carcinoma: glutathione S-transferase genetic polymorphisms as predictive biomarkers of disease outcome. *Int J Clin Oncol.* 2003 Jun;8(3):156-61.

[29] Cabelguenne A, Loriot MA, Stucker I et al. Glutathione-associated enzymes in head and neck squamous cell carcinoma and response to cisplatin-based neoadjuvant chemotherapy. *Int J Cancer.* 2001 Sep 1;93(5):725-30.

[30] Mellish KJ, Kelland LR, Harrap KR. In vitro platinum drug chemosensitivity of human cervical squamous cell carcinoma cell lines with intrinsic and acquired resistance to cisplatin. *Br J Cancer.* 1993 Aug;68(2):240-50.

[31] Meijer C, Mulder NH, Timmer-Bosscha H et al. Relationship of cellular glutathione to the cytotoxicity and resistance of seven platinum compounds. *Cancer Res.* 1992 Dec 15;52(24):6885-9.

[32] Jansen BA, Brouwer J, Reedijk J. Glutathione induces cellular resistance against cationic dinuclear platinum anticancer drugs. *J Inorg Biochem.* 2002 Apr 28;89(3-4):197-202.

[33] Konishi I, Nanbu K, Mandai M et al. Tumor response to neoadjuvant chemotherapy correlates with the expression of P-glycoprotein and PCNA but not GST-pi in the tumor cells of cervical carcinoma. *Gynecol Oncol.* 1998 Sep;70(3):365-71.

[34] Miyatake K, Gemba K, Ueoka H et al. Prognostic significance of mutant p53 protein, P-glycoprotein and glutathione S-transferase-pi in patients with unresectable non-small cell lung cancer. *Anticancer Res.* 2003 May-Jun;23(3C):2829-36.

[35] Filomeni G, Turella P, Dupuis ML et al. 6-(7-Nitro-2,1,3-benzoxadiazol-4-ylthio)hexanol, a specific glutathione S-transferase inhibitor, overcomes the multidrug resistance (MDR)-associated protein 1-mediated MDR in small cell lung cancer. *Mol Cancer Ther.* 2008 Feb;7(2):371-9.

[36] Ishikawa T. The ATP-dependent glutathione S-conjugate export pump. *Trends Biochem Sci.* 1992 Nov;17(11):463-8.

[37] Richardson ME, Siemann DW. Thiol-related mechanisms of resistance in a murine tumor model. *Int J Radiat Oncol Biol Phys.* 1994 May 15;29(2):387-92.

[38] Pompella A, De Tata V, Paolicchi A, Zunino F. Expression of gamma-glutamyltransferase in cancer cells and its significance in drug resistance. *Biochem Pharmacol.* 2006 Jan 12;71(3):231-8.
[39] Nishi M, Abe Y, Fujimori S et al. The modifier subunit of glutamate cysteine ligase relates to cisplatin resistance in human small cell lung cancer xenografts in vivo. *Oncol Rep.* 2005 Aug;14(2):421-4.
[40] Bose Girigoswami K, Bhaumik G, Ghosh R. Induced resistance in cells exposed to repeated low doses of H2O2 involves enhanced activity of antioxidant enzymes. *Cell Biol Int.* 2005 Sep;29(9):761-7.
[41] Rosell R, Cobo M, Isla D et al. Applications of genomics in NSCLC. *Lung Cancer.* 2005 Dec;50 Suppl 2:S33-40.
[42] Xu H, Choi SM, An CS et al. Concentration-dependent collateral sensitivity of cisplatin-resistant gastric cancer cell sublines. *Biochem Biophys Res Commun.* 2005 Mar 11;328(2):618-22.
[43] Chen YJ, Yuan CC, Chow KC et al. Overexpression of dihydrodiol dehydrogenase is associated with cisplatin-based chemotherapy resistance in ovarian cancer patients. *Gynecol Oncol.* 2005 Apr;97(1):110-7.
[44] Huang PY, Liang XM, Lin SX et al. Correlation analysis among expression of ERCC-1, metallothionein, p53 and platinum resistance and prognosis in advanced non-small cell lung cancer. *Ai Zheng.* 2004 Jul;23(7):845-50.
[45] Hospers GA, de Vries EG, Mulder NH. The formation and removal of cisplatin (CDDP) induced DNA adducts in a CDDP sensitive and resistant human small cell lung carcinoma (HSCLC) cell line. *Br J Cancer.* 1990 Jan;61(1):79-82.
[46] Johnson SW, Swiggard PA, Handel LM et al. Relationship between platinum-DNA adduct formation and removal and cisplatin cytotoxicity in cisplatin-sensitive and -resistant human ovarian cancer cells. *Cancer Res.* 1994 Nov 15;54(22):5911-6.
[47] Oldenburg J, Begg AC, van Vugt MJ et al. Characterization of resistance mechanisms to cis-diamminedichloroplatinum(II) in three sublines of the CC531 colon adenocarcinoma cell line in vitro. *Cancer Res.* 1994 Jan 15;54(2):487-93.
[48] Koberle B, Payne J, Grimaldi KA et al. DNA repair in cisplatin-sensitive and resistant human cell lines measured in specific genes by quantitative polymerase chain reaction. *Biochem Pharmacol.* 1996 Dec 13;52(11):1729-34.
[49] Koberle B, Grimaldi KA, Sunters A et al. DNA repair capacity and cisplatin sensitivity of human testis tumour cells. *Int J Cancer.* 1997 Mar 4;70(5):551-5.
[50] Rosell R, Taron M, Barnadas A et al. Nucleotide excision repair pathways involved in Cisplatin resistance in non-small-cell lung cancer. *Cancer Control.* 2003 Jul-Aug;10(4):297-305.
[51] Gillet LC, Scharer OD. Molecular mechanisms of mammalian global genome nucleotide excision repair. *Chem Rev.* 2006 Feb;106(2):253-76.
[52] Aboussekhra A, Biggerstaff M, Shivji MK et al. Mammalian DNA nucleotide excision repair reconstituted with purified protein components. *Cell.* 1995 Mar 24;80(6):859-68.
[53] Li Q, Yu JJ, Mu C et al. Association between the level of ERCC-1 expression and the repair of cisplatin-induced DNA damage in human ovarian cancer cells. *Anticancer Res.* 2000 Mar-Apr;20(2A):645-52.
[54] Metzger R, Leichman CG, Danenberg KD et al. ERCC1 mRNA levels complement thymidylate synthase mRNA levels in predicting response and survival for gastric

cancer patients receiving combination cisplatin and fluorouracil chemotherapy. *J Clin Oncol.* 1998 Jan;16(1):309-16.

[55] Mountzios G, Dimopoulos MA, Papadimitriou C. Excision Repair Cross-Complementation Group 1 Enzyme as a Molecular Determinant of Responsiveness to Platinum-Based Chemotherapy for non Small-Cell Lung Cancer. *Biomark Insights.* 2008;3:219-26.

[56] Bellmunt J, Paz-Ares L, Cuello M et al. Gene expression of ERCC1 as a novel prognostic marker in advanced bladder cancer patients receiving cisplatin-based chemotherapy. *Ann Oncol.* 2007 Mar;18(3):522-8.

[57] Shirota Y, Stoehlmacher J, Brabender J et al. ERCC1 and thymidylate synthase mRNA levels predict survival for colorectal cancer patients receiving combination oxaliplatin and fluorouracil chemotherapy. *J Clin Oncol.* 2001 Dec 1;19(23):4298-304.

[58] Kim MK, Cho KJ, Kwon GY et al. Patients with ERCC1-negative locally advanced esophageal cancers may benefit from preoperative chemoradiotherapy. *Clin Cancer Res.* 2008 Jul 1;14(13):4225-31.

[59] Jun HJ, Ahn MJ, Kim HS et al. ERCC1 expression as a predictive marker of squamous cell carcinoma of the head and neck treated with cisplatin-based concurrent chemoradiation. *Br J Cancer.* 2008 Jul 8;99(1):167-72.

[60] Dabholkar M, Bostick-Bruton F, Weber C et al. ERCC1 and ERCC2 expression in malignant tissues from ovarian cancer patients. *J Natl Cancer Inst.* 1992 Oct 7;84(19):1512-7.

[61] Olaussen KA, Dunant A, Fouret P et al. DNA repair by ERCC1 in non-small-cell lung cancer and cisplatin-based adjuvant chemotherapy. *N Engl J Med.* 2006 Sep 7;355(10):983-91.

[62] Westerveld A, Hoeijmakers JH, van Duin M et al. Molecular cloning of a human DNA repair gene. *Nature.* 1984 Aug 2-8;310(5976):425-9.

[63] Rosell R, Lord RV, Taron M, Reguart N. DNA repair and cisplatin resistance in non-small-cell lung cancer. *Lung Cancer.* 2002 Dec;38(3):217-27.

[64] Sijbers AM, de Laat WL, Ariza RR et al. Xeroderma pigmentosum group F caused by a defect in a structure-specific DNA repair endonuclease. *Cell.* 1996 Sep 6;86(5):811-22.

[65] Usanova S, Piee-Staffa A, Sied U et al. Cisplatin sensitivity of testis tumour cells is due to deficiency in interstrand-crosslink repair and low ERCC1-XPF expression. *Mol Cancer.* 2010;9:248.

[66] Arora S, Kothandapani A, Tillison K et al. Downregulation of XPF-ERCC1 enhances cisplatin efficacy in cancer cells. *DNA Repair* (Amst). 2010 Jul 1;9(7):745-53.

[67] Rosell R, Taron M, Ariza A et al. Molecular predictors of response to chemotherapy in lung cancer. *Semin Oncol.* 2004 Feb;31(1 Suppl 1):20-7.

[68] Camps C, Sarries C, Roig B et al. Assessment of nucleotide excision repair XPD polymorphisms in the peripheral blood of gemcitabine/cisplatin-treated advanced non-small-cell lung cancer patients. *Clin Lung Cancer.* 2003 Jan;4(4):237-41.

[69] Ryu JS, Hong YC, Han HS et al. Association between polymorphisms of ERCC1 and XPD and survival in non-small-cell lung cancer patients treated with cisplatin combination chemotherapy. *Lung Cancer.* 2004 Jun;44(3):311-6.

[70] Taron M, Rosell R, Felip E et al. BRCA1 mRNA expression levels as an indicator of chemoresistance in lung cancer. *Hum Mol Genet.* 2004 Oct 15;13(20):2443-9.

[71] Bavoux C, Hoffmann JS, Cazaux C. Adaptation to DNA damage and stimulation of genetic instability: the double-edged sword mammalian DNA polymerase kappa. *Biochimie*. 2005 Jul;87(7):637-46.
[72] Shachar S, Ziv O, Avkin S et al. Two-polymerase mechanisms dictate error-free and error-prone translesion DNA synthesis in mammals. *EMBO J.* 2009 Feb 18;28(4):383-93.
[73] Raaphorst G, Yang D, Grewaal D et al. Analysis of mechanisms of Cisplatin resistance in 3 pairs of human tumor-cell lines expressing normal and resistant responses to Cisplatin. *Oncol Rep*. 1995 Nov;2(6):1037-43.
[74] Lin X, Trang J, Okuda T, Howell SB. DNA polymerase zeta accounts for the reduced cytotoxicity and enhanced mutagenicity of cisplatin in human colon carcinoma cells that have lost DNA mismatch repair. *Clin Cancer Res*. 2006 Jan 15;12(2):563-8.
[75] Albertella MR, Green CM, Lehmann AR, O'Connor MJ. A role for polymerase eta in the cellular tolerance to cisplatin-induced damage. *Cancer Res.* 2005 Nov 1;65(21):9799-806.
[76] Bassett E, Vaisman A, Havener JM et al. Efficiency of extension of mismatched primer termini across from cisplatin and oxaliplatin adducts by human DNA polymerases beta and eta in vitro. *Biochemistry*. 2003 Dec 9;42(48):14197-206.
[77] Britten RA, Kuny S, Perdue S. Modification of non-conservative double-strand break (DSB) rejoining activity after the induction of cisplatin resistance in human tumour cells. *Br J Cancer.* 1999 Feb;79(5-6):843-9.
[78] Nagatani G, Nomoto M, Takano H et al. Transcriptional activation of the human HMG1 gene in cisplatin-resistant human cancer cells. *Cancer Res.* 2001 Feb 15;61(4):1592-7.
[79] Kunkel TA, Erie DA. DNA mismatch repair. *Annu Rev Biochem.* 2005;74:681-710.
[80] Mello JA, Acharya S, Fishel R, Essigmann JM. The mismatch-repair protein hMSH2 binds selectively to DNA adducts of the anticancer drug cisplatin. *Chem Biol.* 1996 Jul;3(7):579-89.
[81] Aebi S, Kurdi-Haidar B, Gordon R et al. Loss of DNA mismatch repair in acquired resistance to cisplatin. *Cancer Res.* 1996 Jul 1;56(13):3087-90.
[82] Kamal NS, Soria JC, Mendiboure J et al. MutS homologue 2 and the long-term benefit of adjuvant chemotherapy in lung cancer. *Clin Cancer Res*. 2010 Feb 15;16(4):1206-15.
[83] Chu G. Cellular responses to cisplatin. The roles of DNA-binding proteins and DNA repair. *J Biol Chem.* 1994 Jan 14;269(2):787-90.
[84] Sedletska Y, Giraud-Panis MJ, Malinge JM. Cisplatin is a DNA-damaging antitumour compound triggering multifactorial biochemical responses in cancer cells: importance of apoptotic pathways. *Curr Med Chem Anticancer Agents*. 2005 May;5(3):251-65.
[85] Branch P, Masson M, Aquilina G et al. Spontaneous development of drug resistance: mismatch repair and p53 defects in resistance to cisplatin in human tumor cells. *Oncogene*. 2000 Jun 29;19(28):3138-45.
[86] Hengstler JG, Pilch H, Schmidt M et al. Metallothionein expression in ovarian cancer in relation to histopathological parameters and molecular markers of prognosis. *Int J Cancer.* 2001 Mar 20;95(2):121-7.
[87] O'Connor PM, Jackman J, Bae I et al. Characterization of the p53 tumor suppressor pathway in cell lines of the National Cancer Institute anticancer drug screen and

correlations with the growth-inhibitory potency of 123 anticancer agents. *Cancer Res.* 1997 Oct 1;57(19):4285-300.

[88] Minagawa Y, Kigawa J, Itamochi H et al. Cisplatin-resistant HeLa cells are resistant to apoptosis via p53-dependent and -independent pathways. *Jpn J Cancer Res.* 1999 Dec;90(12):1373-9.

[89] Mori T, Okamoto H, Takahashi N et al. Aberrant overexpression of 53BP2 mRNA in lung cancer cell lines. *FEBS Lett.* 2000 Jan 14;465(2-3):124-8.

[90] Kawasaki M, Nakanishi Y, Yatsunami J et al. P53 immunostaining predicts chemosensitivity in non-small cell lung cancer: A preliminary report. *Cancer J Sci Am.* 1996 Jul-Aug;2(4):217-20.

[91] Gregorc V, Darwish S, Ludovini V et al. The clinical relevance of Bcl-2, Rb and p53 expression in advanced non-small cell lung cancer. *Lung Cancer.* 2003 Dec;42(3):275-81.

[92] Huerta S, Heinzerling JH, Anguiano-Hernandez YM et al. Modification of gene products involved in resistance to apoptosis in metastatic colon cancer cells: roles of Fas, Apaf-1, NFkappaB, IAPs, Smac/DIABLO, and AIF. *J Surg Res.* 2007 Sep;142(1):184-94.

[93] Cao X, Bennett RL, May WS. c-Myc and caspase-2 are involved in activating Bax during cytotoxic drug-induced apoptosis. *J Biol Chem.* 2008 May 23;283(21):14490-6.

[94] Burger H, Nooter K, Boersma AW et al. Lack of correlation between cisplatin-induced apoptosis, p53 status and expression of Bcl-2 family proteins in testicular germ cell tumour cell lines. *Int J Cancer.* 1997 Nov 14;73(4):592-9.

[95] De Feudis P, Debernardis D, Beccaglia P et al. DDP-induced cytotoxicity is not influenced by p53 in nine human ovarian cancer cell lines with different p53 status. *Br J Cancer.* 1997;76(4):474-9.

[96] de La Motte Rouge T, Galluzzi L, Olaussen KA et al. A novel epidermal growth factor receptor inhibitor promotes apoptosis in non-small cell lung cancer cells resistant to erlotinib. *Cancer Res.* 2007 Jul 1;67(13):6253-62.

[97] Janson V, Johansson A, Grankvist K. Resistance to caspase-8 and -9 fragments in a malignant pleural mesothelioma cell line with acquired cisplatin-resistance. *Cell Death Dis.* 2010;1:e78.

[98] Tajeddine N, Galluzzi L, Kepp O et al. Hierarchical involvement of Bak, VDAC1 and Bax in cisplatin-induced cell death. *Oncogene.* 2008 Jul 10;27(30):4221-32.

[99] Cetintas VB, Kucukaslan AS, Kosova B et al. Cisplatin resistance induced by decreased apoptotic activity in non-small-cell lung cancer cell lines. *Cell Biol Int.* 2012 Mar 1;36(3):261-5.

[100] Biagosch J, Huber RM, Bergner A. Reduced expression of Bax in small cell lung cancer cells is not sufficient to induce cisplatin-resistance. *Eur J Med Res.* 2010 Oct 25;15(10):448-51.

[101] Chen F, Qu H, Sui G. *Effects of apoptosis protein XIAP inhibitor on the apoptosis and sensitivity of chemotherapy in A549 cell.* Zhongguo Fei Ai Za Zhi. 2008 Jun 20;11(3):368-72.

[102] Cheng YJ, Jiang HS, Hsu SL et al. XIAP-mediated protection of H460 lung cancer cells against cisplatin. *Eur J Pharmacol.* 2010 Feb 10;627(1-3):75-84.

[103] Liu Y, Wu X, Sun Y, Chen F. Silencing of X-linked inhibitor of apoptosis decreases resistance to cisplatin and paclitaxel but not gemcitabine in non-small cell lung cancer. *J Int Med Res.* 2011;39(5):1682-92.
[104] Halasova E, Adamkov M, Matakova T et al. Lung cancer incidence and survival in chromium exposed individuals with respect to expression of anti-apoptotic protein survivin and tumor suppressor P53 protein. *Eur J Med Res.* 2010 Nov 4;15 Suppl 2:55-9.
[105] Zhang LQ, Wang J, Jiang F et al. Prognostic value of survivin in patients with non-small cell lung carcinoma: a systematic review with meta-analysis. *PLoS One.* 2012;7(3):e34100.
[106] Belyanskaya LL, Hopkins-Donaldson S, Kurtz S et al. Cisplatin activates Akt in small cell lung cancer cells and attenuates apoptosis by survivin upregulation. *Int J Cancer.* 2005 Dec 10;117(5):755-63.
[107] Karczmarek-Borowska B, Filip A, Wojcierowski J et al. Survivin antiapoptotic gene expression as a prognostic factor in non-small cell lung cancer: in situ hybridization study. *Folia Histochem Cytobiol.* 2005;43(4):237-42.
[108] Brozovic A, Fritz G, Christmann M et al. Long-term activation of SAPK/JNK, p38 kinase and fas-L expression by cisplatin is attenuated in human carcinoma cells that acquired drug resistance. *Int J Cancer.* 2004 Dec 20;112(6):974-85.
[109] Wang Z, Xu J, Zhou JY et al. Mitogen-activated protein kinase phosphatase-1 is required for cisplatin resistance. *Cancer Res.* 2006 Sep 1;66(17):8870-7.
[110] Bai L, Zhu R, Chen Z et al. Potential role of short hairpin RNA targeting epidermal growth factor receptor in growth and sensitivity to drugs of human lung adenocarcinoma cells. *Biochem Pharmacol.* 2006 Apr 14;71(8):1265-71.
[111] Herbst RS, Giaccone G, Schiller JH et al. Gefitinib in combination with paclitaxel and carboplatin in advanced non-small-cell lung cancer: a phase III trial--INTACT 2. *J Clin Oncol.* 2004 Mar 1;22(5):785-94.
[112] Davies AM, Ho C, Lara PN et al. Pharmacodynamic separation of epidermal growth factor receptor tyrosine kinase inhibitors and chemotherapy in non-small-cell lung cancer. *Clin Lung Cancer.* 2006 May;7(6):385-8.
[113] Lee S, Choi EJ, Jin C, Kim DH. Activation of PI3K/Akt pathway by PTEN reduction and PIK3CA mRNA amplification contributes to cisplatin resistance in an ovarian cancer cell line. *Gynecol Oncol.* 2005 Apr;97(1):26-34.
[114] Ohta T, Ohmichi M, Hayasaka T et al. Inhibition of phosphatidylinositol 3-kinase increases efficacy of cisplatin in in vivo ovarian cancer models. *Endocrinology.* 2006 Apr;147(4):1761-9.
[115] Hovelmann S, Beckers TL, Schmidt M. Molecular alterations in apoptotic pathways after PKB/Akt-mediated chemoresistance in NCI H460 cells. *Br J Cancer.* 2004 Jun 14;90(12):2370-7.
[116] Wangpaichitr M, Wu C, You M et al. Inhibition of mTOR restores cisplatin sensitivity through down-regulation of growth and anti-apoptotic proteins. *Eur J Pharmacol.* 2008 Sep 4;591(1-3):124-7.
[117] Cortes-Sempere M, de Miguel MP, Pernia O et al. IGFBP-3 methylation-derived deficiency mediates the resistance to cisplatin through the activation of the IGFIR/Akt pathway in non-small cell lung cancer. *Oncogene.* 2012 Apr 30.

[118] Nyce JW. Drug-induced DNA hypermethylation: a potential mediator of acquired drug resistance during cancer chemotherapy. Mutat Res. 1997 Apr;386(2):153-61.

[119] Koul S, McKiernan JM, Narayan G et al. Role of promoter hypermethylation in Cisplatin treatment response of male germ cell tumors. *Mol Cancer.* 2004 May 18;3:16.

[120] Okamoto J, Hirata T, Chen Z et al. EMX2 is epigenetically silenced and suppresses growth in human lung cancer. *Oncogene.* 2010 Nov 4;29(44):5969-75.

[121] Beleford D, Rattan R, Chien J, Shridhar V. High temperature requirement A3 (HtrA3) promotes etoposide- and cisplatin-induced cytotoxicity in lung cancer cell lines. *J Biol Chem.* 2010 Apr 16;285(16):12011-27.

[122] Park KS, Kim HK, Lee JH et al. Transglutaminase 2 as a cisplatin resistance marker in non-small cell lung cancer. *J Cancer Res Clin Oncol.* 2010 Apr;136(4):493-502.

[123] Ibanez de Caceres I, Cortes-Sempere M, Moratilla C et al. IGFBP-3 hypermethylation-derived deficiency mediates cisplatin resistance in non-small-cell lung cancer. *Oncogene.* 2010 Mar 18;29(11):1681-90.

[124] Pegram MD, Pienkowski T, Northfelt DW et al. Results of two open-label, multicenter phase II studies of docetaxel, platinum salts, and trastuzumab in HER2-positive advanced breast cancer. *J Natl Cancer Inst.* 2004 May 19;96(10):759-69.

[125] Hurley J, Doliny P, Reis I et al. Docetaxel, cisplatin, and trastuzumab as primary systemic therapy for human epidermal growth factor receptor 2-positive locally advanced breast cancer. *J Clin Oncol.* 2006 Apr 20;24(12):1831-8.

[126] Sandler A, Gray R, Perry MC et al. Paclitaxel-carboplatin alone or with bevacizumab for non-small-cell lung cancer. *N Engl J Med.* 2006 Dec 14;355(24):2542-50.

[127] Reck M, von Pawel J, Zatloukal P et al. Phase III trial of cisplatin plus gemcitabine with either placebo or bevacizumab as first-line therapy for nonsquamous non-small-cell lung cancer: AVAil. *J Clin Oncol.* 2009 Mar 10;27(8):1227-34.

[128] Kelland L. Broadening the clinical use of platinum drug-based chemotherapy with new analogues. Satraplatin and picoplatin. *Expert Opin Investig Drugs.* 2007 Jul;16(7):1009-21.

[129] Vaisman A, Masutani C, Hanaoka F, Chaney SG. Efficient translesion replication past oxaliplatin and cisplatin GpG adducts by human DNA polymerase eta. *Biochemistry.* 2000 Apr 25;39(16):4575-80.

[130] Fokkema E, Groen HJ, Bauer J et al. Phase II study of oral platinum drug JM216 as first-line treatment in patients with small-cell lung cancer. *J Clin Oncol.* 1999 Dec;17(12):3822-7.

[131] Fokkema E, de Vries EG, Meijer S, Groen HJ. Lack of nephrotoxicity of new oral platinum drug JM216 in lung cancer patients. *Cancer Chemother Pharmacol.* 2000;45(1):89-92.

[132] Kawamura-Akiyama Y, Kusaba H, Kanzawa F et al. Non-cross resistance of ZD0473 in acquired cisplatin-resistant lung cancer cell lines. *Lung Cancer.* 2002 Oct;38(1):43-50.

[133] Eckardt JR, Bentsion DL, Lipatov ON et al. Phase II study of picoplatin as second-line therapy for patients with small-cell lung cancer. *J Clin Oncol.* 2009 Apr 20;27(12):2046-51.

In: Lung Cancer: A Comprehensive Overview
Editor: Kathy Gately

ISBN: 978-1-62618-447-3


*Chapter IX*

# Inflammation in Lung Carcinogenesis

***Anne-Marie Baird*[*1,2], Steven G. Gray[2,3] and Ken O'Byrne[2,3]***

[1]Department of Clinical Medicine, Trinity College Dublin, Ireland
[2]Thoracic Oncology Research Group, Institute of Molecular Medicine, Trinity Centre for Health Science, St. James's Hospital, Dublin, Ireland
[3]HOPE Directorate, St. James's Hospital, Dublin, Ireland

## Abstract

It was Dvorak in 1986 that postulated 'tumours are wounds that do not heal' as they share common cellular and molecular mechanisms, which are active in both wounds and in cancer tissue. Inflammation is a crucial part of the innate immune system that protects against pathogens and initiates adaptive immunity. Acute inflammation is usually a rapid and self-limiting process, however it does not always resolve. This leads to the establishment of a chronic inflammatory state and provides the perfect environment for carcinogenesis. Inflammation and cancer have long had an association, going back as far as Virchow in 1863, when leucocytes were noted in neoplastic tissue. It has been estimated that approximately 25% of all malignancies are initiated or exacerbated by inflammation caused by infectious agents. Furthermore, inflammation is linked to all of the six hallmarks of cancer (evasion of apoptosis, insensitivity to anti-growth signals, unlimited replicative potential, angiogenesis, increase in survival factors and invasion and metastasis). It is thought that inflammation may play a critical role in lung carcinogenesis given that individuals with inflammatory lung conditions have an increased risk of lung cancer development. Cigarette smoking can also induce inflammation in the lung and smokers are at a higher risk of developing lung cancer than non-smokers. However, exposure to a number of environmental agents such as radon, have also been demonstrated as a causative factor in this disease. This chapter will focus on inflammation as a contributory factor in non small cell lung cancer (NSCLC), concentrating primarily on the pathological involvement of the pro-inflammatory

* Email: bairda@tcd.ie.

cytokines, TNF-α, IL-1β, and the CXC ($ELR^+$) chemokine family. Targeting of inflammatory mediators will also be discussed as a therapeutic strategy in this disease.

# Introduction

Lung cancer represents a massive global health burden in both smoking and non smoking individuals with a dramatic rise evident in never smokers in particular. Due to difficulties in early detection and with the majority of patients presenting at an advanced stage, lung cancer has a high morbidity, with five year survival rates continuing to remain poor, at approximately 15% [1]. Recently lung cancer has overtaken breast and prostate as the biggest cancer killer in females and males, respectively in a number of countries. Consequently there is an urgent need to identify both new biomarkers in this disease and novel druggable targets to improve treatment options and increase survival rates.

Epidemiological studies have demonstrated a role for inflammation in cancer initiation and progression in a number of solid tumours [2]. Smoking results in inflammation in the lung and individuals who smoke, or have a previous history of inflammatory lung disease, are more likely to develop lung cancer even in the absence of tobacco use [3]. To this end inflammatory mediators may provide a significant innovative therapeutic avenue in this disease.

Inflammation is controlled and initiated by the innate immune system in response to pathogenic insults. The immune system comprises of two main arms: innate and adaptive. The innate immune system consists of the cells and mechanisms that defend the host from infection, in a non-antigen specific manner. Its main functions are the inflammatory and complement response induced by mast cells, macrophages, neutrophils, dendritic cells (DC) and natural killer (NK) cells. The adaptive immune system consists of highly specialised cells that eliminate pathogenic challenges in an antigen specific manner. It consists of T and B lymphocytes and natural killer T (NKT) cells [4]. Malignancy is known to alter immune cell functions, such as suppress cell mediated immunity, which in turn leads to the failure of immune mediated tumour rejection. Immune surveillance can control or eliminate some pre-malignant cells [5], however, with time tumour cells undergo a process known as immune editing [6]. This allows the tumour to escape from immune surveillance and develop a phenotype capable of manipulating or 'hi-jacking' immune cells into secreting chemokines and cytokines [6], also known as the "3 E's" of immune-editing (elimination, equilibrium and escape) [6]. Tumour cells that are not 'eliminated' can rapidly proliferate and become 'resistant' to the immune response. These cells reach an 'equilibrium' phase, 'escaping' from the immune system as such [6]. Humoral immunity may also be affected by cancer, which in some cases leads to an increase in immunoglobulin production and recruitment of mast cells, further potentiating the inflammatory process [7]. While cancer related inflammation is driven by the innate immune system [8], *de novo* carcinogenesis, promoted by chronic inflammation, is in some cases, B lymphocyte dependent as it recruits the innate immune cells [9]. This harmonized response is thought to be performed distantly, as B lymphocytes are not found within the tumour microenvironment [10]. The interplay between both arms of the immune system are important in the process of carcinogenesis [11].

# Cancer Related Inflammation

Inflammation is a crucial part of the innate immune system that protects against pathogens and initiates our adaptive immune response. Acute inflammation is usually a rapid and self-limiting process, however it does not always resolve. This leads to the establishment of a pathological or chronic 'smouldering' inflammatory state, which can contribute to certain diseases, such as cancer [12]. Indeed, a number of epidemiologic studies provide further evidence to a link between a distinct subset of cancers and inflammatory conditions [2, 13-19] (Table 1). In addition to inflammatory conditions, current estimates suggest that approximately 25% of all malignancies are initiated or exacerbated by means of inflammation caused by infectious agents [19, 21] (Table 2). Other studies have suggested that an inflammatory environment can exist within tumours which are not epidemiologically associated with inflammation [22]. Conditions associated with lung cancer will be discussed in a later section.

**Table 1. Inflammatory conditions associated with solid tumours**

| Cancer type | Inflammatory condition |
|---|---|
| Ovarian | Pelvic Inflammatory disease/endometriosis |
| Oesophageal | Barrett's oesophagus |
| Colon | Inflammatory bowel disease/Ulcerative colitis/Crohn's disease |
| Cholangiocarcinoma | Gall stones/Cholecystitis |
| Pancreas | Pancreatitis |
| Prostrate | Prostatitis |

**Table 2. Infectious agents linked to carcinogenesis**

| Cancer type | Infectious agent* |
|---|---|
| Bladder | *Schistosoma haematobium* |
| Cervical | Human Papillomavirus (HPV) |
| Gastric | *Helicobacter pylori* |
| Liver | Hepatitis B and C viruses (HBV/HCV) |
| Kaposi's sarcoma | Human herpes virus type 8 (HHV-8) |
| Hodgkin's lymphoma | Epstein-Barr virus |

* Classified as carcinogenic to humans according to International Agency for Research on Cancer (IARC) [23].

This association between inflammation and cancer is not new and the first connection was made about one hundred and fifty years ago, when Virchow noted leucocytes in cancerous tissue [24]. Dvorak in 1986, went on to describe tumours as 'wounds that do not heal', with both tumours and wounds sharing significant properties such as angiogenesis and stromal remodeling [25]. There are five main areas of evidence which links cancer and inflammation: (a) many chronic inflammatory diseases are associated with an increased risk of cancer, (b) cancers arise at sites of chronic inflammation, (c) many cells associated with chronic inflammatory processes are found at the site of cancer, (d) chemical mediators of inflammation are found to have a role in many cancers, (e) deletion of cellular or chemical mediators of inflammation inhibits cancer spread and development and (f) long-term use of non-steroidal anti inflammatory drugs (NSAIDs) reduce the risk of mortality of some cancers [12, 20, 24, 26-31]. A recent analysis has also noted that risk of distant metastasis is reduced with NSAID use [32]. Is should be noted however that the chemo-preventative properties of NSAIDs is controversial, as some studies have shown reductions in the incidence of breast [33], lung [34, 36], bowel [34, 37] and prostate cancer [34], while others have shown no significant effect in breast [38] or lung [39]. The benefit of NSAIDs may be cancer subtype specific or population dependant and will be discussed later in this chapter.

Additional evidence stems from the strong association of inflammation with all of the six hallmarks of cancer, which consists of limitless replicative potential, insensitivity to negative growth signals, autocrine growth, angiogenesis, invasion and metastasis and survival factors [40, 41]. A number of groups have suggested that an inflammatory microenvironment should become an additional seventh hallmark [29]. Evidence for this can be derived from the following estimated statistics: 5-10% of cancer diagnosis is due to inherited mutations, the remaining 90-95% is attributed to lifestyle factors [42]. These lifestyle factors may be divided into two main pathways, (a) intrinsic and (b) extrinsic [43]. Both pathways are linked to inflammation. The intrinsic pathway is oncogene driven which can result in the up-regulation of inflammatory cascades, while in the microenvironment driven/extrinsic pathway, an inflamed environment can aid in the carcinogenic process [19, 20, 22,29]. Both pathways result in the activation of transcription factors important in the inflammatory response such as the 'master regulator', Nuclear Factor kappa B (NF-κB) and signal transducer and activator of transcription 3 (STAT3) [19, 22, 55]. It is conceivable that reactive oxygen species (ROS) and reactive nitrogen species (RNS) produced as a by-product of chronic inflammation or induced by cigarette smoke, can result in recurring DNA damage through microsatellite and chromosomal instability, resulting in oncogene activation and the down regulation of tumour suppressor genes [20, 22, 45, 36]. This data further underlines cancer related inflammation (CRI) as a hallmark of cancer.

## Lung Cancer and Inflammation

Inflammation plays an important role in lung carcinogenesis [26, 27-50] given that individuals with inflammatory lung conditions have an increased risk of lung cancer development (Table 3). This risk can persist even in the absence of tobacco use, further underscoring the role of chronic inflammation in lung carcinogenesis [51-54]. Breathing, the primary function of the lungs, exposes the lung to various environmental pollutants from chemicals and particulate matter less than 10 microns in diameter ($PM_{10}$) to numerous volatile compounds (Table 4).

These insults can result in inflammation in the lung and, subsequently, the development of inflammatory lung diseases, which can, in a high percentage of cases, progress to lung cancer [48]. Re-enforcing this hypothesis is the number of inflammatory non-malignant lung conditions which have been shown to increase lung cancer risk in non smokers such as pneumonia and TB [3]. Therefore a number of lines of evidence exist to link inflammation and lung carcinogenesis [50].

**Table 3. Inflammatory conditions associated with lung carcinogenesis**

| Condition | Reference(s) |
|---|---|
| Pneumonia | [3, 52, 53] |
| Emphysema | [3, 51. 53, 66] |
| Interstitial lung disease | [56] |
| Asthma | [51, 53, 47, 58] |
| Idiopathic pulmonary fibrosis | [59] |
| Chronic obstructive pulmonary disorder (COPD) | [3, 60] |
| Tuberculosis (TB) | [3, 53, 57, 61,62] |
| Chronic bronchitis | [3, 51] |

**Table 4. Agents linked to lung cancer risk**

| Agent | Reference(s) |
|---|---|
| Cigarette smoke | [63-65] |
| Passive smoke/ETS | [66-69] |
| Exhaust fumes | [69] |
| Radon | [70] |

# Inflammatory Mediators In Lung Cancer

There are a large number of important mediators which are associated with pathological 'smouldering' inflammation in a variety of solid tumours and this is no different in lung cancer. Inflammatory mediators found at cancer sites include Tumour Necrosis Factor alpha (TNF-α), Interleukin 1 beta (IL-1β) and chemokines such as CXCL8 (IL-8). These mediators are associated with leukocyte infiltration, tissue remodelling and neo-angiogenesis [71].

TNF-α and IL-1β are potent pro-inflammatory cytokines, often referred to as the 'alarm' cytokines, as they are the first to act in the inflammatory process, which signifies their importance in inflammatory disease states [72]. TNF-α is released by activated macrophages, B cells and T cells and non-immune cells such as fibroblasts and adipocytes [73]. IL-1β is also produced by DCs and macrophages [74]. TNF-α and IL-1β have a major role in initiating and sustaining the inflammatory response, by inducing the expression of other pro-inflammatory and adhesion molecules, therefore, providing an influx of inflammatory mediators to the site of insult [4]. CXCL8 is an important chemokine in the innate immune response, functioning as both a chemo-attractant and a potent stimulator of the angiogenic response. It is produced by macrophages, activated monocytes and T cells and promotes the recruitment of neutrophils to sites of inflammation [75].

These pro-inflammatory mediators play an important role in pathological inflammation and may participate in lung carcinogenesis. Levels of these cytokines and chemokines, CXCL8, TNF-α and IL-1β, were part of a signature of 11 genes (CLASS-11) identifying patients with a poor prognosis in Stage I adenocarcinoma lung disease [76]. Also, TNF-α was part of a serum algorithm for separating patients with non small cell lung cancer (NSCLC) against cohorts of 'high-risk' individuals [77]. In addition, CXCL8 and CXCL1 were part of an 80 gene biomarker that distinguished smokers with and without lung cancer [78].

Furthermore, polymorphisms of the TNF-α and IL-1β genes are prominent in several cancers, for example gall bladder carcinoma, gastric, cervical and breast [79-83]. In lung cancer, studies have shown that patients with polymorphisms in the IL-1β gene are at a greater risk of developing NSCLC [65, 84-88]. The IL-1β – 31T/C promoter polymorphism would appear to be one of the most important changes [65, 89]. Polymorphisms in the IL-1 receptor antagonist gene have also been linked to lung cancer risk [90]. However, the link with polymorphisms in the TNF- α promoter is not fully understood. A number of studies have found no association with the disease [91, 92], although a Chinese study has reported that the -308 G/A polymorphism promoted lung cancer development and progression [93]. A polymorphism identified in the CXCL8 promoter -251 T/A had no association with lung cancer risk [94]. The association between lung cancer risk and inflammatory gene polymorphisms may vary according to ethnicity.

The involvement of these cytokines and chemokines in lung carcinogenesis will be examined in greater detail in the sections below. Figure 1 provides an overview of inflammation and lung carcinogenesis.

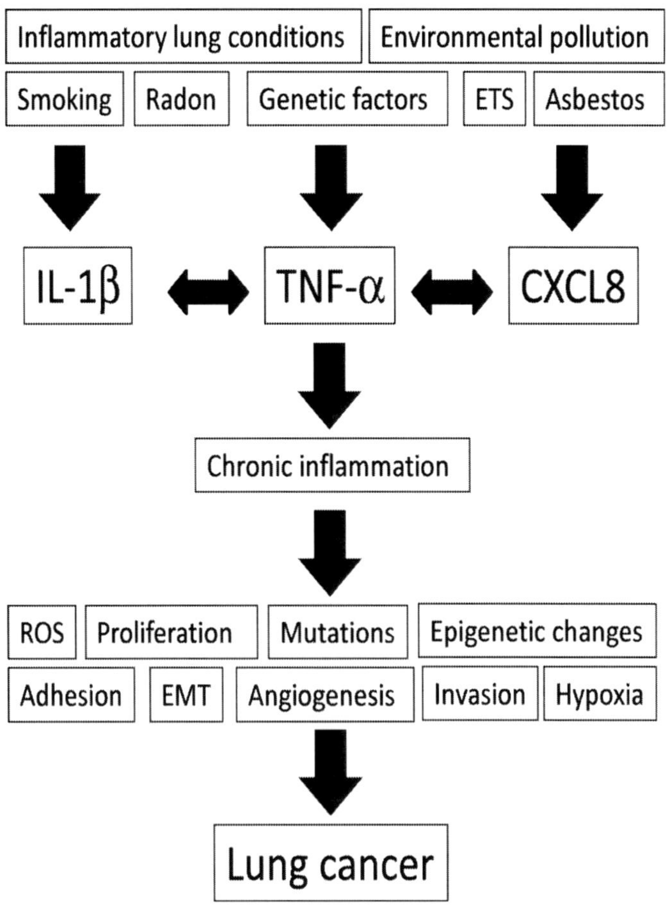


Figure 1. Possible links between chronic inflammation and lung carcinogenesis. ETS – environmental tobacco smoke, ROS – reactive oxygen species, EMT – epithelial *mesenchymal transition.*

## TNF-α

TNF-α is a soluble factor, which was first isolated in bacillus calmette-guerin (BCG) mice treated with endotoxin. This produced haemorrhagic necrosis of tumours, hence the name TNF [95]. It was cloned in 1985 by various groups, demonstrating cytotoxic activity in mouse and human cells [96]. TNF-α is secreted by activated monocytes, macrophages, mast cells and NK, B and T cells. It is associated with chronic inflammation and can induce further cytokine secretion. TNF-α secretion by tumour cells can have two distinct effects. It can result in either anti-tumour (destruction of tissue and tumour blood supply) or pro-tumour effects (tissue remodelling and stromal development) when produced chronically [24, 97, 98]. The disruption of tumour vasculature is thought to involve TNF-α's ability to deactivate integrin αvβ3 resulting in the disruption of the extra-cellular matrix (ECM) [99].

TNF-α belongs to a large super-family of ligands, which are type 2 trans-membrane proteins. It binds as a homo-trimer and signals through two receptors, TNF receptor 1 (TNRR1) and 2 (TNFR2), which initiate intracellular signaling [100]. When TNF-α binds its receptors, it can regulate at least 4 pathways - (a) pro-apoptotic, (b) anti-apoptotic, (c) activator protein 1 (AP-1) and (d) NF-κB activation [101]. TNFR1 is expressed on most cells, whereas TNFR2 is primarily expressed on haematopoietic cells. TNFR1 signalling can trigger STAT3 [102] and Jun N terminal kinase (JNK) activation [103]. Its activation of NF-κB occurs via a number of intermediates, including but not limited to, mitogen activated protein kinase (MAPK) [104]. Although, TNF-α is involved in normal physiological processes it can mediate survival, proliferation and metastases of tumours through the activation of NF-κB [105].

When TNF-α is dysregulated in local environments, this can give rise to several pathological diseases such as rheumatoid arthritis (RA) [106, 107], inflammatory bowel disease (IBD) [107], diabetes [107] and Crohn's disease [108]. There is a wide range of studies that implicate TNF-α in cancer. High levels of TNF-α are linked to poor survival, for example in prostate and breast [24], and is responsible for cancer cachexia in certain mouse tumour models [109]. The TNF gene was expressed in ovarian biopsies [110, 111] and in invasive breast cancer [112]. Furthermore, increased levels of TNF-α can contribute to epithelial mesenchymal transition (EMT) in colon [113], breast [114] and renal [115] cells. TNF-α knock outs (KO) [116, 117] and TNF receptor KO, particularly TNFR1, were resistant to chemically induced skin cancer [117] and chemical carcinogenesis of the liver [118]. Indeed most of the pro–tumour effects of TNF-α are attributable to TNFR1 receptor signalling.

In terms of lung cancer, the lungs of smokers tend to have higher levels of TNF-α than the lungs of non-smokers [119]. Some studies have also found that levels of TNF-α are higher in lung cancer patients compared to cancer free patients [120-123]. For example, De Vita *et al* reported elevated serum levels of TNF-α in patients with metastatic disease and tumour progression. These findings suggest that elevated cytokine levels may be associated with a worse prognosis [122]. It has been demonstrated that TNF-α is required for Lewis lung carcinoma metastasis [124] and studies have shown that TNF-α promotes EMT in both normal bronchial cells [125] and in NSCLC cell lines [126]. Oncogenic Ras is a common mutation in lung cancer [127] and recent evidence has suggested that Ras ($Ras^{V12}$) signalling can alter TNF-α signalling [128]. In *Drosophila*, Ras switches the anti-tumour actions of

TNF-α into pro-tumour activities [128]. This association may also be similar in human cancers.

In our laboratory, we have found that over-expression of TNF-α in a normal bronchial epithelial cell line increased the invasive and adhesive properties of cells when compared with wild type empty vector controls, with changes in the expression of important lung cancer related genes such as *p53* and *c-myc*. Futhermore, gene array studies demonstrated changes in numerous cancer hallmark pathways including matrix metalloproteinases (MMPs), integrins and the metastases mediator gene, S100A4. In addition, basal levels of TNF-α and its two receptors (TNFR1/TNFR2) were higher in NSCLC cells compared with normal cells (unpublished data).

## IL-1β

Interleukins are a group of cytokines secreted by leucocytes; which bring about changes in cellular metabolism and are involved in pathogenic challenges. IL-1β is a pleiotrophic cytokine that primarily affects inflammation and immune responses, but also regulates homeostatic functions [4]. IL-1β and its receptors are expressed in a wide variety of cells and has been implicated in the pathogenesis of acute or chronic inflammatory diseases and malignancies [72], particularly gastric cancers [129]. It was discovered in the late 1960s by a number of groups and is known by a variety of names due to its function. These include; endogenous pyrogen, leukocyte endogenous mediator (LEM), lymphocyte activating factor (LAF) and B cell activating factor [72]. It was cloned in 1984 by Charles Dinarello [130].

IL-1β is secreted by monocytes, macrophages, B cells, DC and endothelial cells. Amongst its targets are B cells, where it promotes maturation and clonal expansion of T helper ($T_H$) cells; and in macrophages and neutrophils, where it acts as a chemo-attractant to promote leukocyte infiltration [4]. Its main function is to promote the movement of inflammatory cells from the blood into inflamed or infected tissues and to stimulate the inflammatory response through NF-κB activation resulting in the activation of pathways such as AP-1, JNK and p38 MAPK [131].

The IL-1 family consists of two agonists, IL-1α and IL-1β, and an Interleukin-1 receptor antagonist (IL-1RA). IL-1β is synthesised as an inactive precursor inside the cell, is processed and then released from the cell by a mechanism involving the IL-1β converting enzyme (ICE) [131]. However, its mechanism of secretion has not yet been fully elucidated [132]. IL-1α is predominantly membrane bound, whereas IL-1β is active in a secreted form. There are two main IL-1 receptors, IL-1R1 and IL-R2. Although IL-1β binds both receptors, it signals through IL-1R1 only as IL-1R2 is considered a decoy receptor [132-134]. IL-1β has a further hierarchy of regulation in the form of receptor accessory proteins (IL-1RacP) of which there are two types, soluble and membrane bound [135]. Membrane bound accessory protein assists in signalling while the soluble form does not [136].

IL-1β initiates inflammation through the recruitment of leukocytes into tissues and induction of other pro-inflammatory genes, such as chemokines/cytokines and MMPs. An important amplification loop in the inflammatory response involves IL-1β and TNF-α, and their ability to stimulate their own expression and that of each other [74]. IL-1β affects the proliferation and differentiation of both innate and adaptive immune cells and is involved in human diseases such as arthritis, pulmonary fibrosis, central nervous system (CNS) issues, diabetes and cardiovascular disease [131].

IL-1β promotes angiogenesis and favours a pro-metastatic environment. It is abundant at tumour sites where it plays a role in carcinogenesis and tumour host interactions [137-139]. Microenvironment derived IL-1β plays a role in the development of chemically induced tumours. In IL-1β deficient mice, tumours began to develop after a prolonged lag period compared to IL-1RA KO mice [140].

Following an initial mutagenic event, local IL-1β can stimulate proliferation of pre-malignant cells, and in turn this extensive proliferation can lead to the generation of malignant cells and enhancement of the invasiveness of a pre-existing tumour by promoting angiogenesis [134]. IL-1β promotes murine tumour growth of Lewis lung carcinoma via the induction of angiogenic factors, through an increase in VEGF and CXCL2 production [141]. Over-expression of IL-1β in 'violent fibrosarcoma' cells resulted in a more invasive tumour [142]. An increased local level of IL-1β usually correlates with tumour invasiveness and a poor prognosis [137, 143].

In IL-1β competent mice, tumours grew more aggressively [144] and had increased experimental liver metastases [145, 146]. The pro-tumour capabilities are re-enforced in these studies as treatment with IL-RA decreases tumour growth and angiogenesis [138, 147], while over-expression of IL-RA inhibited tumour growth and metastasis in a human melanoma xenograft model [148].

IL-1RA would appear to be an important target in IL-1β associated carcinogenesis. Although IL-1α and IL-1β have similar effects, it has been proposed that membrane bound IL-1α expressed on malignant cells stimulates anti-tumour activity [142].

In lung cancer, IL-1β levels are higher in the lungs of smokers [119], levels are also higher in lung cancer patients compared with controls [148-150] and is highly expressed in the microenvironment of murine lung tumours [151]. Elevated serum levels of IL-1β were found in patients with metastatic disease and tumour progression and may be associated with a worse prognosis [122]. Significantly IL-1β has been shown to promote lung cancer and experimental lung metastases through its activation of adhesion, invasion and angiogenesis mediators [74, 137, 143, 152, 153]. IL-1β may contribute to EMT in NSCLC, in part through the down regulation of E-cadherin [154]. IL-1β can activate a number of MMPs in NSCLC cells [155] such as MMP9 [156].

Activation of MMPs may occur through differential signalling pathways such as MAPK to promote invasion [155] and through a c-Src dependent mechanism to promote cell migration [156]. Other signalling mediators in the IL-1β pathway may be cancer promoting such as Interleukin-1 Receptor-Associated Kinase-1 (IRAK1). IRAK1 was increased in NSCLC tumor tissues compared with controls and was associated with worse progression free survival [157]. IL-1β interlinks with a number of immune mediators and most recently has been shown to interact with IL-17 in murine models of lung cancer with varying effects on lung metastases [158].

Studies in our laboratory have demonstrated that, overexpression of IL-1β in normal bronchial epithelial cells produced similar effects as those outlined for TNF-α overexpression above (increased invasion and adhesion) and IL-1RA levels were reduced in NSCLC cell lines compared with normal cell lines (unpublished data).

## Interleukin 8 (CXCL8/IL-8)

The term chemokine refers to a family of low molecular weight (8-10 kDa) chemotactic cytokines. Chemokines are small inducible cytokines, which are chemo-attractants for leukocytes. They cause the directed migration of leukocytes along a chemokine gradient, which was first described by Leber in 1888 who observed the movement of leucocytes towards sites of inflammation [159]. A number of chemokines may also be involved in normal homeostasis, such as leukocyte maturation in the bone marrow and ensuring the renewal of circulating leucocytes [160]. Chemokines are classified by their amino acid composition, functional activity and receptor binding properties and comprise of four sub families defined according to the first two of four conserved cysteine residues (a) C, (b) CC, (c) CXC and (d) CXXXC (151). There are over 50 members of the chemokine ligand family and over 20 functional signalling receptors [75].

The CXC chemokine family contains two subtypes, $ELR^+$ and $ELR^-$, according to a specific Glu-Leu-Arg (ELR) motif preceding the first cysteine residue [74]. The $ELR^+$ chemokines have a number of pleiotrophic effects in immunity such as the regulation of angiogenesis, cell growth and tumour immunity. They act on the nervous system in addition to endothelial cells involved in angiogenesis or angiostasis. Certain chemokine receptor ligand pairs can recruit DCs to the site of inflammation and in homing to lymphoid organs where they present antigens to T and B cells, and are therefore crucial in the initiation of adaptive immune responses [161]. The CXC ($ELR^+$) chemokines are also involved in both physiological and pathological inflammatory conditions. CXCR2 KO mice for example, displayed significant delays in wound healing [162].

A well known family member of the CXC ($ELR^+$) is CXCL8/IL-8. CXCL8 was discovered as a neutrophil activating peptide (NAP1) in 1987 [163, 164]. CXCL8 predominately signals through the G protein coupled receptor (GPCR) CXCR2; however it can also signal through the CXCR1 receptor. Studies have shown that CXCR2 is the primary functional receptor mediating both endothelial cell chemotaxis and angiogenesis [165]. CXCL8 itself is a potent angiogenic factor [166]. Blocking CXCR2 activity, or its downstream effectors, impairs the ability of CXCL8 to promote endothelial tube formation [167]. CXCR2 when activated can regulate several intracellular pathways such as Ras, Phosphatidylinositol 3-kinase (PI3K) and NF-κB [167, 168]. CXC ($ELR^+$) promoters contain a putative *cis* element that recognises NF-κB, resulting in the trans-activation of CXC chemokines [169]. Chemokine receptors are up-regulated on tumour cells which allow the tumour to take advantage of a chemokine rich environment, thereby promoting tumour growth and vascularisation. These mediators can recruit macrophages, which then secrete pro-angiogenic factors [170-172].

Initially, chemokines were thought to play a unique role in attracting specific leucocytes to a site of injury. It has now been shown that they are key players in cancer. They are involved in the neoplastic transformation of cells, promotion of angiogenesis, tumour clonal expansion and changes in the ECM. They also mediate organ specific metastases in cancer 173, 174]. The metastatic destinations of cells are restricted by the expression of chemokines receptors on leucocytes, which may allow the concise control of cell movement and retention at tumour site [175-177].

A variety of CXC chemokines have been detected in neoplastic tissues as products of tumour cells or stromal elements [172]. CXCR2 is involved in skin carcinogenesis [178], while CXCL2 and 3 are up regulated in melanoma [179], as is CXCL1 [180]. CXCL8 stimulates pancreatic cell growth and CXCL8 levels are higher in ovarian cancer cells [111]. CXCL1 is expressed in the colon [181] and promotes tumour growth, leukocyte infiltration and angiogenesis through CXCR2 [182]. CXC expression is increased in adrenal cancer [183] and high CXC expression can mediate tumourigenicity in prostate cancer [184]. CXCL1 and 5 have also been shown to aid in metastasising colon cancer to the liver [185].

High levels of CXCL8 were associated with increased lung cancer risk [186] and were significantly higher in lung cancer patients compared with controls [76, 123, 187, 188]. Smokers also tend to have increased levels of CXCL8 [187-189]. Inhibition of CXCL8 reduced tumourigenesis in a murine model of NSCLC [190] with cancer growth and metastatic potential down-regulated in decreased CXCR2−/− models [191]. In addition, blockade of the CXCR2 receptor leads to a significant inhibition of human melanoma tumour growth and experimental lung metastases in CXCR2−/− mice, as well as a reduction in angiogenesis [191, 192]. It has been found that NSCLC patients with activating mutations in *KRAS* or *EGFR* (Epidermal Growth Factor Receptor) have higher levels of CXCL8 with CXCL8 implicated in oncogenic KRAS-driven NSCLC [187]. Other studies have implicated CXCL8 in the EGFR–PI3K signalling pathway in NSCLC [193].

## Targeting Inflammation as a Therapeutic Option

Five year survival rates remain poor in NSCLC, with the most recent advances in targeted therapy such as Erlotinib and Crizotinib benefiting a small proportion of patients harbouring specific mutations. There is an urgent need to identify novel targets in NSCLC and inflammatory mediators may provide a route to new therapeutic avenues.

The most widely studied anti-inflammatory drugs in cancer patients is NSAIDs which to date has produced somewhat conflicting results. A recent meta analysis found that low dose aspirin reduced the number of cancer related deaths [27]. In terms of lung cancer the results are inconsistent with some analyses showing a reduction in lung cancer risk [194], some showing a protective effect in males only [195] and others showing no change [196]. There are currently a number of studies ongoing but conflicts in overall benefits may be due differences in ethnicity, dosing, history of previous NSAID use and smoking status.

There are a number of anti-inflammatory biologics currently on the market that are almost exclusively used in the treatment of auto-immune conditions. These include anti-TNF-α agents (Adalimumab (Humira), Etanercept (Enbrel), Infliximab (Remicade), Certolizumab (Cimzia)), anti-IL-1β agent (Anakinra (Kineret)) and anti-IL-6 agent (RoActemra (*Tocilizumab*)). Advanced cancer patients (with different primaries) treated with Infliximab showed that it was well tolerated and resulted in disease stabilisation in 7/41 patients [197]. This was also demonstrated in recurrent ovarian cancer patients treated with Etanercept, with 6/30 patients showing pro-longed stable disease [198]. Using high dose Infliximab in renal cell carcinoma, 61% of patients attained stable disease status [199]. Conversely, a new adenovector system, TNFerade, is currently in a number of clinical trials in various solid tumours [200]. It allows for local delivery and stimulates TNF-α production in the tumour. In advanced solid tumours, 4/16 patients had complete regression [201]. Treatment in soft tissue carcinomas with this system resulted in a high number of objective responses [202] and longer survival in a Phase I trial in oesophageal cancer [203]. However, a recent Phase III trial in patients with locally advanced pancreatic cancer ended prematurely based on interim analysis. Results demonstrated an 8% lower risk of death, however based on the numbers enrolled on the trial, this would not have reached statistical significance (www.genvec.com/download/press/2010%2003.29%20GenVec%20PACT%20Press%20Release.pdf).

It is important to note that anti-TNF-α therapies may be more appropriate for non smoking lung cancer patients as some studies have shown an increase in lung cancer diagnoses in heavy and former smokers while on anti-TNF-α treatment for auto immune conditions [204].

Anakinra (Kineret) is an IL-1 receptor antagonist and is currently the only biological agent on the market that targets the IL-1 pathway. Blocking IL-1 signalling through IL-1 receptor antagonist delivery has been shown to reduce angiogenesis and tumour growth [147] and may offer potential to target cancer [138]. IL-1Ra has been shown to reduce the number of lung metastases in a murine B16 melanoma model [205]. In a phase II clinical trial, Anakinra led to an improvement in progression free survival in multiple myeloma patients [206]. Further trials are ongoing in a number of solid tumours using these targeted biological therapies. There is potential that patients could be stratified for treatment according to the expression levels of one or more inflammatory mediators.

# Conclusion

Inflammation is a tightly regulated and controlled process. However chronic or unresolved inflammation can lead to a number of pathological disease states including cancer. To date, a number of biological therapies such as small molecule inhibitors and monoclonal antibodies have shown efficacy against cancer in various *in vitro* and *in vivo* studies and show great promise for the future. It is conceivable that specific inflammatory mediator targeted therapy would provide an important benefit to patients. Further studies are warranted in order to correctly stratify patients for anti-inflammatory based therapies.

# References

[1] Ferlay J, Shin HR, Bray F, et al. Estimates of worldwide burden of cancer in 2008: GLOBOCAN 2008. *Int J Cancer*. 2010 Dec 15;127(12):2893-917.

[2] Youlden DR, Cramb SM, Baade PD. The International Epidemiology of Lung Cancer: geographical distribution and secular trends. *J Thorac Oncol.* 2008 Aug;3(8):819-31.

[3] Doll R, Hill AB. Smoking and carcinoma of the lung. Preliminary report. 1950. *Bull World Health Organ*. 1999;77(1):84-93.

[4] Amos CI, Xu W, Spitz MR. Is there a genetic basis for lung cancer susceptibility? *Recent Results Cancer Res*. 1999;151:3-12.

[5] Simonato L, Agudo A, Ahrens W, et al. Lung cancer and cigarette smoking in Europe: an update of risk estimates and an assessment of inter-country heterogeneity. *Int J Cancer*. 2001 Mar 15;91(6):876-87.

[6] Sun S, Schiller JH, Gazdar AF. Lung cancer in never smokers--a different disease. *Nat Rev Cancer*. 2007 Oct;7(10):778-90.
[7] Yu IT, Chiu YL, Au JS, et al. Dose-response relationship between cooking fumes exposures and lung cancer among Chinese nonsmoking women. *Cancer Res*. 2006 May 1;66(9):4961-7.
[8] Cheng YW, Wu MF, Wang J, et al. Human papillomavirus 16/18 E6 oncoprotein is expressed in lung cancer and related with p53 inactivation. *Cancer Res*. 2007 Nov 15;67(22):10686-93.
[9] Syrjanen K. Detection of Human Papillomavirus in Lung Cancer: Systematic Review and Meta-analysis. *Anticancer Res*. 2012 Aug;32(8):3235-50.
[10] Schabath MB, Wu X, Vassilopoulou-Sellin R, et al. Hormone replacement therapy and lung cancer risk: a case-control analysis. *Clin Cancer Res*. 2004 Jan 1;10(1 Pt 1):113-23.
[11] Blackman JA, Coogan PF, Rosenberg L, et al. Estrogen replacement therapy and risk of lung cancer. *Pharmacoepidemiol Drug Saf*. 2002 Oct-Nov;11(7):561-7.
[12] Hirayama T. Non-smoking wives of heavy smokers have a higher risk of lung cancer: a study from Japan. 1981. *Bull World Health Organ*. 2000;78(7):940-2.
[13] Zhong L, Goldberg MS, Parent ME, Hanley JA. Exposure to environmental tobacco smoke and the risk of lung cancer: a meta-analysis. *Lung Cancer*. 2000 Jan;27(1):3-18.
[14] Hecht SS. Tobacco carcinogens, their biomarkers and tobacco-induced cancer. *Nat Rev Cancer*. 2003 Oct;3(10):733-44.
[15] Darby S, Hill D, Auvinen A, et al. Radon in homes and risk of lung cancer: collaborative analysis of individual data from 13 European case-control studies. *BMJ*. 2005 Jan 29;330(7485):223.
[16] Bailey-Wilson JE, Amos CI, Pinney SM, et al. A major lung cancer susceptibility locus maps to chromosome 6q23-25. *Am J Hum Genet*. 2004 Sep;75(3):460-74.
[17] Brenner DR, McLaughlin JR, Hung RJ. Previous lung diseases and lung cancer risk: a systematic review and meta-analysis. *PLoS ONE*.6(3):e17479.
[18] Goldsby R, Kindt T, Osborne B. Kuby *Immunology*. Fourth ed. New York: W. H. Freeman and Company; 2000.
[19] Shankaran V, Ikeda H, Bruce AT, et al. IFNgamma and lymphocytes prevent primary tumour development and shape tumour immunogenicity. *Nature*. 2001 Apr 26;410(6832):1107-11.
[20] Dunn GP, Old LJ, Schreiber RD. The immunobiology of cancer immunosurveillance and immunoediting. *Immunity*. 2004 Aug;21(2):137-48.
[21] Dalgleish AG, O'Byrne K. Inflammation and cancer: the role of the immune response and angiogenesis. *Cancer Treat Res*. 2006;130:1-38.
[22] Mantovani A, Romero P, Palucka AK, Marincola FM. Tumour immunity: effector response to tumour and role of the microenvironment. *Lancet*. 2008 Mar 1;371(9614):771-83.
[23] de Visser KE, Korets LV, Coussens LM. De novo carcinogenesis promoted by chronic inflammation is B lymphocyte dependent. *Cancer Cell*. 2005 May;7(5):411-23.
[24] Mantovani A. Cancer: inflammation by remote control. *Nature*. 2005 Jun 9;435(7043):752-3.

[25] de Visser KE, Coussens LM. The interplay between innate and adaptive immunity regulates cancer development. *Cancer Immunol Immunother.* 2005 Nov;54(11):1143-52.
[26] Balkwill F, Charles KA, Mantovani A. Smoldering and polarized inflammation in the initiation and promotion of malignant disease. *Cancer Cell.* 2005 Mar;7(3):211-7.
[27] Thun MJ, Henley SJ, Gansler T. Inflammation and cancer: an epidemiological perspective. *Novartis Found Symp.* 2004;256:6-21; discussion 2-8, 49-52, 266-9.
[28] Parkin DM. 11. Cancers attributable to infection in the UK in 2010. *Br J Cancer.* Dec 6;105 Suppl 2:S49-56.
[29] Parkin DM. The global health burden of infection-associated cancers in the year 2002. *Int J Cancer.* 2006 Jun 15;118(12):3030-44.
[30] Kuper H, Adami HO, Trichopoulos D. Infections as a major preventable cause of human cancer. *J Intern Med.* 2000 Sep;248(3):171-83.
[31] Belpomme D, Irigaray P, Hardell L, et al. The multitude and diversity of environmental carcinogens. *Environ Res.* 2007 Nov;105(3):414-29.
[32] Parkin DM, Boyd L, Walker LC. 16. The fraction of cancer attributable to lifestyle and environmental factors in the UK in 2010. *Br J Cancer.* Dec 6;105 Suppl 2:S77-81.
[33] de Martel C, Ferlay J, Franceschi S, et al. Global burden of cancers attributable to infections in 2008: a review and synthetic analysis. *Lancet Oncol.* Jun;13(6):607-15.
[34] Balkwill FR, Mantovani A. Cancer-related inflammation: common themes and therapeutic opportunities. *Semin Cancer Biol.* 2012 Feb;22(1):33-40.
[35] Mantovani A, Allavena P, Sica A, Balkwill F. Cancer-related inflammation. *Nature.* 2008 Jul 24;454(7203):436-44.
[36] Grivennikov SI, Greten FR, Karin M. Immunity, inflammation, and cancer. *Cell.* 2010 Mar 19;140(6):883-99.
[37] Colotta F, Allavena P, Sica A, et al. Cancer-related inflammation, the seventh hallmark of cancer: links to genetic instability. *Carcinogenesis.* 2009 Jul;30(7):1073-81.
[38] Bouvard V, Baan R, Straif K, et al. A review of human carcinogens--Part B: biological agents. *Lancet Oncol.* 2009 Apr;10(4):321-2.
[39] Balkwill F, Mantovani A. Inflammation and cancer: back to Virchow? *Lancet.* 2001 Feb 17;357(9255):539-45.
[40] Dvorak HF. Tumors: wounds that do not heal. Similarities between tumor stroma generation and wound healing. *N Engl J Med.* 1986 Dec 25;315(26):1650-9.
[41] Coussens LM, Werb Z. Inflammation and cancer. *Nature.* 2002 Dec 19-26;420(6917):860-7.
[42] Mills EJ, Wu P, Alberton M, et al. Low-dose aspirin and cancer mortality: a meta-analysis of randomized trials. *Am J Med.* 2012 Jun;125(6):560-7.
[43] Balkwill F, Coussens LM. Cancer: an inflammatory link. *Nature.* 2004 Sep 23;431(7007):405-6.
[44] Mantovani A. Cancer: Inflaming metastasis. *Nature.* 2009 Jan 1;457(7225):36-7.
[45] Mantovani A, Pierotti MA. Cancer and inflammation: A complex relationship. *Cancer Lett.* 2008 Aug 28;267(2):180-1.
[46] Rothwell PM, Price JF, Fowkes FG, et al. Short-term effects of daily aspirin on cancer incidence, mortality, and non-vascular death: analysis of the time course of risks and benefits in 51 randomised controlled trials. *Lancet.* 2012 Apr 28;379(9826):1602-12.

[47] Rothwell PM, Wilson M, Price JF, et al. Effect of daily aspirin on risk of cancer metastasis: a study of incident cancers during randomised controlled trials. *Lancet.* 2012 Apr 28;379(9826):1591-601.
[48] Schreinemachers DM, Everson RB. Aspirin use and lung, colon, and breast cancer incidence in a prospective study. *Epidemiology.* 1994 Mar;5(2):138-46.
[49] Puntoni M, Marra D, Zanardi S, Decensi A. Inflammation and cancer prevention. *Ann Oncol.* 2008 Sep;19 Suppl 7:vii225-9.
[50] Harris RE, Beebe-Donk J, Alshafie GA. Reduced risk of human lung cancer by selective cyclooxygenase 2 (COX-2) blockade: results of a case control study. *Int J Biol Sci.* 2007;3(5):328-34.
[51] Muscat JE, Chen SQ, Richie JP, Jr., et al. Risk of lung carcinoma among users of nonsteroidal antiinflammatory drugs. *Cancer.* 2003 Apr 1;97(7):1732-6.
[52] Gupta RA, Dubois RN. Colorectal cancer prevention and treatment by inhibition of cyclooxygenase-2. *Nat Rev Cancer.* 2001 Oct;1(1):11-21.
[53] Eliassen AH, Chen WY, Spiegelman D, et al. Use of aspirin, other nonsteroidal anti-inflammatory drugs, and acetaminophen and risk of breast cancer among premenopausal women in the Nurses' Health Study II. *Arch Intern Med.* 2009 Jan 26;169(2):115-21; discussion 21.
[54] Feskanich D, Bain C, Chan AT, et al. Aspirin and lung cancer risk in a cohort study of women: dosage, duration and latency. *Br J Cancer.* 2007 Nov 5;97(9):1295-9.
[55] Hanahan D, Weinberg RA. The hallmarks of cancer. *Cell.* 2000 Jan 7;100(1):57-70.
[56] Hanahan D, Weinberg RA. Hallmarks of cancer: the next generation. *Cell.* 2011 Mar 4;144(5):646-74.
[57] Anand P, Kunnumakkara AB, Sundaram C, et al. Cancer is a preventable disease that requires major lifestyle changes. *Pharm Res.* 2008 Sep;25(9):2097-116.
[58] Allavena P, Garlanda C, Borrello MG, et al. Pathways connecting inflammation and cancer. *Curr Opin Genet Dev.* 2008 Feb;18(1):3-10.
[59] Porta C, Riboldi E, Sica A. Mechanisms linking pathogens-associated inflammation and cancer. *Cancer Lett.* 2011 Jun 28;305(2):250-62.
[60] Azad N, Rojanasakul Y, Vallyathan V. Inflammation and lung cancer: roles of reactive oxygen/nitrogen species. *J Toxicol Environ Health B Crit Rev.* 2008 Jan;11(1):1-15.
[61] Wiseman H, Halliwell B. Damage to DNA by reactive oxygen and nitrogen species: role in inflammatory disease and progression to cancer. *Biochem J.* 1996 Jan 1;313 ( Pt 1):17-29.
[62] Smith CJ, Perfetti TA, King JA. Perspectives on pulmonary inflammation and lung cancer risk in cigarette smokers. *Inhal Toxicol.* 2006 Aug;18(9):667-77.
[63] Ballaz S, Mulshine JL. The potential contributions of chronic inflammation to lung carcinogenesis. *Clin Lung Cancer.* 2003 Jul;5(1):46-62.
[64] Engels EA. Inflammation in the development of lung cancer: epidemiological evidence. *Expert Rev Anticancer Ther.* 2008 Apr;8(4):605-15.
[65] Cho WC, Kwan CK, Yau S, et al. The role of inflammation in the pathogenesis of lung cancer. *Expert Opin Ther Targets.* 2011 Sep;15(9):1127-37.
[66] Mayne ST, Buenconsejo J, Janerich DT. Previous lung disease and risk of lung cancer among men and women nonsmokers. *Am J Epidemiol.* 1999 Jan 1;149(1):13-20.
[67] Littman AJ, Jackson LA, Vaughan TL. Chlamydia pneumoniae and lung cancer: epidemiologic evidence. *Cancer Epidemiol Biomarkers Prev.* 2005 Apr;14(4):773-8.

[68] Alavanja MC, Brownson RC, Boice JD, Jr., Hock E. Preexisting lung disease and lung cancer among nonsmoking women. *Am J Epidemiol.* 1992 Sep 15;136(6):623-32.

[69] Kirk GD, Merlo C, O'Driscoll P, et al. HIV infection is associated with an increased risk for lung cancer, independent of smoking. *Clin Infect Dis.* 2007 Jul 1;45(1):103-10.

[70] de Torres JP, Bastarrika G, Wisnivesky JP, et al. Assessing the relationship between lung cancer risk and emphysema detected on low-dose CT of the chest. *Chest.* 2007 Dec;132(6):1932-8.

[71] Daniels CE, Jett JR. Does interstitial lung disease predispose to lung cancer? *Curr Opin Pulm Med.* 2005 Sep;11(5):431-7.

[72] Wu AH, Fontham ET, Reynolds P, et al. Previous lung disease and risk of lung cancer among lifetime nonsmoking women in the United States. *Am J Epidemiol.* 1995 Jun 1;141(11):1023-32.

[73] Santillan AA, Camargo CA, Jr., Colditz GA. A meta-analysis of asthma and risk of lung cancer (United States). *Cancer Causes Control.* 2003 May;14(4):327-34.

[74] Le Jeune I, Gribbin J, West J, et al. The incidence of cancer in patients with idiopathic pulmonary fibrosis and sarcoidosis in the UK. *Respir Med.* 2007 Dec;101(12):2534-40.

[75] Skillrud DM, Offord KP, Miller RD. Higher risk of lung cancer in chronic obstructive pulmonary disease. A prospective, matched, controlled study. *Ann Intern Med.* 1986 Oct;105(4):503-7.

[76] Engels EA, Shen M, Chapman RS, et al. Tuberculosis and subsequent risk of lung cancer in Xuanwei, China. *Int J Cancer.* 2008 Oct 1.

[77] Aoki K. Excess incidence of lung cancer among pulmonary tuberculosis patients. *Jpn J Clin Oncol.* 1993 Aug;23(4):205-20.

[78] Sasco AJ, Secretan MB, Straif K. Tobacco smoking and cancer: a brief review of recent epidemiological evidence. *Lung Cancer.* 2004 Aug;45 Suppl 2:S3-9.

[79] Gandini S, Botteri E, Iodice S, et al. Tobacco smoking and cancer: a meta-analysis. *Int J Cancer.* 2008 Jan 1;122(1):155-64.

[80] Wu KS, Zhou X, Zheng F, et al. Influence of interleukin-1 beta genetic polymorphism, smoking and alcohol drinking on the risk of non-small cell lung cancer. *Clin Chim Acta.* 2010 Oct 9;411(19-20):1441-6.

[81] Lee CH, Ko YC, Goggins W, et al. Lifetime environmental exposure to tobacco smoke and primary lung cancer of non-smoking Taiwanese women. *Int J Epidemiol.* 2000 Apr;29(2):224-31.

[82] Gorlova OY, Zhang Y, Schabath MB, et al. Never smokers and lung cancer risk: a case-control study of epidemiological factors. *Int J Cancer.* 2006 Apr 1;118(7):1798-804.

[83] Silverman DT, Samanic CM, Lubin JH, et al. The Diesel Exhaust in Miners study: a nested case-control study of lung cancer and diesel exhaust. *J Natl Cancer Inst.* Jun 6;104(11):855-68.

[84] Allavena P, Sica A, Solinas G, Porta C, et al. The inflammatory micro-environment in tumor progression: the role of tumor-associated macrophages. *Crit Rev Oncol Hematol.* 2008 Apr;66(1):1-9.

[85] Dinarello CA. Biologic basis for interleukin-1 in disease. *Blood.* 1996 Mar 15;87(6):2095-147.

[86] Strieter RM, Belperio JA, Keane MP. Cytokines in innate host defense in the lung. *J Clin Invest.* 2002 Mar;109(6):699-705.

[87] Apte RN, Voronov E. Is interleukin-1 a good or bad 'guy' in tumor immunobiology and immunotherapy? *Immunol Rev*. 2008 Apr;222:222-41.
[88] Balkwill FR. The chemokine system and cancer. *J Pathol*. 2012 Jan;226(2):148-57.
[89] Seike M, Yanaihara N, Bowman ED, et al. Use of a cytokine gene expression signature in lung adenocarcinoma and the surrounding tissue as a prognostic classifier. *J Natl Cancer Inst*. 2007 Aug 15;99(16):1257-69.
[90] Farlow EC, Vercillo MS, Coon JS, et al. A multi-analyte serum test for the detection of non-small cell lung cancer. *Br J Cancer*. 2010 Oct 12;103(8):1221-8.
[91] Spira A, Beane JE, Shah V, et al. Airway epithelial gene expression in the diagnostic evaluation of smokers with suspect lung cancer. *Nat Med*. 2007 Mar;13(3):361-6.
[92] Sugimoto M, Furuta T, Shirai N, et al. Different effects of polymorphisms of tumor necrosis factor-alpha and interleukin-1 beta on development of peptic ulcer and gastric cancer. *J Gastroenterol Hepatol*. 2007 Jan;22(1):51-9.
[93] Vishnoi M, Pandey SN, Choudhury G, et al. Do TNFA -308 G/A and IL6 -174 G/C gene polymorphisms modulate risk of gallbladder cancer in the north Indian population? *Asian Pac J Cancer Prev*. 2007 Oct-Dec;8(4):567-72.
[94] Zhang J, Dou C, Song Y, et al. Polymorphisms of tumor necrosis factor-alpha are associated with increased susceptibility to gastric cancer: a meta-analysis. *J Hum Genet*. 2008;53(6):479-89.
[95] Sobti RC, Kordi Tamandani DM, Shekari M, et al. Interleukin 1 beta gene polymorphism and risk of cervical cancer. *Int J Gynaecol Obstet*. 2008 Apr;101(1):47-52.
[96] Wang J, Cao C, Luo H, et al. Tumour necrosis factor alpha -308G/A polymorphism and risk of the four most frequent cancers: a meta-analysis. *Int J Immunogenet*. 2011 Aug;38(4):311-20.
[97] Landvik NE, Hart K, Skaug V, et al. A specific interleukin-1B haplotype correlates with high levels of IL1B mRNA in the lung and increased risk of non-small cell lung cancer. *Carcinogenesis*. 2009 May 21.
[98] Zienolddiny S, Ryberg D, Maggini V, et al. Polymorphisms of the interleukin-1 beta gene are associated with increased risk of non-small cell lung cancer. *Int J Cancer*. 2004 Apr 10;109(3):353-6.
[99] Asada M, Yasuda H, Ebihara S, et al. Interleukin-1beta gene polymorphisms associated with risk of lung cancer in Japanese. *Lung Cancer*. 2006 Nov;54(2):261-3.
[100] Landvik NE, Tekpli X, Anmarkrud KH, et al. Molecular characterization of a cancer-related single nucleotide polymorphism in the pro-inflammatory interleukin-1B gene. *Mol Carcinog*. 2012 Mar 29.
[101] Engels EA, Wu X, Gu J, et al. Systematic evaluation of genetic variants in the inflammation pathway and risk of lung cancer. *Cancer Res*. 2007 Jul 1;67(13):6520-7.
[102] Hart K, Haugen A, Zienolddiny S. Allele-specific induction of IL1B -31T/C promoter polymorphism by lung carcinogens. *Mutat Res*. 2008 Jul 9.
[103] Lind H, Zienolddiny S, Ryberg D, et al. Interleukin 1 receptor antagonist gene polymorphism and risk of lung cancer: a possible interaction with polymorphisms in the interleukin 1 beta gene. *Lung Cancer*. 2005 Dec;50(3):285-90.
[104] Flego V, Radojcic Badovinac A, Bulat-Kardum L, et al. Primary lung cancer and TNF-alpha gene polymorphisms: a case-control study in a Croatian population. *Med Sci Monit*. 2009 Jul;15(7):CR361-5.

[105] Wang J, Cao C, Luo H, et al. Tumour necrosis factor alpha -308G/A polymorphism and risk of the four most frequent cancers: a meta-analysis. *Int J Immunogenet.* Aug;38(4):311-20.
[106] Shih CM, Lee YL, Chiou HL, et al. Association of TNF-alpha polymorphism with susceptibility to and severity of non-small cell lung cancer. *Lung Cancer.* 2006 Apr;52(1):15-20.
[107] Wang N, Zhou R, Wang C, et al. -251 T/A polymorphism of the interleukin-8 gene and cancer risk: a HuGE review and meta-analysis based on 42 case-control studies. *Mol Biol Rep.* Mar;39(3):2831-41.
[108] Carswell EA, Old LJ, Kassel RL, et al. An endotoxin-induced serum factor that causes necrosis of tumors. *Proc Natl Acad Sci U S A.* 1975 Sep;72(9):3666-70.
[109] Old LJ. Tumor necrosis factor (TNF). *Science.* 1985 Nov 8;230(4726):630-2.
[110] Lu H, Ouyang W, Huang C. Inflammation, a key event in cancer development. *Mol Cancer Res.* 2006 Apr;4(4):221-33.
[111] Tandle A, Hanna E, Lorang D, et al. Tumor vasculature-targeted delivery of tumor necrosis factor-alpha. *Cancer.* 2009 Jan 1;115(1):128-39.
[112] Ruegg C, Yilmaz A, Bieler G, et al. Evidence for the involvement of endothelial cell integrin alphaVbeta3 in the disruption of the tumor vasculature induced by TNF and IFN-gamma. *Nat Med.* 1998 Apr;4(4):408-14.
[113] Tartaglia LA, Weber RF, Figari IS, et al. The two different receptors for tumor necrosis factor mediate distinct cellular responses. *Proc Natl Acad Sci U S A.* 1991 Oct 15;88(20):9292-6.
[114] Chen G, Goeddel DV. TNF-R1 signaling: a beautiful pathway. *Science.* 2002 May 31;296(5573):1634-5.
[115] Pincheira R, Castro AF, Ozes ON, et al. Type 1 TNF receptor forms a complex with and uses Jak2 and c-Src to selectively engage signaling pathways that regulate transcription factor activity. *J Immunol.* 2008 Jul 15;181(2):1288-98.
[116] MacEwan DJ. TNF receptor subtype signalling: differences and cellular consequences. *Cell Signal.* 2002 Jun;14(6):477-92.
[117] Bazzoni F, Beutler B. The tumor necrosis factor ligand and receptor families. *N Engl J Med.* 1996 Jun 27;334(26):1717-25.
[118] Sethi G, Sung B, Aggarwal BB. TNF: a master switch for inflammation to cancer. *Front Biosci.* 2008;13:5094-107.
[119] Feldmann M. Development of anti-TNF therapy for rheumatoid arthritis. *Nat Rev Immunol.* 2002 May;2(5):364-71.
[120] Locksley RM, Killeen N, Lenardo MJ. The TNF and TNF receptor superfamilies: integrating mammalian biology. *Cell.* 2001 Feb 23;104(4):487-501.
[121] Reich K, Nestle FO, Papp K, et al. Infliximab induction and maintenance therapy for moderate-to-severe psoriasis: a phase III, multicentre, double-blind trial. *Lancet.* 2005 Oct 15-21;366(9494):1367-74.
[122] Yoneda T, Alsina MA, Chavez JB, et al. Evidence that tumor necrosis factor plays a pathogenetic role in the paraneoplastic syndromes of cachexia, hypercalcemia, and leukocytosis in a human tumor in nude mice. *J Clin Invest.* 1991 Mar;87(3):977-85.
[123] Naylor MS, Stamp GW, Foulkes WD, Eccles D, et al. Tumor necrosis factor and its receptors in human ovarian cancer. Potential role in disease progression. *J Clin Invest.* 1993 May;91(5):2194-206.

[124] Szlosarek PW, Grimshaw MJ, Kulbe H, et al. Expression and regulation of tumor necrosis factor alpha in normal and malignant ovarian epithelium. *Mol Cancer Ther.* 2006 Feb;5(2):382-90.
[125] Miles DW, Happerfield LC, Naylor MS, et al. Expression of tumour necrosis factor (TNF alpha) and its receptors in benign and malignant breast tissue. *Int J Cancer.* 1994 Mar 15;56(6):777-82.
[126] Bates RC, Mercurio AM. Tumor necrosis factor-alpha stimulates the epithelial-to-mesenchymal transition of human colonic organoids. *Mol Biol Cell.* 2003 May;14(5):1790-800.
[127] Li CW, Xia W, Huo L, et al. Epithelial-mesenchymal transition induced by TNF-alpha requires NF-kappaB-mediated transcriptional upregulation of Twist1. *Cancer Res.* Mar 1;72(5):1290-300.
[128] Wu ST, Sun GH, Hsu CY, et al. Tumor necrosis factor-alpha induces epithelial-mesenchymal transition of renal cell carcinoma cells via a nuclear factor kappa B-independent mechanism. *Exp Biol Med* (Maywood). Sep 1;236(9):1022-9.
[129] Moore RJ, Owens DM, Stamp G, et al. Mice deficient in tumor necrosis factor-alpha are resistant to skin carcinogenesis. *Nat Med.* 1999 Jul;5(7):828-31.
[130] Arnott CH, Scott KA, Moore RJ, et al. Expression of both TNF-alpha receptor subtypes is essential for optimal skin tumour development. *Oncogene.* 2004 Mar 11;23(10):1902-10.
[131] Knight B, Yeoh GC, Husk KL, et al. Impaired preneoplastic changes and liver tumor formation in tumor necrosis factor receptor type 1 knockout mice. *J Exp Med.* 2000 Dec 18;192(12):1809-18.
[132] Glossop JR, Dawes PT, Mattey DL. Association between cigarette smoking and release of tumour necrosis factor alpha and its soluble receptors by peripheral blood mononuclear cells in patients with rheumatoid arthritis. *Rheumatology* (Oxford). 2006 Oct;45(10):1223-9.
[133] Derin D, Soydinc HO, Guney N, et al. Serum levels of apoptosis biomarkers, survivin and TNF-alpha in nonsmall cell lung cancer. *Lung Cancer.* 2008 Feb;59(2):240-5.
[134] Kayacan O, Karnak D, Beder S, et al. Impact of TNF-alpha and IL-6 levels on development of cachexia in newly diagnosed NSCLC patients. *Am J Clin Oncol.* 2006 Aug;29(4):328-35.
[135] De Vita F, Orditura M, Auriemma A, et al. Serum concentrations of proinflammatory cytokines in advanced non small cell lung cancer patients. *J Exp Clin Cancer Res.* 1998 Dec;17(4):413-7.
[136] Kaminska J, Kowalska M, Kotowicz B, et al. Pretreatment serum levels of cytokines and cytokine receptors in patients with non-small cell lung cancer, and correlations with clinicopathological features and prognosis. M-CSF - an independent prognostic factor. *Oncology.* 2006;70(2):115-25.
[137] Kim S, Takahashi H, Lin WW, et al. Carcinoma-produced factors activate myeloid cells through TLR2 to stimulate metastasis. *Nature.* 2009 Jan 1;457(7225):102-6.
[138] Kamitani S, Yamauchi Y, Kawasaki S, et al. Simultaneous stimulation with TGF-beta1 and TNF-alpha induces epithelial mesenchymal transition in bronchial epithelial cells. *Int Arch Allergy Immunol.*155(2):119-28.
[139] Yamauchi Y, Kohyama T, Takizawa H, et al. Tumor necrosis factor-alpha enhances both epithelial-mesenchymal transition and cell contraction induced in A549 human

alveolar epithelial cells by transforming growth factor-beta1. *Exp Lung Res.* Feb;36(1):12-24.
[140] Sekido Y, Fong KM, Minna JD. Molecular genetics of lung cancer. *Annu Rev Med.* 2003;54:73-87.
[141] Cordero JB, Macagno JP, Stefanatos RK, et al. Oncogenic Ras diverts a host TNF tumor suppressor activity into tumor promoter. *Dev Cell.* Jun 15;18(6):999-1011.
[142] El-Omar EM. The importance of interleukin 1beta in Helicobacter pylori associated disease. *Gut.* 2001 Jun;48(6):743-7.
[143] Auron PE, Webb AC, Rosenwasser LJ, et al. Nucleotide sequence of human monocyte interleukin 1 precursor cDNA. *Proc Natl Acad Sci U S A.* 1984 Dec;81(24):7907-11.
[144] Arend WP, Palmer G, Gabay C. IL-1, IL-18, and IL-33 families of cytokines. *Immunol Rev.* 2008 Jun;223:20-38.
[145] Dinarello CA. The interleukin-1 family: 10 years of discovery. *FASEB J.* 1994 Dec;8(15):1314-25.
[146] Colotta F, Dower SK, Sims JE, Mantovani A. The type II 'decoy' receptor: a novel regulatory pathway for interleukin 1. *Immunol Today.* 1994 Dec;15(12):562-6.
[147] Voronov E, Carmi Y, Apte RN. Role of IL-1-mediated inflammation in tumor angiogenesis. *Adv Exp Med Biol.* 2007;601:265-70.
[148] Jensen LE, Whitehead AS. The 3' untranslated region of the membrane-bound IL-1R accessory protein mRNA confers tissue-specific destabilization. *J Immunol.* 2004 Nov 15;173(10):6248-58.
[149] Jensen LE, Muzio M, Mantovani A, Whitehead AS. IL-1 signaling cascade in liver cells and the involvement of a soluble form of the IL-1 receptor accessory protein. *J Immunol.* 2000 May 15;164(10):5277-86.
[150] Apte RN, Dotan S, Elkabets M, et al. The involvement of IL-1 in tumorigenesis, tumor invasiveness, metastasis and tumor-host interactions. *Cancer Metastasis Rev.* 2006 Sep;25(3):387-408.
[151] Lewis AM, Varghese S, Xu H, Alexander HR. Interleukin-1 and cancer progression: the emerging role of interleukin-1 receptor antagonist as a novel therapeutic agent in cancer treatment. *J Transl Med.* 2006;4:48.
[152] Dinarello CA. The paradox of pro-inflammatory cytokines in cancer. *Cancer Metastasis Rev.* 2006 Sep;25(3):307-13.
[153] Krelin Y, Voronov E, Dotan S, et al. Interleukin-1beta-driven inflammation promotes the development and invasiveness of chemical carcinogen-induced tumors. *Cancer Res.* 2007 Feb 1;67(3):1062-71.
[154] Saijo Y, Tanaka M, Miki M, et al. Proinflammatory cytokine IL-1 beta promotes tumor growth of Lewis lung carcinoma by induction of angiogenic factors: in vivo analysis of tumor-stromal interaction. *J Immunol.* 2002 Jul 1;169(1):469-75.
[155] Apte RN, Douvdevani A, Zoller M, et al. Cytokine-induced tumor immunogenicity: endogenous interleukin-1 alpha expressed by fibrosarcoma cells confers reduced tumorigenicity. *Immunol Lett.* 1993 Dec;39(1):45-52.
[156] Apte RN, Krelin Y, Song X, et al. Effects of micro-environment- and malignant cell-derived interleukin-1 in carcinogenesis, tumour invasiveness and tumour-host interactions. *Eur J Cancer.* 2006 Apr;42(6):751-9.
[157] Nazarenko I, Marhaba R, Reich E, et al. Tumorigenicity of IL-1alpha- and IL-1beta-deficient fibrosarcoma cells. *Neoplasia.* 2008 Jun;10(6):549-62.

[158] Vidal-Vanaclocha F, Amezaga C, Asumendi A, et al. Interleukin-1 receptor blockade reduces the number and size of murine B16 melanoma hepatic metastases. *Cancer Res.* 1994 May 15;54(10):2667-72.
[159] Scherbarth S, Orr FW. Intravital videomicroscopic evidence for regulation of metastasis by the hepatic microvasculature: effects of interleukin-1alpha on metastasis and the location of B16F1 melanoma cell arrest. *Cancer Res.* 1997 Sep 15;57(18):4105-10.
[160] Bar D, Apte RN, Voronov E, Dinarello CA, et al. A continuous delivery system of IL-1 receptor antagonist reduces angiogenesis and inhibits tumor development. *FASEB J.* 2004 Jan;18(1):161-3.
[161] Elaraj DM, Weinreich DM, Varghese S, et al. The role of interleukin 1 in growth and metastasis of human cancer xenografts. *Clin Cancer Res.* 2006 Feb 15;12(4):1088-96.
[162] Alexandrakis MG, Passam FH, Perisinakis K, et al. Serum proinflammatory cytokines and its relationship to clinical parameters in lung cancer patients with reactive thrombocytosis. *Respir Med.* 2002 Aug;96(8):553-8.
[163] Matanic D, Beg-Zec Z, Stojanovic D, et al. Cytokines in patients with lung cancer. *Scand J Immunol.* 2003 Feb;57(2):173-8.
[164] Schmid MC, Avraamides CJ, Foubert P, et al. Combined blockade of integrin-alpha4beta1 plus cytokines SDF-1alpha or IL-1beta potently inhibits tumor inflammation and growth. *Cancer Res.* 2011 Nov 15;71(22):6965-75.
[165] Yano S, Nokihara H, Yamamoto A, et al. Multifunctional interleukin-1beta promotes metastasis of human lung cancer cells in SCID mice via enhanced expression of adhesion-, invasion- and angiogenesis-related molecules. *Cancer Sci.* 2003 Mar;94(3):244-52.
[166] Voronov E, Shouval DS, Krelin Y, et al. IL-1 is required for tumor invasiveness and angiogenesis. *Proc Natl Acad Sci U S A.* 2003 Mar 4;100(5):2645-50.
[167] Heinrich E, Dohadwala M, Charuworn B, Dubinett SM, editors. Inflammation dependent regulation of epithelial-mesenchymal transition in non-small cell lung cancer:the role of interleukin-1beta. *AACR*; 2008; San Diego, CA, USA.
[168] Petrella BL, Armstrong DA, Vincenti MP. Interleukin-1 beta and transforming growth factor-beta 3 cooperate to activate matrix metalloproteinase expression and invasiveness in A549 lung adenocarcinoma cells. *Cancer Lett.* 2012 Jul 13.
[169] Cheng CY, Kuo CT, Lin CC, Hsieh HL, et al. IL-1beta induces expression of matrix metalloproteinase-9 and cell migration via a c-Src-dependent, growth factor receptor transactivation in A549 cells. *Br J Pharmacol.* 2010 Aug;160(7):1595-610.
[170] Behrens C, Feng L, Kadara H, et al. Expression of interleukin-1 receptor-associated kinase-1 in non-small cell lung carcinoma and preneoplastic lesions. *Clin Cancer Res.* 2010 Jan 1;16(1):34-44.
[171] Carmi Y, Rinott G, Dotan S, et al. Microenvironment-derived IL-1 and IL-17 interact in the control of lung metastasis. *J Immunol.* 2011 Mar 15;186(6):3462-71.
[172] Jin T, Xu X, Hereld D. Chemotaxis, chemokine receptors and human disease. *Cytokine.* 2008 Aug 20.
[173] Baggiolini M. Chemokines and leukocyte traffic. *Nature.* 1998 Apr 9;392(6676):565-8.
[174] Sozzani S, Bosisio D, Mantovani A, Ghezzi P. Linking stress, oxidation and the chemokine system. *Eur J Immunol.* 2005 Nov;35(11):3095-8.
[175] Devalaraja RM, Nanney LB, Du J, et al. Delayed wound healing in CXCR2 knockout mice. *J Invest Dermatol.* 2000 Aug;115(2):234-44.

[176] Baggiolini M, Imboden P, Detmers P. Neutrophil activation and the effects of interleukin-8/neutrophil-activating peptide 1 (IL-8/NAP-1). *Cytokines.* 1992;4:1-17.
[177] Yoshimura T, Matsushima K, Tanaka S, et al. Purification of a human monocyte-derived neutrophil chemotactic factor that has peptide sequence similarity to other host defense cytokines. *Proc Natl Acad Sci U S A.* 1987 Dec;84(24):9233-7.
[178] Addison CL, Belperio JA, Burdick MD, Strieter RM. Overexpression of the duffy antigen receptor for chemokines (DARC) by NSCLC tumor cells results in increased tumor necrosis. *BMC Cancer.* 2004 Jun 23;4:28.
[179] Strieter RM, Polverini PJ, Arenberg DA, et al. Role of C-X-C chemokines as regulators of angiogenesis in lung cancer. *J Leukoc Biol.* 1995 May;57(5):752-62.
[180] Heidemann J, Ogawa H, Dwinell MB, et al. Angiogenic effects of interleukin 8 (CXCL8) in human intestinal microvascular endothelial cells are mediated by CXCR2. *J Biol Chem.* 2003 Mar 7;278(10):8508-15.
[181] Strieter RM, Burdick MD, Mestas J, et al. Cancer CXC chemokine networks and tumour angiogenesis. *Eur J Cancer.* 2006 Apr;42(6):768-78.
[182] Strieter RM, Burdick MD, Gomperts BN, et al. CXC chemokines in angiogenesis. *Cytokine Growth Factor Rev.* 2005 Dec;16(6):593-609.
[183] Raman D, Baugher PJ, Thu YM, Richmond A. Role of chemokines in tumor growth. *Cancer Lett.* 2007 Oct 28;256(2):137-65.
[184] Mantovani A, Bonecchi R, Locati M. Tuning inflammation and immunity by chemokine sequestration: decoys and more. *Nat Rev Immunol.* 2006 Dec;6(12):907-18.
[185] Balkwill F. Cancer and the chemokine network. *Nat Rev Cancer.* 2004 Jul;4(7):540-50.
[186] Arya M, Patel HR, Williamson M. Chemokines: key players in cancer. *Curr Med Res Opin.* 2003;19(6):557-64.
[187] Strieter RM, Belperio JA, Phillips RJ, Keane MP. Chemokines: angiogenesis and metastases in lung cancer. *Novartis Found Symp.* 2004;256:173-84; discussion 84-8, 259-69.
[188] Zlotnik A. Involvement of chemokine receptors in organ-specific metastasis. *Contrib Microbiol.* 2006;13:191-9.
[189] Balkwill F. Chemokine biology in cancer. *Semin Immunol.* 2003 Feb;15(1):49-55.
[190] Gomperts BN, Strieter RM. Chemokine-directed metastasis. *Contrib Microbiol.* 2006;13:170-90.
[191] Cataisson C, Ohman R, Patel G, et al. Inducible cutaneous inflammation reveals a protumorigenic role for keratinocyte CXCR2 in skin carcinogenesis. *Cancer Res.* 2009 Jan 1;69(1):319-28.
[192] Owen JD, Strieter R, Burdick M, et al. Enhanced tumor-forming capacity for immortalized melanocytes expressing melanoma growth stimulatory activity/growth-regulated cytokine beta and gamma proteins. *Int J Cancer.* 1997 Sep 26;73(1):94-103.
[193] Dhawan P, Richmond A. Role of CXCL1 in tumorigenesis of melanoma. *J Leukoc Biol.* 2002 Jul;72(1):9-18.
[194] Wen Y, Giardina SF, Hamming D, et al. GROalpha is highly expressed in adenocarcinoma of the colon and down-regulates fibulin-1. *Clin Cancer Res.* 2006 Oct 15;12(20 Pt 1):5951-9.
[195] Loukinova E, Dong G, Enamorado-Ayalya I, et al. Growth regulated oncogene-alpha expression by murine squamous cell carcinoma promotes tumor growth, metastasis,

leukocyte infiltration and angiogenesis by a host CXC receptor-2 dependent mechanism. *Oncogene*. 2000 Jul 20;19(31):3477-86.
[196] Schteingart DE, Giordano TJ, Benitez RS, et al. Overexpression of CXC chemokines by an adrenocortical carcinoma: a novel clinical syndrome. *J Clin Endocrinol Metab*. 2001 Aug;86(8):3968-74.
[197] Moore BB, Arenberg DA, Stoy K, et al. Distinct CXC chemokines mediate tumorigenicity of prostate cancer cells. *Am J Pathol*. 1999 May;154(5):1503-12.
[198] Rubie C, Frick VO, Wagner M, et al. ELR+ CXC chemokine expression in benign and malignant colorectal conditions. *BMC Cancer*. 2008;8:178.
[199] Orditura M, De Vita F, Catalano G , et al. Elevated serum levels of interleukin-8 in advanced non-small cell lung cancer patients: relationship with prognosis. *J Interferon Cytokine* Res. 2002 Nov;22(11):1129-35.
[200] Sunaga N, Imai H, Shimizu K, et al. Oncogenic KRAS-induced interleukin-8 overexpression promotes cell growth and migration and contributes to aggressive phenotypes of non-small cell lung cancer. *Int J Cancer*. Apr 15;130(8):1733-44.
[201] Pine SR, Mechanic LE, Enewold L, et al. Increased levels of circulating interleukin 6, interleukin 8, C-reactive protein, and risk of lung cancer. *J Natl Cancer Inst*. 2011 Jul 20;103(14):1112-22.
[202] Takizawa H, Tanaka M, Takami K, et al. Increased expression of inflammatory mediators in small-airway epithelium from tobacco smokers. *Am J Physiol Lung Cell Mol Physiol*. 2000 May;278(5):L906-13.
[203] Arenberg DA, Kunkel SL, Polverini PJ, et al. Inhibition of interleukin-8 reduces tumorigenesis of human non-small cell lung cancer in SCID mice. *J Clin Invest*. 1996 Jun 15;97(12):2792-802.
[204] Singh S, Varney M, Singh RK. Host CXCR2-dependent regulation of melanoma growth, angiogenesis, and experimental lung metastasis. *Cancer Res*. 2009 Jan 15;69(2):411-5.
[205] Keane MP, Belperio JA, Xue YY, Burdick MD, et al. Depletion of CXCR2 inhibits tumor growth and angiogenesis in a murine model of lung cancer. *J Immunol*. 2004 Mar 1;172(5):2853-60.
[206] Zhang Y, Wang L, Zhang M, et al. Potential mechanism of interleukin-8 production from lung cancer cells: an involvement of EGF-EGFR-PI3K-Akt-Erk pathway. *J Cell Physiol*. Jan;227(1):35-43.
[207] Xu J, Yin Z, Gao W, et al. Meta-analysis on the association between nonsteroidal anti-inflammatory drug use and lung cancer risk. *Clin Lung Cancer*. 2012 Jan;13(1):44-51.
[208] McCormack VA, Hung RJ, Brenner DR, et al. Aspirin and NSAID use and lung cancer risk: a pooled analysis in the International Lung Cancer Consortium (ILCCO). *Cancer Causes Control*. 2011 Dec;22(12):1709-20.
[209] Oh SW, Myung SK, Park JY, et al. Aspirin use and risk for lung cancer: a meta-analysis. *Ann Oncol*. 2011 Nov;22(11):2456-65.
[210] Brown ER, Charles KA, Hoare SA, et al. A clinical study assessing the tolerability and biological effects of infliximab, a TNF-alpha inhibitor, in patients with advanced cancer. *Ann Oncol*. 2008 Jul;19(7):1340-6.
[211] Madhusudan S, Muthuramalingam SR, Braybrooke JP, et al. Study of etanercept, a tumor necrosis factor-alpha inhibitor, in recurrent ovarian cancer. *J Clin Oncol*. 2005 Sep 1;23(25):5950-9.

[212] Harrison ML, Obermueller E, Maisey NR, et al. Tumor necrosis factor alpha as a new target for renal cell carcinoma: two sequential phase II trials of infliximab at standard and high dose. J Clin Oncol. 2007 Oct 10;25(29):4542-9.
[213] MacGill RS, Davis TA, Macko J, et al. Local gene delivery of tumor necrosis factor alpha can impact primary tumor growth and metastases through a host-mediated response. Clin Exp Metastasis. 2007;24(7):521-31.
[214] McLoughlin JM, McCarty TM, Cunningham C, et al. TNFerade, an adenovector carrying the transgene for human tumor necrosis factor alpha, for patients with advanced solid tumors: surgical experience and long-term follow-up. Ann Surg Oncol. 2005 Oct;12(10):825-30.
[215] Mundt AJ, Vijayakumar S, Nemunaitis J, et al. A Phase I trial of TNFerade biologic in patients with soft tissue sarcoma in the extremities. Clin Cancer Res. 2004 Sep 1;10(17):5747-53.
[216] Chang KJ, Reid T, Senzer N, et al. Phase I evaluation of TNFerade biologic plus chemoradiotherapy before esophagectomy for locally advanced resectable esophageal cancer. Gastrointest Endosc. 2012 Jun;75(6):1139-46 e2.
[217] Lees CW, Ironside J, Wallace WA, Satsangi J. Resolution of non-small-cell lung cancer after withdrawal of anti-TNF therapy. N Engl J Med. 2008 Jul 17;359(3):320-1.
[218] Lavi G, Voronov E, Dinarello CA, et al. Sustained delivery of IL-1 Ra from biodegradable microspheres reduces the number of murine B16 melanoma lung metastases. J Control Release. 2007 Nov 6;123(2):123-30.
[219] Lust JA, Lacy MQ, Zeldenrust SR, et al. Induction of a chronic disease state in patients with smoldering or indolent multiple myeloma by targeting interleukin 1{beta}-induced interleukin 6 production and the myeloma proliferative component. Mayo Clin Proc. 2009 Feb;84(2):114-22.

In: Lung Cancer: A Comprehensive Overview
Editor: Kathy Gately
ISBN: 978-1-62618-447-3


*Chapter X*

# The Link between Chronic Obstructive Pulmonary Disease and Lung Cancer: Novel Molecular Insights

***Nikoletta Rovina* and Fotis Vlastos***
Pulmonary and Critical Care Medicine, Sotiria Hospital,
University of Athens, Athens, Greece

## Abstract

The combined effect of environmental inhaled factors (mainly, cigarette smoke) and a genetic predisposition may result in two leading causes of morbidity and of mortality worldwide, namely lung cancer and Chronic Obstructive Pulmonary Disease (COPD). Cigarette smoke exposure induces oxidative stress and a chronic inflammatory response in the airways of smokers, which may persist long after smoking cessation. Several studies have identified common genes implicating in the pathobiology of these diseases. There is evidence that an overlapping genetic susceptibility may be mediated through receptors expressed on the bronchial epithelium that implicate molecular pathways underlying both COPD and lung cancer pathophysiology. Furthermore, it appears that aberrant inflammatory and/or immune-modulatory pathways leading to excess matrix metalloproteinases, growth factors and airway remodelling in COPD may also be promoting malignant transformation of the bronchial epithelium. In support of these findings, COPD is by far the greatest risk factor for lung cancer amongst smokers found in 50–90% of patients with lung cancer.

The understanding of the common signalling pathways involved in COPD and lung cancer may have several clinical implications. New treatments targeting the underlying disease process in COPD and therefore reducing the risk of developing lung cancer in these patients may be developed. Finally, the identification of genes/biomarkers of susceptibility for lung cancer among COPD patients may provide markers for the early diagnosis of lung cancer.

* Email: nikrovina@med.uoa.gr.

**Keywords:** Chronic Obstructive Pulmonary Disease, lung cancer, chronic inflammation, oxidative stress, smoking exposure

# Introduction

The burden of tobacco smoke exposure is considerable. In a worldwide scale, 57% of men and 10% of women are reported to consume tobacco products, especially cigarettes [1]. Cigarette smoke exposure in combination with a genetic predisposition results in two of the leading causes of morbidity and mortality worldwide, namely lung cancer and chronic obstructive pulmonary disease (COPD), a disease state characterised by airflow limitation that is not fully reversible, it is usually progressive, and associated with an abnormal inflammatory response of the lungs. Although the concept that lung cancer and COPD share a common 'familial component' was first suggested by Cohen et al. in 1977 [2] interest in this hypothesis has only recently re-emerged [3, 4]. Based on studies conducted in twins, it has been suggested that the heritability of lung cancer is estimated to be 15–25%, while a reduced forced expiratory volume in 1 second (FEV1) is estimated to be 40–77% [5, 6]. This observation suggests that among smokers, genetic factors appear to play a greater role in the susceptibility to COPD than in lung cancer.

Each year, 1.2 millions of lung cancer cases are registered and 90% of them concern current or ex-smokers [7]. Epidemiological studies show that although tobacco smoke exposure accounts for over 80% of COPD and lung cancer cases, only 10–15% of smokers develop lung cancer while 20–30% develop clinically significant COPD, implying a clear role for genetic factors [8-10]. The presence of COPD increases the risk of lung cancer up to 4.5-fold among long-term smokers. COPD is by far the greatest risk factor for lung cancer amongst smokers and is found in 50–90% of patients with lung cancer [11]. Even a small reduction in forced expiratory volume in 1 second ($FEV_1$), a marker of airflow obstruction, is a significant predictor of lung cancer, especially among women [11].

In addition, lung cancer is also a leading cause of morbidity and mortality in patients with COPD as Wasswa-Kintu et al., showed that 33% of patients died of lung cancer over a 14.5-year follow-up [12]. Furthermore 50–70% of patients diagnosed with lung cancer have spirometric evidence of COPD [13]. Non-small cell lung carcinoma (NSCLC) accounts for 85% of all lung cancer cases in the United States [14] and importantly, the COPD-related cancer type (squamous cell carcinoma) [15] still represents the most common histological subtype of lung cancer in European men [16]. Despite significant advances in the diagnosis of lung cancer, and in the understanding of the mechanisms involved in the pathophysiology of lung cancer there has been little improvement in 5-year survival rates, indicating that new approaches are needed [17, 18].

Although the causal relationship between tobacco smoking and lung cancer has been well established, the crucial molecular mechanisms remain unknown. It has only been in the last 2 years that genes conferring 'susceptibility' to COPD have been shown to be relevant in susceptibility [19-20]. It has recently been suggested that with a greater understanding of COPD may come a greater understanding of lung cancer biology [21].

# Hazardous Effects of Cigarette Smoking

A carcinogen is defined every agent (chemical, physical or viral) that is related to the appearance of cancer. The main stream of tobacco smoke contains gases and nearly $10^{10}$ particles/mL [22]. Ninety-nine percent of tobacco smoke consists of gases such as nitrogen, oxygen, carbon dioxide, carbon monoxide, hydrazine, nitric oxides, benzene, formaldehyde, acetaldehyde and 1,3-butadiene (Table 1). Despite the fact that the administration of these gases to laboratory animals hardly ever induces carcinogenesis [23] for some of these 400 to 500 compounds a tumorigenic potential has been proposed, as is the case for 1,3 butadiene [24]. The particulate phase of smoke (tar phase) contains small particles with a diameter of about 0.4 μm. More than 3,500 biologically active substances are included in the particulate phase of smoke, and these are among the most mutagenic and carcinogenic agents of smoke.

The particulate phase of smoke is divided in four fractions: a) The neutral fraction that contains aromatic hydrocarbons, the most extensively studied carcinogenic components of smoke, b) The basic fraction, with the dependence-inducing nicotine and its toxic metabolites, the nitrosamines, c) The acid fraction, that includes agents considered as auxiliaries to carcinogenesis, such as phenols and catechols and d) The insoluble fraction, rich in metals (chromium, nickel, cadmium, the radioactive polonium). Carcinogenicity due to metals is in general attributed to the production of the reactive oxygen species (ROS). The carcinogenic effects of tobacco constituents are enhanced by other environmental factors such as professional exposure, diet and others [23, 24].

The International Agency for Research on Cancer (IARC) has ranked the carcinogenic substances in four classes, depending on their degree of involvement in the carcinogenesis process. While tobacco smoking figures in the first class among cancer causative agents, its mainstream carcinogenic agents are ranked in the classes 2A and 2B and are considered as potentially carcinogenic [25].

**Table 1. Toxic and carcinogenic chemicals in the gas phase of tobacco smoke**

| |
|---|
| *1. Hydrocarbons* |
| Methyl-propane, Methyl-butane, Hexane, Ethylene, Acetylene, Propylene, Butadiene, Isoprene, Pentadienes, Methyl-pentadienes, Ethyl-pentadienes |
| *2. Aldehydes and Ketones* |
| Formaldehyde, Acetaldehyde, Acrolein, Crotonaldehyde, Methacrolein, Propionaldehyde, Isobutyraldehyde, Acetone, Propanone, Butanone |
| *3. Nitriles and Amines* |
| Methyl nitrile, Ethyl nitrile, Acetonitrile, Acrylonitrile, Benzonitrile, Methacrylonitrile, Ethylamine, Benzylamine, Phenylamine |
| *4. Aromatic Hydrocarbons* |
| Benzene, Toluene, Ethyl-benzene, Xylenes, Styrene |
| *5. Heterocyclic compounds of oxygen* |
| Furan, Methyl furans, Dimethyl furans |
| *6. Other volatile non-organic compounds* |
| Hydrogen sulfide, Methyl mercaptan, Ethyl mercaptan, Sulfur dioxide, Hydrogen cyanide, Ammonia, Nitrogen dioxide, Nitric oxide, Carbon dioxide, Carbon monoxide |

Nicotine itself is not considered as carcinogenic nevertheless, it is the main biochemical inducer for dependence, therefore a crucial factor for the chronicity of exposure to smoke.

The majority of smoke carcinogens are the result of the incomplete pyrolysis (combustion) of organic compounds in the dried leaves of tobacco and other organic constituents of cigarette. Table B summarizes the main toxic substances of cigarette combustion that are inhaled by the smoker.

## Carcinogenic Compounds in the Side-Stream Smoke

Many of the carcinogenic compounds contained in the tobacco smoke's mainstream are found also in the surrounding air of the smoker. This diffusion is due either to cigarette's side-stream or to burning of cigarette's paper [26]. Among these compounds are included aromatic hydrocarbons, nitrosamines, organic and inorganic agents. The dilution of these agents into the environmental air of the smoker lowers significantly the inhaled doses for the non-smokers and the subsequent carcinogenic risk [27]. Nevertheless, the incidence of lung cancer among non-smokers has been reported between16-24% and is attributed to environmental tobacco smoke and to air pollution [28]. Biomarkers of exposure to tobacco smoke, such as NNK and its compounds with glucuronic acid, were found in the urines of non-smokers exposed to environmental smoke for a long period [29]. Many studies concerning biomarkers of exposition to smoke confirmed the presence of these markers in passive smokers. Comparative studies of molecular abnormalities in smokers and non-smokers lung cancer patients' tissues showed similar genetic lesions [30].

## Chronic Inflammation in COPD and Lung Cancer

### Evidence for a Molecular Link between Lung Cancer and COPD

The close association between COPD and lung cancer identified by epidemiological studies has led to several hypotheses linking COPD and lung cancer at the molecular level [31-33]. A widely held hypothesis suggests that a genetically determined aberrant (or exaggerated] inflammatory-repair response to smoking (or other aero-pollutants) might link COPD with lung cancer Figure 1 [33, 34]. However, the mechanism by which chronic lower airway inflammation is linked to lung carcinogenesis is still not completely understood [35]. Inflammatory mediators in the microenvironment of bronchioalveolar stem cells (BASCs) may promote neoplasia by inducing proneoplastic mutations, proliferation, resistance to apoptosis, angiogenesis, invasion, metastasis, and secretion of immunosuppressive factors. In fact, inflammatory cells such as macrophages and T lymphocytes can communicate with the neoplastic cells through a reciprocal and self-perpetuating interaction, resulting in increased growth and resistance to immune destruction [36]. All these changes confer a survival advantage to the neoplastic cell. Furthermore, oxidative stress provided by exogenous cigarette smoke itself and from endogenous cellular sources may lead to the activation of many intracellular pathways including kinases, transcription factors and epigenetic events that modulate the inflammatory response and cell cycling/proliferation [33, 34, 36].

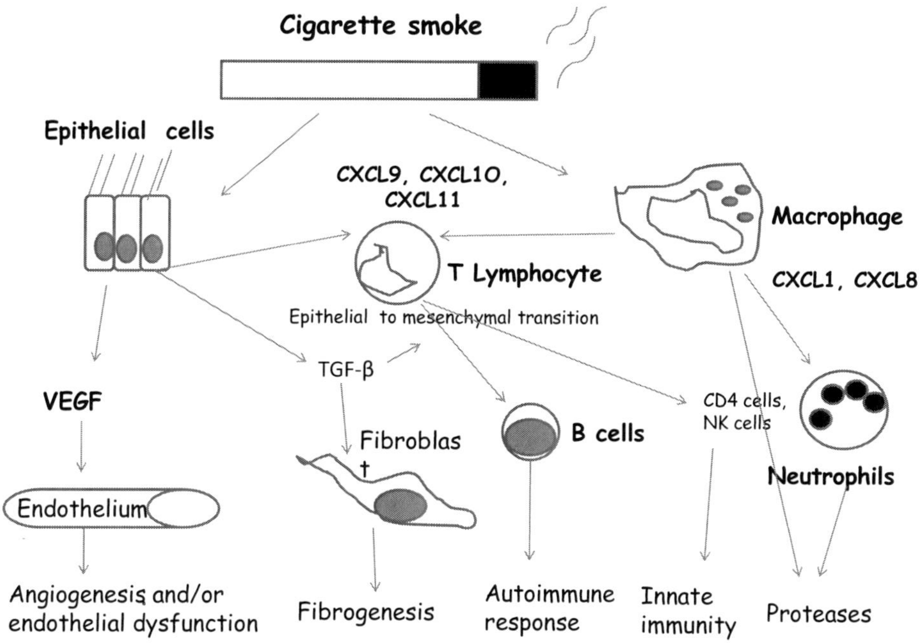


Figure 1. Cells and mediators involved in the pathogenesis of COPD and lung cancer.

COPD is a chronic inflammatory disease of the lower airways characterized by the accumulation of macrophages, CD4+ and CD8+ T cells, dendritic cells, B cells and neutrophils, particularly in smaller airways and lung parenchyma. The severity of COPD is associated with the degree of infiltration by these inflammatory cells [37]. A causal relationship between inflammation and cancer infiltration of leucocytes in malignant tissues has been described, suggesting that cancers arise at regions of chronic inflammation. The longer the inflammation persists, the higher the risk of associated carcinogenesis [38]. Host immune cells mediate antitumor effects by eradicating aberrant cells, a process which is termed as immune-surveillance. However, these cells including macrophages, neutrophils, and T lymphocytes (CD4+ and CD8+) can communicate with cancer cells through a reciprocal and self-perpetuating interaction resulting in increased growth and resistance to immune destruction by sculpting/mounting tumor immunogenicity or attenuating anti-tumor immune response in local milieu [39, 40]. Indeed, the ability of alveolar macrophages to induce T cell and anti-tumor immune responses is significantly compromised in many patients with lung cancer. Hence, the studies on ligands and signaling pathways of communication between cancer and immune/inflammatory cells may provide therapeutic options for not only augmenting antitumor immune response but also blocking or overcoming immune-sculpting at the same time.

Recently, it has been shown that adaptive immune response also participates in the pathogenesis of COPD since mature lymphoid follicles with a germinal center and separated T and B cells zone occur in lungs of patients with COPD [41-43]. These lymphoid follicles are rarely found in the lungs of non smokers, but they are present in the airways and are correlated with the severity of COPD [41]. This may be due to the large antigen load associated with bacterial and viral infections in lower respiratory tract during severe stages of COPD [41]. Another possibility underlying these findings may attribute to increased exposure to neoantigens from degraded extracellular matrix (ECM) or carbonyl modifying proteins by cigarette smoke leading to autoimmune impairment in advanced stages of COPD [43, 44].

The perpetuating chronic inflammation seen in lungs of patients with COPD [45] can induce immune escape of cancer cells especially in a tumor-promoting microenvironment. For example, it has been shown that COPD-like airway inflammation induced by non-typeable *Haemophilus influenza* promotes lung carcinogenesis in mice [46]. Furthermore, repeated lung injury and repair triggered by chronic inflammation enhances cell turnover, and potential genetic error, epithelial-to-mesenchymal transition and can ultimately lead to lung tumorigenesis. Interestingly, patients with COPD who are treated with inhaled corticosteroids and/or statins have reduced incidence of lung cancer and death suggesting inhibition of inflammation can retard lung tumorigenicity [47, 48]. Statins have been shown to have anti-oxidant and anti-apoptotic effects, which could also be relevant to minimizing airway remodelling [48]. Although observational, there is considerable clinical data suggesting patients with COPD do better when taking statins. Clinical data to support the above hypothesis include reduction in lung function decline and lower lung cancer incidence in those taking statins [48]. These studies highlight the key role of inflammation in both diseases.

The exaggerated inflammatory response leads to aberrant airway epithelial and matrix remodelling characterized by excessive growth factor release and elevated matrix metalloproteinases (MMP) [48, 31-33]. The exaggerated release of growth factors and MMPs may promote malignant transformation in the respiratory epithelium through epithelial mesenchymal transition (EMT). EMT has recently been identified in COPD and is a known precursor to many forms of epithelial cancers including lung cancer [49-51]. Integrins are heterodimeric transmembrane receptors, and are involved in a variety of cellular functions as well as in lung inflammation. Integrin αvβ6 is located in epithelial cells, and its expression is increased during lung inflammation or injury. Integrin αvβ6 plays an important role in maintaining normal lung homeostasis and preventing lung destruction since ablation of integrin αvβ6 leads to airspace enlargement in mice by regulating the TGF-β/MMP-12 pathway. The inhibition of MMP-12 by integrin αvβ6 is dependent on its ability to bind and activate latent TGF-β [52]. However, the levels of TGF-β 1 mRNA and protein are up-regulated in the airway and alveolar epithelial cells in patients with COPD, and the levels of TGF-β1 mRNA are positively correlated with the smoking history and degree of small airway obstruction suggesting the pro-fibrogenic, pro-remodeling, and a cell-specific role of TGF-β in COPD [53]. During late stage lung cancer, TGF-β promotes tumor spreading by enhancing invasion and angiogenesis [54]. Given that TGF-β has a potential role as an inhibitor of normal epithelial cell proliferation and repair, its activation may prevent proliferative response to environmental carcinogens, such as cigarette smoke, under normal conditions.

Also of interest is the likely role of inflammation in promoting the elevation of inflammatory cytokines such as interleukin-6 (IL-6), interleukin-8 (IL-8) and tumour necrosis factor-a (TNF-a) [35, 36, 55]. In this respect, elevated IL-6 has been implicated in the development of both COPD [56] and lung cancer [56, 57]. Recent data have shown that anti-IL-6 based treatment suppresses tumorigenesis [58]. At a sub-cellular level, it has been shown that many of the intracellular signalling pathways implicated in COPD are also important in lung cancer. These include the GTPase signalling pathways, [59, 60], PI3K [31], NF-kB [31, 35, 36] and STAT3 signalling molecules [31, 35, 60]. These pathways are probably activated as part of an inflammatory-repair process that promotes EMT and involves embryological pathways [51, 61].

In animal models, the guanine triphosphatase (GTPase) binding proteins, (e.g. Ras, Rho and Rac) have been linked to the development of lung cancer, with NF-kB mediating this effect in a COPD mouse model [62]. *In vitro* studies show that inhibition of GTPases can reverse EMT and restore epithelium to its normal morphology [62].

## Genetics of COPD and Lung Cancer

In contrast to the *ex vivo* studies, the *in vitro* studies, using cell cultures, have already offered important information related to the molecular mechanisms implicated in the carcinogenic transformation of physiologic bronchial epithelium under the effect of tobacco smoke. The transcription factor activator protein-1 (AP-1) heterodimerises with proteins belonging to c-Jun, c-Fos and Fra-1 families and has been shown to be activated by smoke [63]. This activation may act as endocellular sensor and participates in the conversion of the cellular program as a response to external stimuli. This effect of smoke seems to be induced through the EGFR receptor.

The tumor-suppressor gene *p53* is an important gene in carcinogenesis due to its crucial role in the regulation of the cell cycle. Therefore, it may be an important target for the toxic effects of smoke. Mutations of *p53* have been observed in the majority of lung cancer patients [64]. The spectrum of these mutations has been correlated to various tumors. For instance, lung cancer in smokers is related to transversions from G:C to T:A [65]. Mutations at codons 157, 158, 248, 249 and 273 are more frequent in patients with lung cancer in comparison to mutations at other loci of gene *p53* [66]. These characteristic mutations of *p53*are found in lung tissues in vicinity to lung tumor in smokers, as well as in plasma DNAof healthy smokers. The number of these mutations is analogous to smoking history [67]. Cigarette smoking significantly increases lung cancer risk in carriers of a germline p53 mutation [68] and some p53 SNPs have been associated with an increased risk of developing COPD [69]. The tumour suppressor gene p21 WAP/CIP1 is transcriptionally activated by p53 to induce cell cycle arrest and DNA repair. p21 WAP/CIP1 protein expression is increased in alveolar macrophages and bronchial epithelial cells of patients with COPD and is highly responsive to oxidative stress resulting in cytoplasmic translocation and inhibition of apoptosis in these cells [70].

The short arm of chromosome 3 was considered as place of genetic lesions linked to lung carcinogenesis. In particular, deletions in the region 3p21 were correlated to smoking-related carcinogenesis. In a relative PCR-based study, loss of heterozygosity (LOH) was discovered in region 3p21 in the 44.2% of non-small cell lung cancer and in the 30.2% of small cell lung cancer tissues. The incidence of this LOH was higher in current and ex-smokers in comparison with never smokers, as well as in patients with mutations at *p53*. Among patients with squamous lung cancer, a significant correlation was reported between increased rate of LOH in the region 3p21 and increased concentration of DNA adducts. This increased rate of LOH in the region 3p21 was correlated to the early onset of smoking [71].

In contrast to *p53*, lung cancer patients with *K-ras* mutationsdo not seem to be more frequent in smokers in comparison to non-smokers [72].

**Table 2. Proposed chromosomal loci and/or genes associated with COPD and lung cancer**

| Study type | COPD | Lung cancer |
|---|---|---|
| Genome-wide association study | 1q23 (IL6R)<br>4q22 (FAM13A)<br>4q24 (GSTCD)<br>4q31 (HHIP/GYPA)<br>5q33 (HTR4/ADAM19)<br>6p21 (BAT3/AGER)<br>6q24 (GPR126)<br>15q25 (CHRNA) | 1q21 (CRP)<br>4q22 (FAM13A)<br><br>4q31(HHIP†/GYPA)<br>5q33 (ADAM19)<br>6p21 (BAT3)<br>5p15 (CRR9/TERT)<br>15q25 (CHRNA) |
| Candidate genes | GSTM1 (null genotype)<br>TGF-b1 (rs 1800470)<br>TNF-a (rs 1800629)<br>SOD3 (rs 1799896) | GSTM1 (null genotype)<br>XRCC3 (T241M)<br>XPD (K571Q)<br>TP53 (R72P)<br>OGG1 (S326C) |

Deregulation in the activity of telomerase is thought to take place early in the process of carcinogenesis [73]. The gradual shortening of telomeres length regulates the process of apoptosis. The telomerase activity maintains the length of telomeres and, thereby, lengthens the cell life. Tobacco smoke is considered as an activator of telomerase. In a relative study, in cell cultures of non-smokers, healthy smokers and smokers with lung cancer, the telomerase activity was found significantly higher for smokers, and it was proportionate to their tobacco consumption [74].

Recently published genome-wide association studies (GWA) of lung cancer [75, 76], lung function [77] and COPD [78, 79] have identified several chromosomal regions and candidate genes including 1q21-23 (*CRP, IL-6R*), 4q22 (*FAM13A*), 4q24 (*GSTCD*), 4q31 (*HHIP, GYPA*), 5p15 (*CRR9*), 5q32-33 (*HTR4, ADAM19*), 6p21 (*BAT3,AGER*), 6q24 (*GPR126*) and 15q25 (*CHRNA*). Interestingly, several of these disease loci from the GWA studies of lung cancer, lung function and COPD overlap (Table 2). Although these genes were first identified through GWA studies, involving thousands of subjects, an overlapping role in COPD and lung cancer was only established in a case–control study where these genetic associations were examined in all affected (phenotypic) groups: smokers with normal lung function, smokers with COPD (GOLD 2 + criteria) and smokers with histology confirmed primary lung cancer (subgrouped by COPD sub-phenotype) [80].

## Epigenetic Phenomena and Cigarette Smoke

Epigenetic molecular events are heritable biochemical changes in DNA without alteration in the physiologic sequence of nuclear acids. The addition of methyl groups in particular sites of promoter regions (CpG islands) of tumor suppressor genes induces their respective transcriptional silence, a fact that may favor carcinogenesis. [81]. Exposure to toxic agents may enhance epigenetic phenomena. During recent years, many studies reported epigenetic changes in the genome of smokers and of patients with COPD and lung cancer. Figure 2. Genes involved in the modulation of oxidant and noxious compounds are likely to be important in gene environment interactions in COPD and lung cancer [30, 82]. In both lung cancer and COPD, environmental factors (mainly tobacco smoking) interact with multiple polymorphic genes to influence susceptibility to disease. Thus, only a fraction of smokers (around 15%) will develop lung cancer and/or COPD in their lifetime [82, 83], which suggests a different individual susceptibility to the risk of lung cancer and COPD or time of disease onset. Metabolism of noxious substances present in tobacco smoke by xenobiotic metabolizing enzymes is usually benign but in some instances the metabolic process can transform harmless substances into toxic chemicals [84], suggesting that differences in xenobiotic metabolism may contribute to the risk of developing both COPD and squamous cell lung carcinoma [85]. The major xenobiotic metabolizing enzymes, including both phase I (microsomal epoxide hydrolases, flavin monooxygenases and myeloperoxidase) and phase II enzymes (conjugation enzymes, including several transferases such as glutathione S-transferases (GSTs) and arylamine N-acetyltransferases) are expressed in human lung tissues [86]. The combination of several genetic polymorphisms in CYPs, EPHX, HO1 and GST enzymes that activate or detoxify the tobacco smoke carcinogens might modulate squamous cell lung carcinoma [87]. The gene *p16 INK4A* plays a central role in the regulation of the cell cycle. It encodes a protein that binds with and inhibits the kinases of cyclin D (CdK4, CdK6), which in turn activates the retinoblastoma protein (Rb) [88]. Therefore, protein p16 may be of great importance for the normal procedure of cell cycle. The methylation of the promoter region of this gene may induce and maintain the carcinogenetic process. This kind of methylation has been reported in patients with lung cancer [89].

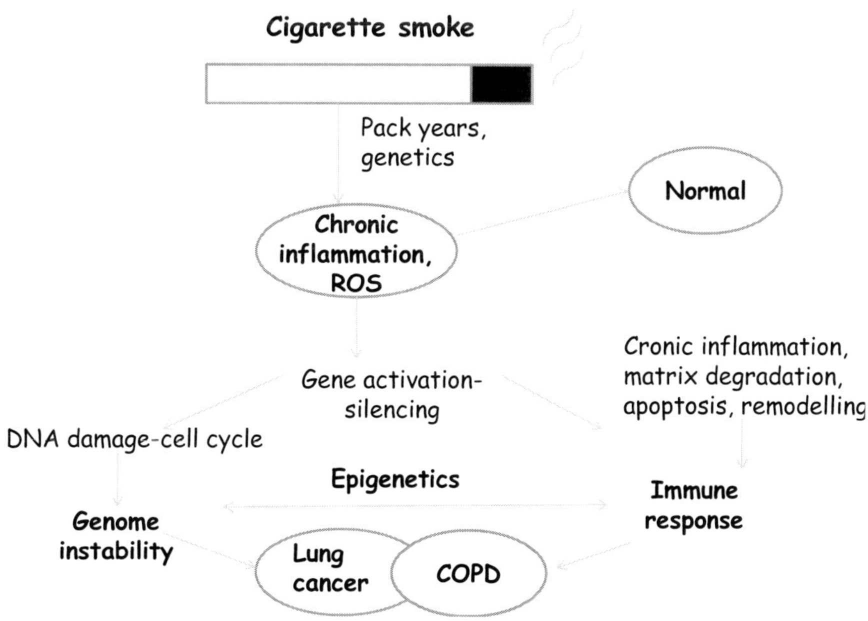


Figure 2. A combination of immune-inflammatory signals and epigenetic events may underlie the risk of patients with COPD developing lung cancer.

In a study including 122 smokers and non-smokers with NSCLC, the gene *p16*was found methylated in 52.5% of patients, mainly smokers [90]. In the same study, comparable results have been reported concerning the gene *MGMT* (O6-methylguanine-DNA-methyltransferase). This gene encodes a protein that participates in the DNA repair process.

Abnormal methylation has been reported for a large number of tumor suppressor genes that are involved in lung carcinogenesis. Squamous cell lung carcinoma results from the accumulation of multiple independent genetic and epigenetic abnormalities, including DNA sequence alterations, copy number changes, and aberrant promoter hypermethylation [91]. Together, these abnormalities result in the activation of oncogenes and inactivation of tumour suppressor genes [92]. Loss of heterozygosity (i.e., deletion of one copy of allelic DNA sequences) and microsatellite alterations in widely dispersed, apparently clonally independent foci also occur in normal and hyperplastic bronchial epithelium and these changes may persist for many years after smoking cessation [93]. In a methylation study including 7 relevant genes [*p16*, *RASSF1A* (RAS association domain family 1), *APC*, *RARβ*, *CDH13*, *MGMT* and*GSTP1*], the methylation index was found significantly higher in smokers [91]. The methylation of tumor suppressor genes has been studied extensively as a potential biomarker of carcinogenesis onset in a variety of biologic materials (sputum, induced sputum, bronchial secretions, broncho-alveolar lavage, blood) in healthy smokers and patients with COPD or lung cancer [89, 92, 93].

## Conclusion

Epidemiological and genetic profiling of lung cancer and COPD suggest that they are not discrete diseases related only through smoking exposure, but that many of the smokers who are susceptible to COPD are also susceptible to lung cancer. Given the apparent overlap in susceptibility loci, it appears plausible that some of the genetic factors implicated in COPD might also be relevant in lung cancer. In addition to the genetic overlap from epidemiological studies, there is growing evidence suggesting that inflammatory and/or immune-modulating pathways involved in intracellular signalling are also shared between COPD and lung cancer. These data suggest a plausible inflammatory or immune-modulatory link, possibly orchestrated by the epithelial response to chronic smoke exposure. Thus, understanding the cellular and molecular mechanisms underlying these processes will provide novel aspects in the treatment of cigarette smoke-induced lung chronic inflammatory diseases including COPD and lung cancer.

## References

[1] Mackay J, Eriksen M. The tobacco atlas. *World Health Organization*, Geneva, 2002;24–27.

[2] Cohen BH, Diamond EL, Graves CVG *et al.* A common familial component in lung cancer and chronic obstructive pulmonary disease. *Lancet* 1977; September:523–526.

[3] Petty TL. Are COPD and lung cancer two manifestations of the same disease? *Chest* 2005;128:1895–1897.

[4] Punturieri A, Szabo E, Croxton TL *et al.* Lung cancer and chronic obstructive pulmonary disease: needs and opportunities for integrated research. *JNCI* 2009;101:554–9.

[5] Lichtenstein P, Holm NV, Verkasalo PK *et al.* Environmental and heritable factors in the causation of cancer: analyses of cohorts of twins from Sweden, Denmark and Finland. *N. Eng. J. Med.*2000;343: 78–85.

[6] Chen Y. Genetic epidemiology of pulmonary function. *Thorax* 1999; 54:818–24.

[7] International Agency for Research on Cancer Tobacco smoke and involuntary smoking. IARC monographs on the evaluation of carcinogenic risks to humans. IARC, Lyon, FR. 2004; 83:1179-1187.

[8] Løkke A, Lange P, Scharling H *et al.* Developing COPD: a 25 year follow up study of the general population. *Thorax* 2006;61:935–9.

[9] Egleston BL, Meireles SI, Flieder DB, et al: Population-based trends in lung cancer incidence in women. *Semin. Oncol.* 2009; 36: 506–515.

[10] Scagliotti GV, Longo M, Novello S: Nonsmall cell lung cancer in never smokers. *Curr. Opin. Oncol.* 2009; 21: 99–104.

[11] Young RP, Hopkins RJ, Christmas T, et al: COPD prevalence is increased in lung cancer, independent of age, sex and smoking history. *Eur. Respir. J.* 2009; 34: 380–386.

[12] Wasswa-Kintu S, Gan WQ, Man SF, et al: Relationship between reduced forced expiratory volume in one second and the risk of lung cancer: a systematic review and meta-analysis. *Thorax* 2005; 60: 570–575.

[13] Yao H, Rahman I: Current concepts on the role of inflammation in COPD and lung cancer. *Curr. Opin. Pharmacol* 2009; 9: 375–383.

[14] Molina JR, Yang P, Cassivi SD, et al: Non-small cell lung cancer: epidemiology, risk factors, treatment, and survivorship. *Mayo Clin. Proc.* 2008; 83: 584–594.

[15] Papi A, Casoni G, Caramori G, et al: COPD increases the risk of squamous histological subtype in smokers who develop non-small cell lung carcinoma. *Thorax* 2004; 59: 679–681.

[16] Janssen-Heijnen ML, Coebergh JW: Trends in incidence and prognosis of the histological subtypes of lung cancer in North America, Australia, New Zealand and Europe. *Lung Cancer* 2001; 31: 123–137.

[17] Carney DN: Lung cancer – time to move on from chemotherapy. *N. Engl. J. Med.* 2002; 346:126–128.

[18] Young RP, Hopkins RJ, Hay BA *et al.* Lung cancer gene associated with COPD: triple whammy or possible confounding effect? *Eur. Respir. J.* 2008; 32: 1158–64.

[19] Young RP, Whittington CF, Hopkins RJ *et al.* Chromosome 4q31 locus in COPD also associated with lung cancer. *Eur. Respir. J.* 2010; 36: 1375–82.

[20] Young RP, Hopkins RJ, Hay BA *et al.* FAM13A locus in COPD independently associated with lung cancer—evidence of a molecular genetic link between COPD and lung cancer. *Appl. Clin. Genet.* 2011; 4: 1–13.

[21] Strange C. COPD and lung cancer: are they both airways diseases? *Chest* 2010; 138: 1289–90. Smith CJ, Perfetti TA, Rumble MA et al. «IARC Group 2A Carcinogens» Reported in Cigarette Mainstream Smoke. *Food and Chemical Toxicology* 2000, 38, 371-383.

[22] Mossman BT and Eastman A. Carcinogenesis in the respiratory tract. In: Macdowell EM (ed). Lungcarcinomas. *Churchill Livingstone* 1987; 129-161.

[23] Church D, Fand Pryor WA. Free-radical chemistry of cigarette smoke and its toxicological implications. *Environment health perspective* 1985; 64:111-126.

[24] Hecht SS. Tobacco carcinogens, their biomarkers, and tobacco-induced cancer. *Nat. Rev. Cancer* 2003; 3: 733–44.

[25] Smith CJ, Perfetti TA, Rumble MA et al. «IARC Group 2A Carcinogens» Reported in Cigarette Mainstream Smoke. *Food and Chemical Toxicology* 2000;38:371-383.

[26] GuerinMR, JenkinsRA, TomkinsBA. The chemistry of environmental tobacco smoke: composition and management. Chelsea (MA): LewisPublishers;1992.

[27] Blot WJ, McLaughlin JK. Passive smoking and lung cancer risk: what is the story now? *J. Natl. Cancer Inst.* 1998;90:1416–7.

[28] Vineis P, Hoek G, Krzyzanowski M, et al. Lung cancers attributable to environmental tobacco smoke and air pollution in non-smokers in different European countries: a prospective study. *Environ. Health.* 2007;15:7.

[29] Hecht SS. A biomarker of exposure to environmental tobacco smoke (ETS) and Ernst Wynder's opinion about ETS and lung cancer. *Prev. Med.* 2006;43(4):256-60.

[30] Husgafvel-Pursiainen K. Genotoxicity of environmental tobacco smoke: a review. *Mutation Research* 2004;567:427–445.

[31] Yang IA, Relan V, Wright CM *et al.* Common pathogenic mechanisms and pathways in the development of COPD and lung cancer. *Expert Opin. Ther. Targets* 2011; 15: 439–56.

[32] Lee G, Walser TC, Dubinett SM. Chronic inflammation, chronic obstructive pulmonary disease, and lung cancer. *Curr. Opin. Pulm. Med.* 2009; 15: 303–7.

[33] Brody JS, Spira A. Chronic obstructive pulmonary disease, inflammation and lung cancer. *Proc. Am. Thorac. Soc.* 2006; 3:535–8.

[34] Balkwill F, Mantovani A: Cancer and inflammation: implications for pharmacology and therapeutics. *Clin. Pharmacol. Ther.* 2010; 87: 401–406.

[35] Reiman JM, Kmieciak M, Manjili MH, Knutson KL: Tumor immunoediting and immunosculpting pathways to cancer progression. *Semin. Cancer Biol.* 2007; 17: 275–287.

[36] Chung KF, Adcock IM: Multifaceted mechanisms in COPD: inflammation, immunity, and tissue repair and destruction. *Eur. Respir J.* 2008; 31: 1334–1356.

[37] National Institutes of Health, National Heart, Lung and Blood Institute. Global Initiative for Chronic Obstructive Lung Disease (GOLD): Global strategy for the diagnosis, management and prevention of chronic obstructive pulmonary disease. NHLBI/WHO workshop report. NIH Publication No 2701A, March 2001. www goldcopd com (accessibility verified May 15, 2010).

[38] Balkwill F, Mantovani A: Inflammation and cancer: back to Virchow? *Lancet* 2001; 357: 539–545.

[39] Salvi SS, Barnes PJ: Chronic obstructive pulmonary disease in non-smokers. *Lancet* 2009; 374: 733–743.

[40] Seibold MA, Schwartz DA: The lung: the natural boundary between nature and nurture. *Annu. Rev. Physiol.* 2011 Mar 17;73:457-78.

[41] Hogg JC, Chu F, Utokaparch S, et al. The nature of small-airway obstruction in chronic obstructive pulmonary disease. *N. Engl. J. Med.* 2004;350:2645–2653.2653 [PubMed: 15215480].
[42] Hogg JC. Timens W: The Pathology of Chronic Obstructive Pulmonary Disease. *Annu. Rev. Pathol.* 2009;4:435–459.459 [PubMed: 18954287].
[43] van der Strate BW, Postma DS, Brandsma CA, et al. Cigarette smoke-induced emphysema: A role for the B cell? *Am. J. Respir. Crit. Care Med.* 2006;173:751–758.
[44] Lee SH, Goswami S, Grudo A, et al. Antielastin autoimmunity in tobacco smoking-induced emphysema. *Nat. Med.* 2007;13:567–569.
[45] Reiman JM, Kmieciak M, Manjili MH, et al. Tumor immunoediting and immunosculpting pathways to cancer progression. *Semin. Cancer Biol.* 2007;17:275–287.
[46] Moghaddam SJ, Li H, Cho SN, et al. Promotion of Lung Carcinogenesis by COPD-like Airway Inflammation in a K-ras Induced Mouse Model. *Am. J. Respir. Cell Mol. Biol.* 2009;40:443–453.
[47] Parimon T, Chien JW, Bryson CL, et al. Inhaled corticosteroids and risk of lung cancer among patients with chronic obstructive pulmonary disease. *Am. J. Respir. Crit. Care Med.* 2007;175:712–719.
[48] Young RP, Hopkins R, Eaton TE. Pharmacological actions of statins: potential utility in COPD. *Eur. Respir. Rev.* 2009; 18: 222–32.
[49] Dasari V, Gallup M, Lemjabbar H *et al.* Epithelial-mesenchymal transition in lung cancer: is tobacco the 'smoking gun'? *Am. J. Respir. Cell Mol. Biol.* 2006; 35: 3–9.
[50] Shintani Y, Maeda M, Chaika N *et al.* Collagen 1 promotes epithelial-to-mesenchymal transition in lung cancer cells via transforming growth factor-b signalling. *Am. J. Respir. Cell Mol. Biol.* 2008; 38: 95–104.
[51] Kalluri R, Weinberg RA. The basics of epithelial-mesenchymal transition. *J. Clin. Invest.* 2009; 119: 1420–8.
[52] Morris DG, Huang X, Kaminski N, et al. Loss of integrin alpha (v)beta6-mediated TGF-beta activation causes MMP12-dependent emphysema. *Nature* 2003;422:169–173.
[53] Takizawa H, Tanaka M, Takami K, et al. Increased expression of transforming growth factor-beta1 in small airway epithelium from tobacco smokers and patients with chronic obstructive pulmonary disease (COPD). *Am. J. Respir. Crit. Care Med.* 2001;163:1476–1483.
[54] Fong YC, Hsu SF, Wu CL, et al. Transforming growth factor-beta1 increases cell migration and beta1 integrin up-regulation in human lung cancer cells. *Lung Cancer* 2009;64:13–21.
[55] Cosio MG, Saetta M, Agusti A. Immunologic Aspects of Chronic Obstructive Pulmonary Disease. *N. Engl. J. Med.* 2009; 360: 2445–54.
[56] Dowlati A, Levitan N, Remick SC. Evaluation of interleukin-6 in bronchoalveolar lavage fluid and serum of patients with lung cancer. *J. Lab. Clin. Med.* 1999; 134: 405–9.
[57] Begany T. Mounting evidence that IL-6 contributes to lung cancer. *Pulm. Rev.* 2005; November: 17.
[58] Ancrile B, Lim K-H, Counter CM. Oncogenic Ras-induced secretion of IL-6 is required for tumorigenesis. *Mol. Interv.* 2008; 8: 22–7.

[59] Asnaghi L, Vass WC, Quadri R *et al.* E-Cadherin negatively regulates neoplastic growth in non-small cell lung cancer: role of GTPases. *Oncogene* 2010; 29: 2760–71.

[60] Qu P, Roberts J, Li Y *et al.* Stat3 downstream genes serve as biomarkers in human lung carcinomas and chronic obstructive pulmonary disease. *Lung Cancer* 2009; 63: 341–7.

[61] ShiW, Chen F, Cardoso WV. Mechanisms of lung development—contribution to adult lung disease and relevance to chronic obstructive pulmonary disease. *Proc. Am. Thorac. Soc.* 2009; 6: 558–63.

[62] Zondag GCM, Evers EE, ten Klooster JP *et al.* Oncogenic Ras down regulates Rac activity, which leads to increased Rho activity and epithelial-mesenchymal transition. *J. Cell Biol.* 2000; 149:775–82.

[63] Young RP, Hopkins RJ, Hay BA *et al.* A gene based risk score for lung cancer susceptibility in smokers and ex-smokers. *Postgrad. Med. J.* 2009; 85: 515–24.

[64] Hwang SJ, Cheng LS, Lozano G, et al. Lung cancer risk in germline p53 mutation carriers: association betweenan inherited cancer predisposition, cigarette smoking, and cancer risk. Hum Genet 2003; 113: 238–243.

[65] Pfeifer GP, Hainaut P. On the origin of G – transversions in lung cancer. *Mutat Res* 2003;526:39–43.

[66] Pfeifer GP, Denissenko MF, Olivier M, et al. Tobacco smoke carcinogens, DNA damage and p53 mutations in smoking-associated cancers. *Oncogene* 2002;21:7435–51.

[67] Nobutoshi HN, Mechanic LE, Glenwood E. Quantitative Detection of p53 Mutations in Plasma DNA from Tobacco Smokers. *Cancer Res.* 2006; 66(16): 8309-17.

[68] Arif E, Vibhuti A, Deepak D, et al. COX2 and p53 risk alleles coexist in COPD. *Clin. Chim. Acta* 2008; 397: 48–50.

[69] Lee YL, Chen W, Tsai WK, et al. Polymorphisms of p53 and p21 genes in chronic obstructive pulmonary disease. *J. Lab. Clin. Med.* 2006; 147: 228–233.

[70] Tomita K, Caramori G, Lim S, et al. Increased p21(CIP1/WAF1) and B cell lymphoma leukemia-x(L) expression and reduced apoptosis in alveolar macrophages from smokers. *Am. J. Respir. Crit. Care Med.* 2002; 166: 724–731.

[71] HiraoT, Nelson HH, Ashok T et al. Tobacco Smoke-induced DNA Damage and an Early Age of Smoking Initiation Induce Chromosome Loss at 3p21 in Lung Cancer. *Cancer Research* 2001;61:612-615.

[72] Vahakangas KH, Bennett WP, Castren K, et al. p53 and K-ras mutations in lung cancers from former and never-smoking women. *Cancer Res.* 2001 Jun 1;61(11):4350-6.

[73] Yashima K, Litzky LA, Kaiser L, et al. Telomerase expression in respiratory epithelium during the multistage pathogenesis of lung carcinomas, *Cancer Research* 1997;57:2373–2377.

[74] Yim HW, Slebos R, Randell S. Smoking is associated with increased telomerase activity in short-term cultures of human bronchial epithelial cells. *Cancer Letters* 2007;246:24–33.

[75] Amos CI,Wu X, Broderick P *et al.* Genome-wide association scan of tag SNPs identifies a susceptibility locus for lung cancer at 15q25.1. *Nat. Genet.* 2008; 40: 616–22.

[76] Repapi E, Sayers I, Wain LV *et al.* Genome-wide association study identifies five loci associated with lung function. *Nat. Genet.*2009; 42: 36–44.

[77] Hancock DB, Eijgelsheim M, Wilk JB *et al.* Meta-analyses of genome-wide association studies identify multiple loci associated with pulmonary function. *Nat. Genet.* 2009; 42: 45–52.
[78] Pillai SG, Ge D, Zhu G *et al.* A genome-wide association study in chronic obstructive pulmonary disease (COPD): identification of two major susceptibility loci. *PLoS Genet.* 2009; 5: e1000421.
[79] Cho MH, Boutaoui N, Klanderman BJ *et al.* Variants in FAM13A are associated with chronic obstructive pulmonary disease. *Nat. Genet.* 2010; 42: 200–2.
[80] Young RP, Hopkins R, Black PN *et al.* Functional variants of antioxidant genes in smokers with COPD and in those with normal lung function. *Thorax* 2006; 30: 394–9.
[81] Jones PA, Baylin SB. The fundamental role of epigeneticevents in cancer. *Nat. Rev. Genet.* 2002;3:415 – 428.
[82] Caramori G, Adcock I. Gene-environment interactions in the development of chronic obstructive pulmonary disease. *Curr. Opin. Allergy Clin. Immunol.* 2006; 6: 323–328.
[83] Spitz MR, Wei Q, Dong Q, Amos CI, Wu X: Genetic susceptibility to lung cancer: the role of DNA damage and repair. *Cancer Epidemiol. Biomarkers Prev.* 2003; 12: 689–698.
[84] Zhang JY, Wang Y, Prakash C. Xenobiotic metabolizing enzymes in human lung. *Curr. Drug Metab.* 2006; 7: 939–948.
[85] Rotunno M, Yu K, Lubin JH, et al. Phase I metabolic genes and risk of lung cancer: multiple polymorphisms and mRNA expression. *PLoS One* 2009; 4:e5652.
[86] Ye Z, Song H, Higgins JP, et al. Five glutathione s-transferase gene variants in 23,452 cases of lung cancer and 30,397 controls: meta-analysis of 130 studies. *PLoS Med.* 2006; 3(4): 524-534.
[87] Gresner P, Gromadzinska J, Wasowicz W. Polymorphism of selected enzymes involved in detoxification and biotransformation in relation to lung cancer. *Lung Cancer* 2007; 57:1–25.
[88] WeinbergRA. The retinoblastoma protein and cell cycle control. *Cell* 1995;81:323 – 330.
[89] Belinsky SA, Nikula KJ, PalmisanoWA ET AL. Aberrant Methylation of p16 (INK4a) is an early event in lung cancer and a potential biomarker for early diagnosis. *Proc. Natl. Acad. Sci. USA* 1998;95:11891 – 11896.
[90] Liu LY, Lan Q, Siegfried J et al. Aberrant Promoter Methylation of p16 and MGMT Genes in Lung Tumors from Smoking and Never-Smoking Lung Cancer Patients. *Neoplasia* 2006;8:46 – 51.
[91] Toyooka S, Maruyama R, Toyooka KO, et al. Smoke exposure, histologic type and geography-related differences in the methylation profiles of non-small cell lung cancer. *Int. J. Cancer.* 2003;103(2):153-60.
[92] Belinsky SA, Liechty KC, Gentry FD, et al. Promoter hypermethylation of multiple genes in sputum precedes lung cancer incidence in a high-risk cohort. *Cancer Res.* 2006;66(6):3338-44.
[93] Belinsky SA, Klinge DM, Dekker JD, Smith MW, Bocklage TJ, Gilliland FD, Crowell RE, Karp DD, et al. Gene promoter methylation in plasma and sputum increases with lung cancer risk. *Clin. Cancer Res.* 2005 Sep 15;11(18):6505-11.

In: Lung Cancer: A Comprehensive Overview
Editor: Kathy Gately

ISBN: 978-1-62618-447-3


*Chapter XI*

# Diagnosis, Treatment and Follow-Up of Neoplastic Pericardial Disease in Lung Cancer

***Chiara Lestuzzi*[1], *Massimiliano Berretta*[2], *Alessandra Bearz*[2] *and Witold Tomkowski*[3]**
[1]Cardiology, CRO, National Cancer Institute, Aviano (PN), Italy
[2]Oncology, CRO, National Cancer Institute, Aviano (PN), Italy
[3]Cardio-Pulmonary Intensive Care,
National Tb and Lung Diseases Research Institute, Warsaw, Poland

## Abstract

Lung cancer is the most frequent cause of neoplastic pericardial effusion. The main path of pericardial metastases is the retrograde lymphatic way. Lymphatic obstruction often leads to a rapid accumulation of a large amount of pericardial fluid, and eventually to cardiac tamponade. Cardiac tamponade is diagnosed on the basis of clinical (engorged jugular veins, pulsus paradoxus) and echocardiographic (right atrial wall collapse, dilated vena cava) findings. Not all the pericardial effusions in lung cancer patients are neoplastic: up to 30% may be due to other causes. To confirm the diagnosis of pericardial metastases the gold standard is the detection of neoplastic cells within the pericardial fluid. Cytological diagnosis is most reliable when a large amount of fresh fluid is available. Immunocytochemistry and cell block analysis in addition to visual analysis of smears may improve the diagnostic power of cytopathologic analysis. In equivocal cases, the dosage of carcinoembryonic antigen (CEA) and serum cytocheratin 19 fragments (CYFRA 21-1) in the pericardial fluid may be very useful both in the diagnosis of neoplastic pericarditis and in the differential diagnosis among different neoplasms. The cut-off value for CEA is 5ng/ml and for CYFRA 21-1 is 90 ng/ml. The main advantage of the use of neoplastic markers is that they require a small amount of fluid only and the results are available in a timely manner. As regards the therapeutic approach, several treatments have been proposed: mechanical (extended pericardial drainage, pericardial window, intrapericardial administration of sclerosing agents) or administration of antineoplastic drugs (locally, intravenous or both). The main problem in neoplastic pericarditis is the high rate of recurrence of effusion after drainage. This problem should be considered on the medium to long term period, according to the more prolonged survival of lung cancer patients treated with the new targeted therapies. On the basis of the most recent reports, the combined administration of local (intrapericardial) platinum and systemic antineoplastic therapy gives the highest rate of response and the longest relapse-free survival. Local chemotherapy has favourable pharmacokinetics (with high intrapericardial concentration, slow absorption and few systemic effects) and is usually well tolerated even by patients with a poor performance status. The surgical approach (pericardial window) and local radiation therapy may be used in cases of refractory to chemotherapy.

## Introduction

Malignant pericarditis in association with a primary tumor is one of the most frequent causes of recurrent pericardial effusion and cardiac tamponade, and may be the initial sign of malignant disease [1, 2]. The most common primary malignant tumors reported to involve the pericaridium are: carcinoma of the lung (18 to 37%), carcinoma of the breast (7 to 25%), malignant melanoma (up to 71%), lymphoma and leukaemia [3].

The prevalence of neoplastic pericarditis varies according to the population considered and to the methods used to diagnose it. In autopsy studies it has been reported in <4% of the general population, in about 10% of cancer patients, and among these in 19%-40% of patients dying of lung cancer [4, 5]. Even if autopsy studies tend to overestimate the clinical problem (they usually study terminally ill patients; they detect even microscopic metastases and small effusions without clinical relevance), neoplastic pericarditis in lung cancer is still rather frequent [6]. It occasionally is the first clinical presentation of neoplasm and may lead to a dramatic worsening of clinical conditions when it causes cardiac tamponade. Currently, large pericardial effusions and cardiac tamponades are more frequent in neoplastic pericarditis (mostly in lung cancer) compared to other causes of pericarditis [7-9]. This is probably due to the retrograde lymphatic pathway of pericardial metastasis, which causes the obstruction of lymphatic vessels and reduces the reasbsorption of pericardial fluid [10-12]. Several forms of malignant involvement of the pericardium can be observed: small elastic effusion, large effusion, which can become decompensated to tamponade and constriction due to thickened pericardium (the so-called tumor encasement of the heart) that either adheres to the myocardium or not [13-15].

## Diagnosis

The chest roentgenogram is abnormal in the majority of patients with malignant pericardial effusion. Typical features are cardiac enlargement, mediastinal widening, hilar mass and pleural effusion (Figure 1). Computed tomography (CT) and magnetic resonance imaging (MRI) can detect and assess the presence of both pericardial effusion, intrapericardial masses and pericardial thickening; they also can detect the site of the primary tumor when pericarditis is the first clinical finding (Figure 2). Electrocardiograms are usually abnormal. The most frequent abnormalities are tachycardia, low QRS voltage, ST and T wave changes. Electrical alternans (i.e. an alternation of the configuration of the electrocardiographic complexes) may be present in very large effusions with exaggerated movements of the heart (the so-called swinging heart) (Figure 3) [1, 3, 11, 16-18]. Echocardiography is the method of choice among the diagnostic procedures in patients with suspected malignant pericardial effusion. It can assess (like computer tomography and MRI) the size of effusion, presence or absence of metastatic intra-pericardial masses and thickness of pericardial layers. The presence of spontaneous echo-contrast (due to the echogenicity of cell-rich effusions) is rather frequent in neoplastic pericarditis and can suggest the diagnosis (Video 1). Echocardiography also provides essential information about the hemodynamic impairment, as will be discussed in greater detail below.

The most frequent symptoms and clinical signs are dyspnea, tachycardia, cough, jugular venous distension. Less frequent symptoms include: orthopnea, weakness, dysphagia, syncope, palpitations, pericardial friction rubs, hiccups, decreased heart sounds and hepatomegaly.

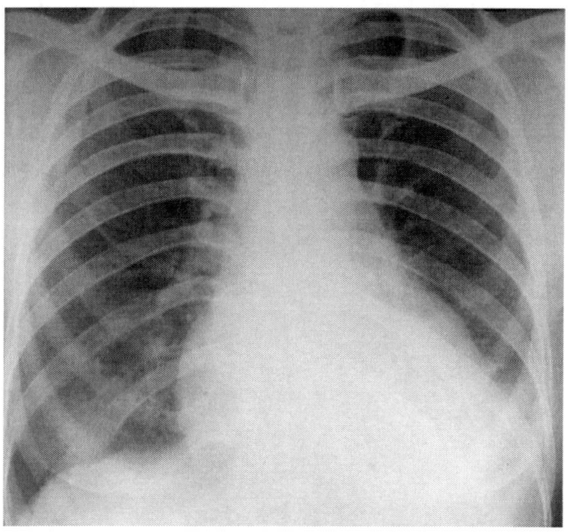

Figure 1. Chest X ray of a large pericardial effusion. The cardiac shadow is enlarged and round-shaped.

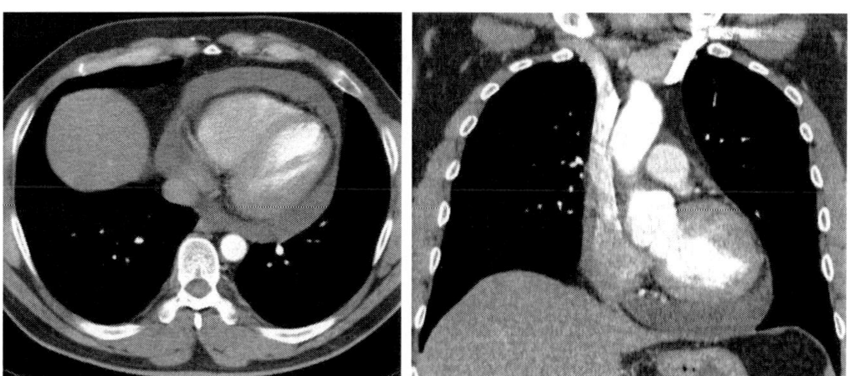

Figure 2. Computed Tomography of a large pericardial effusion surrounding the heart. A) transversal plane. B) frontal plane: the effusion accumulates mostly over the diaphragm.

Pleural effusion, oliguria, edema can also be present [1, 3, 4, 11]. Ewert's sign (a dullness in the left lung base secondary to the compression from the large pericardial effusion observed during percussion of the anterior thorax) can be important in physical examination. Bronchial breathing and broncophony may also be present in cases of large pericardial effusion.

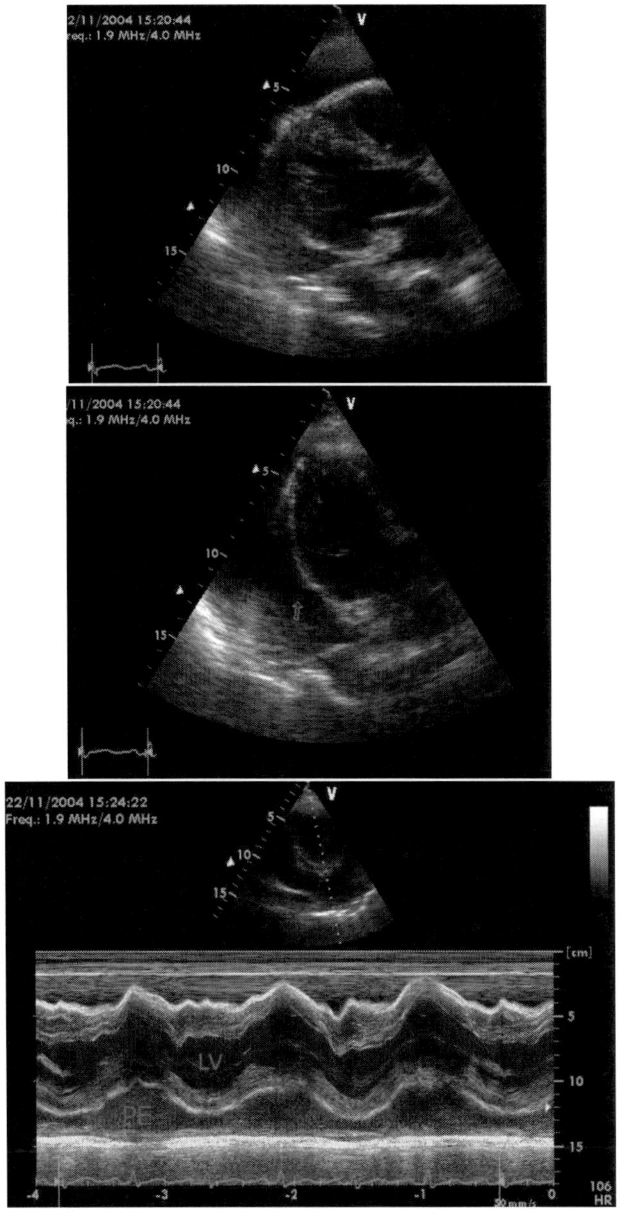


Figure 3. Echocardiogram of a patient with large effusion and "swinging heart". A and B, parasternal axis view showing the exaggerated movement of the heart (arrow) in different beats. C: mono-dimensional image showing the abnormal movement of the whole heart, and the concomitant changes in ECG amplitude (bottom). PE= pericardial effusion. LV= left ventricle.

With the majority of patients with malignant pericardial effusion, symptoms and signs are not evident until cardiac decompensation occurs. The rate of fluid accumulation,either slow and gradual or rapid, is essential to their appearance. If the accumulation of effusion is slow and gradual, onset of symptoms may be delayed and become evident only when the volume exceeds 1-2 liters. Rapid accumulation of malignant pericardial effusion and slow accumulation of large volumes of fluid may cause acute cardiac tamponade, which is a life-threatening condition requiring urgent treatment.

Clinically, cardiac tamponade is a hemodynamic syndrome due to the compression of cardiac chambers by the pericardial effusion. It is characterized by engorged jugular veins, pulsus paradoxus (a decrease of $\geq$15 mmHg of systolic blood pressure during quiet inspiration), tachycardia and in the most severe cases hypotension, syncope or shock. With the progressive increase in intrapericardial pressure the hemodynamic impairment worsens and causes abnormalities detectable earlier in the catheterization laboratory (equalization of right atrial and pericardial pressure), then by echocardiography (right chamber collapse) and only in the later stages clinically [19-24]. Being a clinical syndrome that is linked to increased intrapericardial/intracardiac pressure, it is somehow independent from the grade of pericardial effusion. A reduced intravascular volume, and/or a rapid increase of intrapericardial fluid may lead to cardiac tamponade with even small effusions [25]. On the other hand, as reported above, a slowly accumulating effusion may become very large before causing tamponade. The clinical signs of cardiac tamponade are not always all present and not always reliable. Jugular veins may not be evident in hypovolemic patients even in presence of large effusions, and may be engorged in patients with obstruction of superior vena cava even without tamponade. Pulsus paradoxus is frequent in patients with obstructive lung disease and tachycardia may be due to anemia, and so on [26]. In a study conducted by Levine et al., only 50% of the patients with cardiac tamponade had clinical diagnostic signs [27].

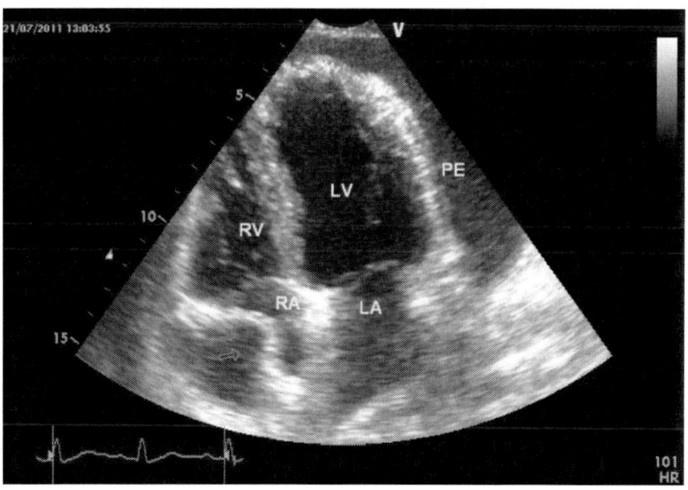


Figure 4. Typical echocardiographic appearance of large neoplastic pericardial effusion with signs of cardiac tamponade. Large pericardial effusion with neoplastic epicardial masses at the apex. The right atrial free wall is collapsed in diastole (arrow). LA= left atrium, LV= left ventricle, PE= pericardial effusion, RA= right atrium, RV= right ventricle.

In constrictive pericarditis, diastolic filling is restricted by an inelastic pericardium after an initial expansion of the myocardium, even without any effusion (as in the case of tumor encasement) or with minimal effusion (effusive- constrictive pericarditis). The jugular venous pressure is always elevated in constrictive pericarditis with a deep, steep *y* descent. Evidence of the Kussmaul sign (an elevation in the jugular venous pressure during inspiration) is typical of pericardial constriction and less frequent in cardiac tamponade.

Echocardiographic signs of hemodynamic impairment are collapsing right chambers, changes in mitral flow velocities, dilation of the inferior vena cava [29-30] (Figure 4; video 1). Echocardiographic signs are not always sensitive and specific: in a study by Mercé et al., 90% of patients with cardiac tamponade and 34% without underwent a collapse of one or more cardiac chambers; sensitivity and specificity of venous flow analysis was better: 75% and 91%, respectively [31]. The typical echocardiographic sign of pericardial constriction is the sudden left shift of the interventricular septum during inspiration. During inspiration the decrease in intrathoracic pressure enhances the venous return and consequently the filling of the right ventricle. In constrictive pericarditis the thickened rigid pericardium does not allow the expansion of the right ventriclular free wall during inspiration. As a consequence, the interventricular septum shifts toward the left ventricle, but the total cardiac volume does not change. Conversely, during expiration , the septum shifts toward the right ventricle as its filling decreases.

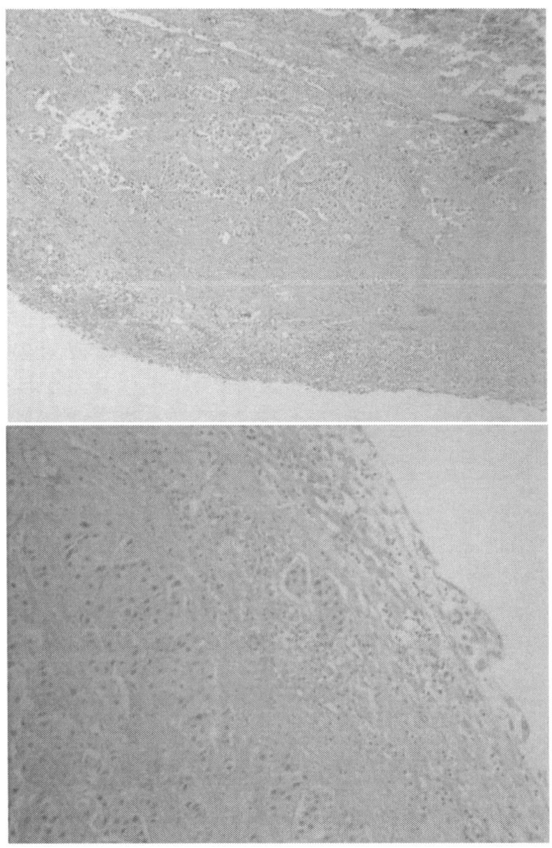

Figure 5. Pathologic specimens of neoplastic pericarditis from small cell lung carcinoma. Hematoxiline.

The diagnosis of malignant involvement of the pericardium is based on the presence of metastases within the pericardial sac. Proper diagnostic procedure is mandatory, because in 30% to 50% of patients with lung cancer and pericardial effusion, pericarditis is caused by non-malignant disease: viral or opportunistic infections (many patients are immunocompromised by therapy or by the disease itself), inflammation (mostly after radiation therapy), lymphatic drainage impairment by mediastinal masses and haemorrhages [11].

The diagnosis should then be confirmed by pathology. Fluid cytology is positive in 87% of patients with known pericardial involvement in malignant disease, and in 44-65% of those without a previous diagnosis of systemic cancer [32, 33]. Pericardial biopsy is positive in 27-56 % of patients with malignant pericardial disease and is less sensitive than the cytology of the pericardial fluid [9, 34-37]. Pericardial fluid cytology and/or pericardial tissue histology are the methods of choice in diagnostic procedures, in patients with suspicion of malignant involvement of the pericardium (rapidly growing effusion, intrapericardial masses, haemorrhagic fluid) particularly if there is no known primary tumor (Figure 5).

However, cytology may be difficult because mesothelial cells exhibit a spectrum of cytomorphologic features, sometimes mimicking carcinoma [38, 39]. In the case of mesothelioma, the cytologic diagnosis is even more difficult because hyperplastic or reactive mesothelial cells may mimic malignant mesothelioma. Differentiation from metastatic adenocarcinoma may be challenging and, on the other hand, effusion may have no cytologic evidence; the sensitivity has been reported to be 38%-50% [40, 41]. To improve the reliability of cytologic examinations, all the drained fluid (not only a small specimen) should be sent to the cytopathology laboratory immediately after drainage in the fresh state or refrigerated and stored at 2-8° [42, 43].

Cell block preparations, in addition to smears, and immunohistochemical markers may improve the sensitivity and specificity of the diagnosis [44-46]. Recently, Claudin 4 has been reported as highly sensitive and specific in recognizing neoplastic effusions due to carcinomas. The problem with this marker is that it is not tumor-specific; however, it is useful in patients with known lung carcinoma, or in differentiating between mesothelioma and carcinoma [47-48].

In cytology-negative samples or whenever the diagnosis is equivocal, the dosage of tumor markers, such as carcinoembryonic antigen (CEA), serum cytokeratin 19 fragments (CYFRA 21-1) and Neuron Specific Enolase (NSE) may be useful [49-54]. Paganuzzi et al., found that a high value of CYFRA 21-1 with low CEA in pleural fluid can identify patients with mesothelioma [55]. Even if the majority of these studies were focused on pleural effusions (that are much more common and more easily drained) the same results have been obtained in pericardial effusions. CEA is still the most accurate single diagnostic marker, followed by CYFRA 21-1, and the combination of a CEA > 6 ng/mL and CYFRA 21-1 > 60 ng/mL resulted in a sensitivity of 97.6% and a specificity of 91.4% in the most recent report [56].

Since only a small amount of fluid is required for the analysis, we suggest routine checks of CEA (easily available in every hospital), and possibly CYFRA 21-1 in a sample of the drained fluid. The remaining fluid should be sent immediately to the pathology laboratory for centrifugation and cytological diagnosis, or refrigerated at 4°C.

# Treatment

There are three possible goals in treating neoplastic pericarditis:

A. Relief of symptoms (cardiac tamponade, dyspnea). This seems reasonable in terminally ill patients, with a life expectancy of a few weeks and without any possibility of a cure that would improve survival. This goal may be obtained draining the fluid percutaneously or by surgical methodologies.
B. Long term prevention of recurrences of symptomatic effusion, regardless to the survival time. This is often the only goal in patients with a medium-term poor prognosis. The most used approaches are the injection of sclerosing agents into the pericardial space or the creation of a pleuro-pericardial window
C. Long term prevention of recurrence and an attempt to prolong survival by actually curing the pericardial neoplasm. This goal is particularly meaningful in patients without other sites of metastasis, or in cancers with otherwise good prognosis.

## A) Patients with Cardiac Tamponade

Treatment of cardiac tamponade in the course of malignant pericardial effusion is mandatory and urgent because it can cause death. Proper treatment of malignant pericardial effusion improves prognosis of malignant disease and prolongs survival. No consensus has been achieved regarding the optimal management and treatment of patients with decompensated heart functions due to neoplastic effusion. No randomised trials comparing efficacy and safety of different methods have been performed. The best method of management and treatment of cardiac tamponade should be based on local technical possibilities and experience. Relief of symptoms and signs of cardiac tamponade can be obtained by pericardiocentesis or surgical methods.

Pericardiocentesis (percutaneous drainage using the Seldinger technique) is useful to rapidly relieve symptoms and is recognised as a convenient, relatively safe and effective procedure connected with a low incidence of complications. The patient should be positioned at a 45° angle from the supine position. Echocardiography is used first to identify the best site for puncture (i.e. the approach where the distance between parietal and visceral pericardium is wider, minimizing the risk of accidental cardiac puncture), and to select the direction of the drainage needle. The area should be properly treated to allow maximum antisepsis. After anesthetizing the skin and subcutaneous tissue with 5-10 ml of 1-2% lidocaine, a needle of appropriate length (connected to a 10 ml syringe filled with lidocaine) is insercted following the direction previously identified by echocardiography. Maintaining suction (in order to avoid intravenous injection of the anesthetic) and injecting every few millimeters a small amount of lidocaine, the needle is gently pushed until the parietal pericardium is punctured and pericardial fluid can be drained. Since the pericardial fluid is usually bloody, the needle should be connected to another syringe filled with saline, and a few milliliters of saline should be rapidly injected (under echocardiographic monitoring from a different approach). The appearance of echographic contrast (i.e. echogenic microbubbles) within the pericardium confirms the correct placement of the needle. If fluoroscopy rather than echocardiography is used to monitor the procedure, one ml of iodine contrast medium may be injected. The needle can be retracted and a 18-gauge Seldinger needle is inserted in the same manner, again checking the position of the tip of the needle injecting a few ml of saline or contrast medium when reaching the pericardium. A guidewire is then inserted through the needle and a small skin incision is made to enlarge the puncture site. The needle is removed, a dilator is inserted over the guidewire into the pericardium, to enlarge the pericardial puncture site, and then removed. Finally a pig-tail catheter is inserted using the guidewire (Figure 6, video 2). After draining as much effusion as possible, the catheter should be washed with a small amount of heparinized solution, closed and fixed to the skin to avoid accidental displacement. The preferred approach is subcostal, for several reasons: a) due to gravity the pericardial fluid accumulates mostly near the diaphragm (Figure 2b), b) there is no risk of causing pneumothorax, c) the long-term maintenance of a pericardial catheter is safer because it is partially tunnelled, and d) the subcostal approach is more comfortable for the patient should the catheter be left in place for several days. Nevertheless, in particular cases (loculated effusions, obese patients, atypical position of the heart due to previous pneumonectomy and so on) a different approach (mostly apical through an intercostal puncture) may be indicated [59-61]. Pericardiocentesis guided by echocardiography is the most widely used procedure and can be performed in the majority of hospitals [57-62]. With special echocardiographic transducers the whole procedure may be followed in real-time improving the safety. Pericardiocentesis guided by fluoroscopy or computed tomography is optional. Blinded pericardiocentesis should never be performed [58]. Pericardial drainage is obligatory, when technically possible, in all patients with large pericardial effusion because of the risk of sudden hemodynamic impairment, and for diagnostic purposes as well [57, 58]. Without any additional treatment, the rate of recurrence is high (up to 40%). For this reason, we suggest the catheter not be removed at least until a cytologic diagnosis has been obtained and until it is evident that no further interventions are required. The catheter, filled with heparin solution, closed and maintained sterile (with the usual care devoted to permanent central venous lines) may be left in place for weeks without problems (personal experience of the authors).

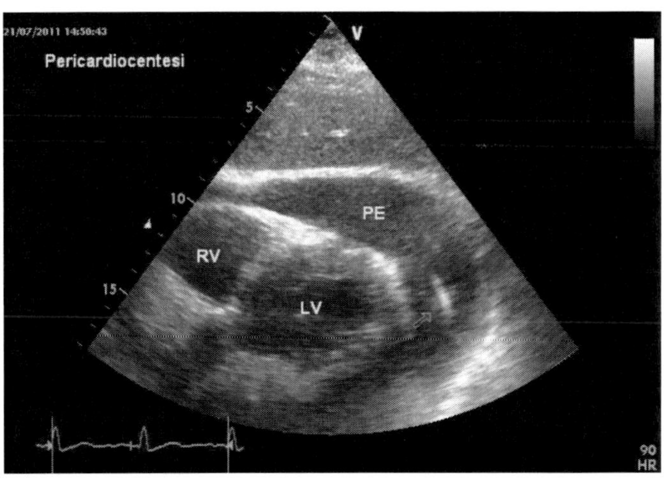


Figure 6. Echocardiographic-guided pericardiocentesis. From the subcostal approach the separation between the pericardial layers is evaluated before puncture, and the position of the catheter within the pericardial space (arrow) is checked after puncture.

## B) Prevention of Recurrence of Symptomatic Effusion

Three possibilities are used here: the catheter may be left in place, permanently or intermittently opened, until the daily drained fluid is reduced to <25-30ml (extended drainage), and/or used to instill sclerosing agents into the pericardium (sclerosing therapy). An alternative drainage method is the creation of a pericardial window, that can be obtained both through a surgical approach, and with a balloon inserted with the Seldinger technique [63, 64]. This technique decompresses the pericardium by draining the fluid in a larger cavity (pleura or peritoneum) but also causes an inflammatory process that promotes adhesion between parietal and visceral pericardium, as confirmed by a small autopsy study [65].

Extended drainage has a success rate (in terms of prevention of clinically significant relapse of effusion) of about 75% and is the preferred first-line treatment for some physicians. The long term results are probably due to the adherence between the pericardial layers, which prevent the accumulation of fluid. [22].

Sclerosing therapy has been widely used to favour adherence between the pericardial layers.

The first agents used for sclerotherapy were antibiotics, such as powdered tetracycline and doxycycline, according to previous favorable experiences in pleural effusions. The rationale was to induce irritation, inflammation and subsequent fibrosis, but the exact mechanism of action of these agents is not yet clear. Acytostatic activity has been suggested as contributing to the therapeutic effect of tetracycline [66]. The largest study examining tetracycline or doxycycline sclerosis reported an outcome of 93 cancer patients (69 with positive and 21 negative cytology, 3 not determined), of whom 85 received sclerosis.

The procedure was complicated by pain in 17 (20%), fever in 7 (8%), atrial fibrillation or flutter in 6 (7%) and was effective in 75 (81%) [67]. Antibiotics are no longer used as sclerosing agents in neoplastic pericarditis since other compounds, with both sclerosing and weak antineoplastic effects, have been proven to be at least equally effective with a lower morbidity [68]. The first drug tested was bleomycin *(BLM)*, already used in pleural and peritoneal effusions for chemical pleurodesis. In one report, 5/7 patients with lung carcinoma treated by intrapericardial BLM had a stable control of effusion [69].

Triethylenethiophosphoramide (Thiotepa) is another anticancer agent with sclerosing properties used for local therapy with good results and few side effects. Thiotepa was used by Martinoni et al., in 33 patients (16 breast cancer, 15 lung cancer, 4 different tumors) with cytology positive effusions, without recurrence in 30 patients at a follow-up of 22 to 1108 days (median 115 days). All patients also received systemic CT and the overall survival was longer in the breast cancer subgroup compared to the lung cancer group (median 272 *vs* 85 days) [70].

Surgical management plays an essential role in the treatment of recurrences of malignant pericardial effusion. Subxyphoid pericardiotomy can be performed using local anesthesia in the majority of patients. This procedure is safe and well tolerated. Variants of subxyphoid pericardiotomy include: formation of a pericardioperitoneostomy using subxyphoid or laparoscopic approaches and video-assisted pericardioscopy [71]. Reaccumulation rate of malignant pericardial effusion was observed in 11% of patients treated with subxyphoid pericardiotomy [35]. Complications including arrhythmias, myocardial laceration, pneumothorax, operative morbidity and surgical mortality were observed in a relatively small percentage of patients [35, 71-76]. In a retrospective study of 127 patients with underlying malignancies and pericardial effusion (55% percent malignant, comprising 71% of adenocarcinomas of the lung, breast, esophagus, and unknown primary site), subxyphoid pericardiotomy proved to be a safe and effective intervention that successfully relieved pericardial effusions in 99% of cases with recurrence and reoperation rates of 9% and 7%, respectively [76]. Pleuropericardiotomy involves thoracotomy with resection of part of the parietal pericardium, allowing drainage of malignant pericardial fluid into the pleural space. This procedure is associated with higher complication rates and offers no advantage over subxyphoid pericardiotomy [35, 76].

As mentioned previously, percutaneous balloon pericardial window, performed under local anesthesia, creates a pleuro-pericardial direct communication which allows fluid drainage into pleural space. In patients with large malignant pericardial effusion and recurrent cardiac tamponade, percutaneous balloon pericardial window techniques seem to be very effective (97%) and relatively safe [77]. In a retrospective analysis of 50 patients with cancer (30 lung cancer) treated with double-balloon pericardiostomy, Wang et al., reported a 90% success rate (prevention of recurring effusion) using this method, but a median survival rate of 4 months overall, with a significantly shorter survival in the cytology positive subgroup. No subgroup analysis (lung vs other cancer) was carried out [78].

Gross, describing the outcome of 43 solid cancer patients treated with different surgical approaches (21 subxiphoid pericardial window, 14 pleuropericardial window and 8 pericardiodesis with thiotepa), reported 2.1% mortality (myocardial rupture during finger exploration of the pericardial space), and 6.4% morbidity. Most of the patients had concomitant chemotherapy or radiotherapy (RT) and the median overall survival was 5.2 months in patients with breast cancer and 3.2 months in the others [64].

## C) Attempt to Cure the Metastatic Site

This can be obtained with the use of systemic or local antineoplastic treatments or both.

### *Systemic Antineoplastic Therapy*

Systemic antineoplastic therapy has been shown to be effective in previously published studieswhere pericardial effusion is due to lymphoma and breast carcinoma, but its efficacy in lung carcinoma is apparently lower. This can be explained by the lower chemosensitivity of lung cancer compared with breast cancer and haematologic malignancies. It is possible that with the introduction of new targeted therapies the role of systemic therapy will become more relevant [35, 79-82].

### *Local Chemotherapy*

The rationale behind local chemotherapy is to obtain a higher concentration of the antineoplastic drug at the site of the tumor. Of the few pharmacokinetic studies performed examining the effect of intrapericardial chemotherapy, all confirm this hypothesis by intrapleural and intraperitoneal CT [83-87]. In fact, after local injection, the drug concentration is high in the effusion for at least 48-72 hours, while blood concentration is very low. The opposite is true for systemic CT, which results in high concentrations of drugs in the blood and low concentrations in the effusion. As a result of this pharmacokinetic behaviour, local CT is usually well tolerated even by severely compromised patients, with very few side effects (the most frequent being transitory atrial fibrillation). An additional advantage of local chemotherapy is the beneficial action on the lymphatic metastases [88]. The use of intrapericardial cisplatin (DDP) in lung cancer pericarditis was first reported in 1985 in a single case treated with 10 mg over 5 continuous days. The same methodology was used by others in a few small series of mostly lung cancer patients and positive results were achieved [89-91]. In a study of 9 patients with various tumors, Tomkowski et al., had 2 long-lasting responses in lung adenocarcinoma also treated with systemic CT, but most of the patients died of cancer within 3 months, and in all of the 7 patients who had an autopsy, neoplastic pericardial involvement was found even without pericardial effusion [92]. Maisch et al. used 30 mg/sm of DDP in a single administration (removing the drug after 24 h) in 42 patients with various tumors also undergoing systemic CT, and observed a relapse in 1/22 lung cancer cases [93]. Bischiniotis et al used 10 mg of DDP over 3 continuous days in 25 cases of lung adenocarcinoma, obtaining a complete disappearance of effusion in 13 cases and residual small (< 0.5 cm) effusions in 9 cases; a surgical approach was necessary in 1 case of DDP failure and in 1 case of tumor encasement of the heart [94].

Currently, DDP (at 0.3%-1% dilution), in a cumulative dosage of 30-50 mg (10 mg repeated on 5 consecutive days or 50 mg in single bolus) is the most widely used local chemotherapy. Studies have shown good tolerability with a low rate of significant side effects. Recurrent pericardial effusion was rarely observed and complete response was achieved in the majority (85%- 90%) of cases. Signs of constrictive pericarditis and sclerosis (fibrosis) of the pericardium were observed only in a few patients treated with intrapericardial administration of cisplatin. Very low rates of pericardial fibrosis seem to be an advantage of this method. Some physicians remove the drug after 24 hours while others leave the drug in the pericardial sac and repeat drainage only if fluid reaccumulates. There are no studies comparing the efficacy of one schedule over the other.

According to pharmacokinetic studies the drug is reabsorbed over 72 hours or more. Depending on the clinical presentation the following approach could be undertaken: In the case of rapidly accumulating effusions: 10 mg in 10-20 ml over 3-5 running days, draining as much fluid as possible before each instillation. This method allows for very high concentrations of the drug in the pericardial sac for several days, avoiding the risk of recurring tamponade. The disadvantage is the necessity of daily opening and manipulation of the catheter.

In the case of slowly accumulating effusions: 30-50 mg in 50-100 ml in single bolus, then close the catheter and re-open only if significant fluid accumulates. This method allows for a high concentration of the drug in the pericardial sac for several days, and is useful for treatments on an ambulatory basis. In fact, the patient can present every 4-7 days to check the evolution. The disadvantage is the need to inject larger amount of fluid in a single bolus (which can be dangerous in case of effusive-constrictive pericarditis).

### *Local Radiation Therapy*

Radiation therapy seems to be very effective (93%) in controlling malignant pericardial effusion in patients with radiosensitive tumors such as lymphoma, leukemia, breast cancer [95]. Radiotherapy of the heart can itself cause serious complications such as myocarditis and pericarditis [76]. External beam radiotherapy in the lung cancer setting may be used in selected cases, such as tumor encasement of the heart (Figure 7). The instillation of radioactive compounds (such as $^{32}P$ colloid), even if proven effective in some early studies, has been abandoned because of the concern about radiation risk and the availability and cost of the radioactive compound [96, 97].

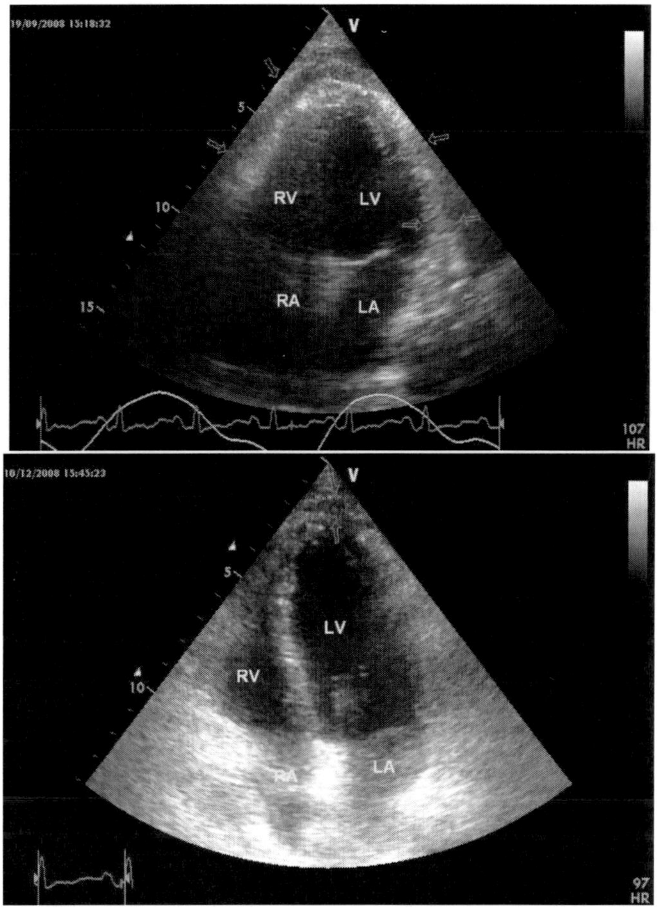


Figure 7. Tumor encasement of the heart with constrictive pericarditis treated with radiation therapy. (A) A 2 cm thick echogenic mass cover the epicardial surface (arrows). Clinically, there is a pericardial constriction syndrome. (B) After direct radiation therapy (25 Grays over 13 fractions) the tumor encasement has disappeared, and only a residual pericardial thickening is visible at the cardiac apex (arrows). At 3 months follow-up the patient is asymptomatic.

### *Comparison of Different Treatments*

Overall, there are four main approaches in treating neoplastic pericarditis: reduction of the effusion burden (with extended drainage or promoting pericardial sclerosis), systemic chemotherapy, local chemo- or radiation therapy, and a combination of local and systemic antineoplastic therapy. It is hard to compare the efficacy of these methods according to literature reports, because the diagnosis is often not well defined (large pericardial effusion in a patient with cancer classified as "malignant" even without cytology or neoplastic marker confirmation, as discussed above). Also often the results are obtained with a single method or compare just two methods, and the efficacy criteria, which are necessarily arbitrary, change in different reports and few prospective randomized studies have been published. Moreover, many of the earlier reports consider an intervention successful if the patient survived for 30 days without recurrence of symptoms or tamponade. In a classic review from 1994, Vaitkus et al., suggested to classify the response as "successful" if the patient survived the procedure, the symptoms did not recur, and no other interventions directed at the pericardium were required, regardless of the length of "survival". Since then, the assessment of efficacy has been assessed at the last follow-up in most papers [76]. As discussed above, the assessment of efficacy on the basis of clinical signs is not always reliable. Moreover, the decision to undertake subsequent interventions may depend on both the physician and the patient. In more recent reports the classification of a "successful" intervention includes the amount of drained fluid and the entity of pericardial effusion at echocardiography. The results would be better evaluated with objective outcomes, such as a complete response, partial response, stable disease and progression, as in the case of solid tumors. However, effusions are considered "not measurable" in oncologic staging [98, 99]. Nevertheless, a semi-quantitative assessment of pericardial effusion is possible by measuring the daily drained fluid from the catheter or by echocardiography [100]. Recently, a scoring system based on echocardiographic findings, considering both effusion and masses, has been proposed. The outcome was classified as a complete response (no more signs of pericarditis), partial response (reduction of disease score), no response and progression (Table 1).

A retrospective study done on 60 patients (30 with positive cytology only) treated either with *intrapericardial sclerosis with thiotepa or surgery* (pericardial window or partial pericardiectomy) showed no advantage of one procedure over another in preventing effusion recurrence, but pericardiocentesis was more cost-effective.

**Table 1. Scoring system used to assess local outcome**

| | | |
|---|---|---|
| Pericardial effusion | 1 | Mean separation between parietal and visceral pericardium <1 cm |
| | 2 | Mean separation between parietal and visceral pericardium 1-2 cm |
| | 3 | Mean separation between parietal and visceral pericardium >2cm |
| Pericardial Masses | 1 | Single mass < 2x 2 cm |
| | 2 | Multiple masses <2 x 2 cm *or* single mass > 2 x 2 cm *or* mass with superficial infiltration of the underlying myocardium |
| | 3 | Tumor encasement of the heart *or* transmural infiltration of the myocardium |
| Complete response (CR) | | Complete disappearance of pericardial effusion and masses, with apparently normal pericardium (i.e. score =0) *or*<br>No residual neoplasm at postmortem exam |
| Partial response (PR) | | Stable reduction of pericardial effusion and masses (reduced total score) *or*<br>Adhesive pericarditis (thickened pericardium without effusion) *or*<br>No effusion at echo but detection of microscopic neoplastic infiltration at postmortem exam |
| No response (NR) | | No changes in pericardial effusion and mass score *or*<br>Necessity of periodical drainage of small quantity of fluid |
| Progressing disease (PD) | | Increase of pericardial effusion and/or masses score *including* infiltration of the underlying myocardium and/or tumor encasement of the heart (even if pericardial effusion disappears) *or*<br>Necessity of frequent drainage of large amount of fluid *or*<br>Detection of diffuse neoplastic pericardial disease at autopsy |

In this study, the morbidity and recurrence was higher using a surgical approach rather than pericardiocentesis. The overall median survival time was 97 days., Patients with breast cancer had longer survival rates than those with lung cancer. No subgroup analysis was associated with systemic CT [101]. In the management of patients with large malignant pericardial effusion and/or recurrent cardiac tamponade, thoracotomy with pericardiectomy appears to be disadvantageous compared with less invasive approaches [76].

In a prospective randomized study, the outcomes of 79 lung cancer patients with pericardial effusion (58 with positive cytology) treated either with intrapericardial BLM or pericardial drainage (24 patients receiving systemic CT) were compared. There were 9 early deaths within 30 days (5 in the drainage arm and 4 in the BLM arm), 1 case of constrictive pericarditis and 1 of cardiac dysfunction, both in the BLM group. The median effusion failure-free survival was 30 days in the drainage alone arm and 57 days in the BLM arm ($P$ = 0.03 by log-rank test), but in the subgroup analysis this advantage was more evident in the cytology negative patients. The actual efficacy of sclerosing therapy was not fully evaluable in this heterogeneous group of patients [102].

In a multicenter study of 119 lung cancer patients, the outcome of *4 different treatments* (extended drainage or sclerosis, systemic antineoplastic therapy, local chemo-radiotherapy and combined local plus systemic therapy) were analyzed using the scoring system reported in Table 1 [103]. A complete response was achieved in 37/53 of patients with combined, in 12/22 with local, in 5/27 with systemic chemotherapy, respectively, and in 4/17 after drainage/sclerosis (p<0.001). Overall response was achieved in 51/53 with combined, 18/22 and 16/27 with local or systemic chemotherapy, respectively, and in 5/17 with drainage/sclerosis only (p<0.001) (Figure 8). Survival was significantly better after combined chemotherapy (p<0.001) and 12/53 patients (23%) in this subgroup survived for more than 1 year.

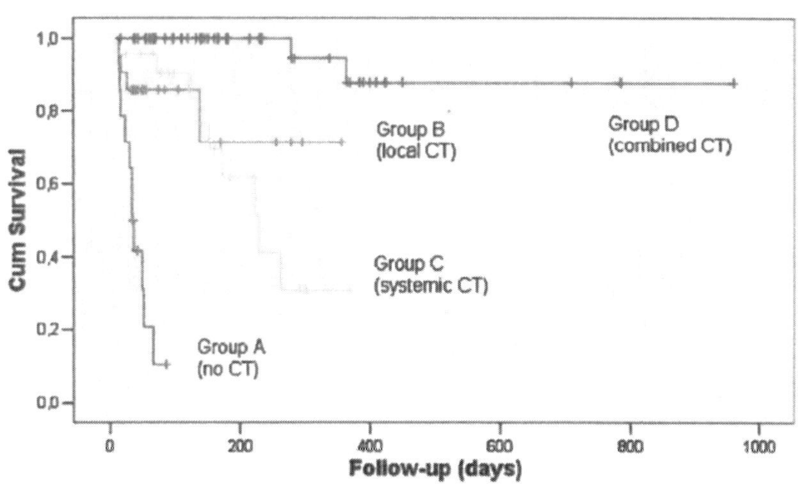


Figure 8. Kaplan-Meier curves of observation with stable reduction of pericardial effusion or masses (complete response, partial response or adhesive pericarditis) in the four groups of treatment. Overall Log-Rank test: p<0.001. Combined chemotherapy vs Systemic chemotherapy: p<0.001; Combined chemotherapy vs Local chemotherapy: p=0.002; Local chemotherapy vs Systemic chemotherapy: p=NS. CT=chemotherapy (Reprinted with Elsevier's permission from Lestuzzi C. et al. Neoplastic pericardial disease in lung cancer: impact on outcomes of different treatment strategies. A multicenter study. Lung Cancer 2011; 72:340-47).

As regards intrapericardial treatments, it might be argued that BLM, Thiotepa and DDP act as either sclerosing or as antineoplastic agents. The sclerosing properties of BLM are well known, and this drug is currently used for this purpose even in benign conditions as lymphatic malformations [104]. The use of Thiotepa in local treatment of pericardial effusion has been justified because of its sclerosing or antineoplastic properties [70, 105]. Its efficacy was greater in breast cancer (a tumor where it is currently used for systemic CT) compared to the lung cancer patients in the study of Martinoni [70].

DDP is a powerful antineoplastic agent, currently used for systemic CT in NSCLC. It has vesicanting properties at concentrations >0.5 mg/ml, but with currently used doses in local CT intrapericardial concentration is below this limit. Actually, the most frequent side effects of typical sclerosing agents (pain, fever and adhesive or constrictive pericarditis at long-term follow-up) have been seldomly reported after intrapericardial injection of DDP. According to these facts, its local effect in the particular setting of lung cancer neoplastic pericarditis is probably due mostly to the antineoplastic activity rather than to a sclerosing effect. In our study (the largest study published to date), in 75 lung cancer patients who received intrapericardial CT, the overall response rate was higher with intrapericardial platinum (65 patients) than with other agents (10 patients: 5 BLM, 2 Thiotepa, 3 teniposide): 98% vs 80%, $\chi^2=7.69$, $p<0.01$ [103]. Moreover, in the subgroup of lung cancer patients (all treated with intrapericardial Thiotepa and systemic CT) of Martinoni's study the event-free survival was shorter in comparison with our patients treated with intrapericardial platinum [70, 13]. Also according to other studies intrapericardial administration of cisplatin seems to have the tendency to prolong survival of patients with malignant pericardial involvement by lung cancer, mainly adenocarcinoma [91, 106].

# Conclusion

Neoplastic pericarditis is still a potentially harmful complication in lung cancer patients. The diagnosis should be confirmed by cytology (possibly with the aid of immunohistochemistry).

Attention to the rise of neoplastic markers (CEA, CYFRA 21-1) in the pericardial fluid, may also help with the diagnosis. The optimal treatment is based on a combination of local chemotherapy and systemic antineoplastic therapy. Local chemotherapy alone is recommended for patients with a poor health status, as it is well tolerated and at least as effective as systemic antineoplastic therapy alone, as regards local disease.

Pericardiocentesis should be attempted not only in cases of cardiac tamponade, but in every case where it is technically feasible.

# References


[1] Spodick DH. Neoplastic pericardial disese. In: Spodick DH: The pericardium: A comprehensive textbook. New York, Marcel Dekker, 1997. P 301-313.

[2] Klatt EC, Heitz DR: Cardiac metastases. *Cancer* 1990: 1456-59.

[3] Maghfoor I, Doll DC, Yarbro JW. Effusions. In: Abeloff MD, Armitage JO, Lichter AS, Niederhuber JE: Clinical Oncology. New York, *Churchill Livingstone*, 2000. 922-949.
[4] Butany J, Leong SW, Carmichael K, et al. A 30-year analysis of cardiac neoplasms at autopsy. *Can. J. Cardiol*. 2005:675–680.
[5] Abraham KP, Reddy V, Gattuso P. Neoplasms metastatic to the heart: review of 3314 consecutive autopsies. *Am. J. Cardiovasc. Pathol.* 1990:195–198.
[6] Lestuzzi C. Neoplastic pericardial disease: Old and current strategies for diagnosis and management. *World J. Cardiol.* 2010: 270-279.
[7] Hancock EW. Neoplastic pericardial disease. *Cardiol. Clin*. 1990:673-82.
[8] Sagristà-Sauleda J, *Mercé J, Permanye*r-Miralda G, et al. Clinical clues to the causes *of large peric*ardial effusions. *Am. J. Med.* 2000: 95-101.
[9] Fraser RS, Viloria JB, Wang NS. Cardiac tamponade as a presentation of extracardiac malignancy. *Cancer*. 1980:1697-1704.
[10] Kline IK. Cardiac lymphatic involvement by metastatic tumor. *Cancer* 1972: 799-808.
[11] Press OW, Livingston R. Management of malignant pericardial effusion and tamponade. *JAMA*. 1987:1088-92.
[12] Tamura A, Matsubara O, Yoshimura N, et al. Cardiac metastasis of lung cancer. A study of metastatic pathways and clinical manifestations. *Cancer*. 1992:437-42.
[13] Mohiuddin AB: Constrictive pericarditis: An analysis of 17 cases. Dis *Chest* 1967:298-303.
[14] Elguezabal A, Parry JP, Depace NL. Massive metastatic cardiac tumour encasement with pericardial constriction. 7 *Med. Soc. NJ* 1980:820-4.
[15] Tsolakis EJ, Charitos CE, Mitsibounas D, et al. Cardiac tamponade rapidly evolving toward constrictive pericarditis and shock as a first manifestation of noncardiac cancer. *J. Card Surg*. 2004:134-5.
[16] Niarchos AP. Electrical alternans in cardiac tamponade. *Thorax*. 1975:228-33.
[17] Surawicz B, Fisch C. Cardiac alternans: diverse mechanisms and clinical manifestations. *J. Am. Coll. Cardiol.* 1992:483-99.
[18] Olearczyk BM, Chongkrairatanakul T, Menzies DJ. The swinging heart: cardiac alternans an*d right ventricular* collapse in classic tamponade. *Can. J. Cardiol.* 2009:240.
[19] Reddy PS, Curtiss EI, Uretsky BF. Spectrum of hemodynamic changes in cardiac tamponade. *Am. J. Cardiol. 1990;6*6(20):1487-91.
[20] Klopfenstein HS, Cogswell TL, Bernath GA, et al. Alterations in intravascular volume affect the relation between right ventricular diastolic collapse and the hemodynamic severity of cardiac tamponade. *J. Am. Coll Cardiol.* 1985:1057-63.
[21] Singh S, Wann LS, Schuchard GH, et al. Right ventricular and right atrial collapse in patients with cardiac tamponade--a combined echocardiographic and hemodynamic study. *Circulation*. 1984:966-71.
[22] Sagristà-Sauleda J, Mercé AS, Soler-Soler J. Diagnosis and management of pericardial effusion. *World J. Cardiol.* 2011:135-43.
[23] Refaat MM, Katz WE. Neoplastic pericardial effusion. *Clin Cardiol.* 2011:593-8.
[24] Reddy PS, Curtiss EI, Uretsky BF. Spectrum of hemodynamic changes in cardiac tamponade. *Am. J. Cardiol*. 1990:1487-1491.

[25] Guberman BA, Fowler NO, Engel PJ, et al. Cardiac tamponade in medical patients. *Circulation* 1978: 265-72.
[26] Shabetai R. Pericardial effusion: haemodynamic spectrum. *Heart.* 2004: 255–256.
[27] Levine MJ, Lorell BH, Diver DJ, et al. Implications of echocardiographically assisted diagnosis of pericardial tamponade in contemporary medical patients: detection before hemodynamic embarrassment. *J. Am. Coll. Cardiol.* 1991:59-65.
[28] Khandaker MH, Espinosa RE, Nishimura RA, Sinak LJ, Hayes SN, Melduni RM, Oh JK. Pericardial disease: diagnosis and management. *Mayo Clin. Proc.* 2010:572–593.
[29] Kronzon I, Cohen ML, Winer HE. Diastolic atrial compression: a sensitive ehocardiographic sign of cardiac tamponade. *J. Am. Coll Cardiol*, 1983: 770–775.
[30] Gonzalez MS, Basnight MA, Appleton CP. Experimental pericardial effusion: relation of abnormal respiratory variation in mitral flow velocity to hemodynamics and diastolic right heart collapse. *J. Am. Coll Cardiol.* 1991:239-248.
[31] Mercé J, Sagristà-Sauleda J, Permanyer-Miralda G, et al. Correlation between clinical and Doppler echocardiographic findings in patients with moderate and large pericardial effusion: implications for the diagnosis of cardiac tamponade. *Am. Heart J.* 1999:759-64.
[32] Zipf RE Jr, Johnston WW. The role of cytology in the evaluation of pericardial effusions. *Chest.* 1972:593-6.
[33] Meyers DG, Bouska DJ. Diagnostic usefulness of pericardial fluid cytology. *Chest.* 1989:1142-3..
[34] Susini G, Pepi M, Sisillo E, et al. Percutaneous pericardiocentesis versus subxyphoid pericardiotomy in cardiac tamponade due to postoperative pericardial effusion. *J. Cardiothorac Vasc. Anesthes* 1993: 178-183.
[35] Wilkes JD, Fidias P, Vaickus L, et al. Malignancy related pericardial effusion: 127 cases from Roswell Park Cancer Institute. *Cancer* 1995: 1377-1387.
[36] Bardales RH, Stanley MW, Schaefer RF, et al. Secondary pericardial malignancies. A critical appraisal of the role of cytology, pericardial biopsy, and DNA ploidy analysis. *Am. J. Clin. Pathol.* 1996:29-34.
[37] Malamou-Mitsi VD, Zioga AP, Agnantis NJ. Diagnostic accuracy of pericardial fluid cytology: An analysis of 53 specimens from 44 consecutive patients. *Diagn Cytopathol.* 1996: 197-204.
[38] Gavin FM, Gray C, Sutton J, et al. Morphometric differences between cytologically benign and malignant serous effusions. *Acta Cytol.* 1988:175-182.
[39] Naylor B. Pleural, peritoneal, and pericardial fluids. In: Bibbo M editor. Comprehensive cytopathology. 2nd ed. Philadelphia, WB Saunders; 1997: 551-621.
[40] Tao LC. Aspiration biopsy cytology of mesothelioma. *Diagn Cytopathol.* 1989:14-21.
[41] Rakha EA, Patil S, Abdulla K, et al. The sensitivity of cytologic evaluation of pleural fluid in the diagnosis of malignant mesothelioma. *Diagn Cytopathol.* 2010: 874-9.
[42] Fetsch PA, Abati A. Immunocytochemistry in effusion cytology: a contemporary review. *Cancer.* 2001:293-308.
[43] Manosca F, Schinstine M, Fetsch PA, et al. Diagnostic effects of prolonged storage on fresh effusion samples. *Diagn Cytopathol.* 2007:6-11.
[44] Nathan NA, Narayan E, Smith MM, et al. Cell block cytology. Improved preparation and its efficacy in diagnostic cytology. *Am. J. Clin. Pathol.* 2000:599-606.

[45] Shield PW, Koivurinne K. The value of calretinin and cytokeratin 5/6 as markers for mesothelioma in cell block preparations of serous effusions. *Cytopathology.* 2008:218-223.
[46] Lyons-Boudreaux V, Mody DR, Zhai J, et al. Cytologic malignancy versus benignancy: how useful are the "newer" markers in body fluid cytology?. *Arch. Pathol. Lab. Med.* 2008:23-28.
[47] Facchetti F, Lonardi S, Gentili F, et al. Claudin 4 identifies a wide spectrum of epithelial neoplasms and represents a very useful marker for carcinoma versus mesothelioma diagnosis in pleural and peritoneal biopsies and effusions. *Virchows Arch.* 2007:669-80.
[48] Lonardi S, Manera C, Marucci R, et al. Usefulness of Claudin 4 in the cytological diagnosis of serosal effusions. *Diagn Cytopathol.* 2011:313-7.
[49] Szturmowicz M, Tomkowski W, Fijalkowska A, et al. The role of carcinoembryonic antigen (CEA) and neuron-specific enolase (NSE) evaluation in pericardial fluid for the recognition of malignant pericarditis. *Int. J. Biol. Markers* 1997: 96-101.
[50] Salama G, Miédougé M, Rouzaud P, et al. Evaluation of pleural CYFRA 21-1 and carcinoembryonic antigen in the diagnosis of malignant pleural effusions. s. 1998:472-476.
[51] Lee JH, Chang JH. Diagnostic utility of serum and pleural fluid carcinoembryonic antigen, neuron-specific enolase, and cytokeratin 19 fragments in patients with effusions from primary lung cancer. *Chest.* 2005:2298-2303.
[52] Alataş F, Alataş O, Metintaş M, et al. Diagnostic value of CEA, CA 15-3, CA 19-9, CYFRA 21-1, NSE and TSA assay in pleural effusions. *Lung Cancer.* 2001:9-16.
[53] Szturmowicz M, Tomkowski W, Fijalkowska A, et al. Diagnostic utility of CYFRA 21-1 and CEA assays in pericardial fluid for the recognition of neoplastic pericarditis. *Int. J. Biol. Markers.* 2005:43-49.
[54] Gu P, Huang G, Chen Y, et al. Diagnostic utility of pleural fluid carcinoembryonic antigen and CYFRA 21-1 in patients with pleural effusion: a systematic review and meta-analysis. *J. Clin. Lab. Anal.* 2007:398-405.
[55] Paganuzzi M, Onetto M, Marroni P, et al. Diagnostic value of CYFRA 21-1 tumor marker and CEA in pleural effusion due to mesothelioma. *Chest.* 2001:1138-1142.
[56] Huang WW, Tsao SM, Lai CL, et al. Diagnostic value of Her-2/neu, Cyfra 21-1, and carcinoembryonic antigen levels in malignant pleural effusions of lung adenocarcinoma. *Pathology.* 2010:224-228.
[57] Tomkowski W, Szturmowicz M, Fijalkowska A, et al. New approaches to the management and treatment of malignant pericardial effusion. *Support Care Cancer* 1997: 64-66.
[58] Fagan SM, Chan KI. Pericardiocentesis. Blind no more! *Chest* 1999: 275-276.
[59] Callagan JA, Seward JBN, Nishimura RA, et al. Two dimensional echocardiographically guided pericardiocentesis: Experience in 117 consecutive patients. *Am. J. Cardiol* 1985: 476-479.
[60] TsangTS, Barnes ME, Gersh BJ et al. Outcomes of clinically significant idiopathic pericardial effusion requiring intervention. *Am. J. Cardiol.* 2002:704–707.
[61] Maisch B, Seferović PM, Ristić AD, et al.; Task Force on the Diagnosis and Management of Pericardial Diseases of the European Society of Cardiology. Guidelines on the diagnosis and management of pericardial diseases executive summary; The Task

force on the diagnosis and management of pericardial diseases of the European society of cardiology. *Eur. Heart J.* 2004:587-610.

[62] Tsang TS, Seward JB, Barnes ME, et al. Outcomes of primary and secondary treatment of pericardial effusion in patients with malignancy. *Mayo Clin Proc.* 2000:248-253.

[63] Ready A, Black J, Lewis R et al. Laparoscopic pericardial fenestration for malignant pericardial effusion. *Lancet.* 1992:1609.

[64] Gross JL, Younes RN, Deheinzelin D, et al. Surgical management of symptomatic pericardial effusion in patients with solid malignancies. *Ann. Surg. Oncol.* 2006:1732-1738.

[65] Sugimoto JT, Little AG, Ferguson MK, et al. Pericardial window: mechanisms of efficacy. *Ann. Thorac. Surg.* 1990:442-445.

[66] Sauter C. Cytostatic activity of oxidized tetracycline in vitro: relevance for the treatment of malignant effusions?. *Br. J. Cancer.* 1988:514-515.

[67] Maher EA, Shepherd FA, Todd TJ. Pericardial sclerosis as the primary management of malignant pericardial effusion and cardiac tamponade. *J. Thorac. Cardiovasc. Surg.* 1996:637-643.

[68] Liu G, Crump M, Goss PE, et al. Prospective comparison of the sclerosing agents doxycycline and bleomycin for the primary management of malignant pericardial effusion and cardiac tamponade. *J. Clin. Oncol.* 1996:3141-3147.

[69] Yano T, Yokoyama H, Inoue T, et al. A simple technique to manage malignant pericardial effusion with a local instillation of bleomycin in non-small cell carcinoma of the lung. *Oncology.* 1994:507-509.

[70] Martinoni A, Cipolla CM, Cardinale D, et al. Long-term results of intrapericardial chemotherapeutic treatment of malignant pericardial effusions with thiotepa. *Chest.* 2004:1412-1416.

[71] Wall TC, Campbell PT, O'Connor CM, et al. Diagnosis and management (by subxyphoid pericardiotomy) of large pericardial effusions causing cardiac tamponade. *Am. J. Cardiol.* 1992:1075-1078.

[72] Krause TJ, Margiotta M, Chandler JJ. Pericardio-peritoneal window for malignant pericardial effusion. *Surg. Gynecol. Obstet.* 1991: 487-488.

[73] Griffin S, Fountain W. Pericardio-peritoneal shunt for malignant pericardial effusion. *J. Cardiovasc. Surg.* 1989: 1153-1154.

[74] Ready A, Black J, Lewis R, et al. Laparoscopic pericardial fenestration for malignant pericardial effusion. *Lancet* 1992:1609.

[75] Shapira OM, Aldea GS, Fonger JD, et al. Video-assisted thoracic surgical techniques in the diagnosis and management of pericardial effusion in patients with advanced lung cancer. *Chest* 1993:1262-1263.

[76] Vaitkus PT, Herrmann HC, LeWinter MM. Treatment of malignant pericardial effusion. *JAMA* 1994; 272:59-64.

[77] Ziskind AA, Pearce AC, Lemmon AC, et al. Percutaneous balloon pericardiotomy for the treatment of cardiac tamponade and large pericardial effusions: description of the technique and report of the first 50 cases. *J. Am. Coll. Cardiol.* 1993: 1-5.

[78] Wang HJ, Hsu KL, Chiang FT, et al. Technical and prognostic outcomes of double-balloon pericardiotomy for large malignancy-related pericardial effusions. *Chest.* 2002;122:893-899.

[79] Zaharia L, Gill PS. Primary cardiac lymphoma. *Am. J. Clin. Oncol.* 1991:142-145.

[80] Reynolds PM, Byrne MJ. The treatment of malignant pericardial effusion in carcinoma of the breast. *Aust. N. Z. J. Med.* 1977:169-171.

[81] Primrose WR, Clee MD, Johnston RN. Malignant pericardial effusion managed with Vinblastine. *Clin. Oncol.* 1983:67-70.

[82] Kikuchi N, Satoh H, Kodama T, et al. Response to gefitinib in pericardial effusion due to lung cancer. *Acta Medica* (Hradec Kralove). 2003:215-6.

[83] Figoli F, Zanette ML, Tirelli U, et al. Pharmacokinetics of VM 26 given intrapericardially or intravenously in patients with malignant pericardial effusion. *Cancer Chemother Pharmacol.* 1987:239-242.

[84] Moriya T, Takiguchi Y, Tabeta H, et al. Controlling malignant pericardial effusion by intrapericardial carboplatin administration in patients with primary non-small-cell lung cancer. *Br. J. Cancer.* 2000:858-862.

[85] Lerner-Tung MB, Chang AY, Ong LS, et al. Pharmacokinetics of intrapericardial administration of 5-fluorouracil. *Cancer Chemother Pharmacol.* 1997:318-320.

[86] Casper ES, Kelsen DP, Alcock NW, et al. Ip cisplatin in patients with malignant ascites: pharmacokinetic evaluation and comparison with the iv route. *Cancer Treat Rep.* 1983:235-23.

[87] Wang X, Zhou J, Wang Y, et al. A phase I clinical and pharmacokinetic study of paclitaxel liposome infused in non-small cell lung cancer patients with malignant pleural effusions. *Eur. J. Cancer.* 2010:1474-1480.

[88] Liu J, Meisner D, Kwong E, et al. Translymphatic chemotherapy by intrapleural placement of gelatin sponge containing biodegradable Paclitaxel colloids controls lymphatic metastasis in lung cancer. *Cancer Res.* 2009:1174-1181.

[89] Markman M, Howell SB. Intrapericardial instillation of cisplatin in a patient with a large malignant effusion. *Cancer Drug Deliv.* 1985;2:49-52.

[90] Fiorentino MV, Daniele O, Morandi P, et al. Intrapericardial instillation of platin in malignant pericardial effusion. *Cancer.* 1988:1904-1906.

[91] Tomkowski WZ, Filipecki S. Intrapericardial cisplatin for the management of patients with large malignant pericardial effusion in the course of the lung cancer. *Lung Cancer.* 1997:215-222.

[92] Tomkowski W, Szturmowicz M, Fijalkowska A, et al. Intrapericardial cisplatin for the management of patients with large malignant pericardial effusion. *J. Cancer Res. Clin. Oncol.* 1994:434-436.

[93] Maisch B, Ristić AD, Pankuweit S, et al. Neoplastic pericardial effusion. Efficacy and safety of intrapericardial treatment with cisplatin. *Eur. Heart J.* 2002:1625-1631.

[94] Bischiniotis TS, Lafaras CT, Platogiannis DN, et al. Intrapericardial cisplatin administration after pericardiocentesis in patients with lung adenocarcinoma and malignant cardiac tamponade. *Hellenic J. Cardiol..* 2005:324-329.

[95] Cham WC, Freiman AH, Carstens PH, et al. Radiation therapy of cardiac and pericardial metastases. *Radiology* 1975:701-704

[96] Dempke W, Firusian N. Treatment of malignant pericardial effusion with 32P-colloid. *Br. J. Cancer.* 1999:1955-1957.

[97] Martini N, Freiman AH, Watson RC, et al. Intrapericardial installation of radioactive chromic phosphate in malignant effusion. *AJR Am. J. Roentgenol.* 1977:639-641.

[98] Therasse P. Evaluation of response: new and standard criteria. *Ann. Onc. Med.* 2002: 127-9.

[99] Cademartiri F, Luccichenti G, Maffei E, et al. Imaging for oncologic staging and follow-up: review of current methods and novel approaches. *Acta Biomed.* 2008:85-91.

[100] Leibowitz D, Perlman G, Planer D, et al. Quantification of pericardial effusions by echocardiography and computed tomography. *Am. J. Cardiol.* 2011:331-5.

[101] Girardi LN, Ginsberg RJ, Burt ME. Pericardiocentesis and intrapericardial sclerosis: effective therapy for malignant pericardial effusions. *Ann. Thorac. Surg.* 1997:1422-1427; discussion 1427-1428.

[102] Kunitoh H, Tamura T, Shibata T, et al.; JCOG Lung Cancer Study Group, Tokyo, Japan. A randomised trial of intrapericardial bleomycin for malignant pericardial effusion with lung cancer (JCOG9811). *Br. J. Cancer.* 2009:464-9.

[103] Lestuzzi C, Bearz A, Lafaras C, et al. Neoplastic pericardial disease in lung cancer: impact on outcomes of different treatment strategies. A multicenter study. *Lung Cancer* 2011:340-47.

[104] Churchill P, Otal D, Pemberton J, et al. Sclerotherapy for lymphatic malformations in children: a scoping review. *J. Pediatr Surg.* 2011: 912-22. Review.

[105] Martinoni A, Cipolla CM, Civelli M, et al. Intrapericardial treatment of neoplastic pericardial effusions. *Herz.* 2000:787-93.

[106] Tomkowski WZ, Filipecki S: Intrapericardial administration of cisplatin in treatment of metastatic pericardial involvement in adenocarcinoma of the lung. *Monaldi Arch. Chest Dis.* 1997: 221-224.

In: Lung Cancer: A Comprehensive Overview
Editor: Kathy Gately
ISBN: 978-1-62618-447-3


*Chapter XII*

# The Role of Claudin Proteins in Lung Tumorigenesis

***Zhe Lu[1,3], Qun Lu[1,2], Lei Ding[4] and Yan-Hua Chen[1,2*]***
[1]Department of Anatomy and Cell Biology,
[2]Leo W. Jenkins Cancer Center, Brody School of Medicine,
East Carolina University, Greenville, NC, US
[3]Department of Basic Medicine, Hangzhou Normal University,
Hangzhou, China
[4]Department of Oncology, Beijing Shijitan Hospital,
Capital Medical University, Beijing, China

## Abstract

Tight junctions (TJs), or zonula occludens, are the most apical component of the junctional complex and provide one form of cell-cell adhesion in epithelial and endothelial cells. Nearly 90% of malignant tumors are derived from the epithelium. Loss of cell-cell adhesion is one of the major steps in cancer progression to metastasis. At least three main TJ family proteins have been discovered: occludin, claudin, and junctional adhesion molecule (JAM). Claudins are the most important structural and functional components of TJ integral membrane proteins with at least 24 members in mammals. They are crucial for the paracellular flux of ions and small molecules. Several claudins, such as claudin-1, -2, -3, -4, -5, -7 and -18, were detected in normal human airway epithelial cells, whereas other claudins, including claudin-6, -9, -10, -11, -15, and -16, were not detected in the lung. Claudins are important in maintaining the normal structure of epithelial cells by regulating airway TJ permeability and epithelial cell polarity.

Recent studies have found that claudins are closely associated with lung tumorigenesis. Altered expression and distribution of different claudins have been reported in various human lung cancer tissues, indicating that they could be a useful prognostic predictor and potential drug treatment target for patients with lung cancer. Post-translational modifications of claudins can also alter TJ structure and function,

* Email: cheny@ecu.edu.

leading to tumorigenesis. In this chapter, we discuss the conceptual framework of TJs with an emphasis on claudins, their crosstalks with different carcinogenic signaling pathways such as ERK/MAPK and PI3K pathways, and their potential implications in lung cancer. Therapeutic approaches that target TJ proteins are emerging. It is hoped that there will be an increased understanding of the potential roles of TJ proteins in tumorigenesis, thus providing effective targeted therapy for certain types of lung cancer.

## Introduction

Tight junctions (TJs), or zonula occludens (ZO), were originally identified in the early 1960s by Farquhar and Palade [1]. They are one mode of cell-cell adhesion in epithelial cellular sheets that is only present in vertebrates. They form a circumferential belt around an epithelial cell, separating the cell membrane into the apical (the side toward the lumen) and basolateral (the side facing the extracellular matrix) domains. At the TJs, the outer leaflets of the cell membrane of the two adjoining cells fuse at various points, forming a branching network of sealing strands around the epithelium of skin, gut, and airways, separating the external environment from the internal environment [2].

TJs serve as a "fence function" as well as a "barrier function" [3]. As a boundary between the apical and the basolateral cell membranes, TJs maintain the asymmetric distribution of proteins and lipid molecules between these two domains and generate the apical-basal polarity of the cell membrane, which is known as "fence function" [2]. TJs can also prevent or slow the diffusion of ions and small molecules across an epithelium via the paracellular pathway, known as "barrier function", which is important for the fluid and electrolyte balance in the body. The efficiency of TJs in preventing ion passage increases exponentially with the number of strands. Various TJs can be classified either as "tight" or "leaky" based on their charge and size selectivity in permeability. Tight epithelia have TJs that prevent most molecules from passing through the paracellular pathway; for example, TJs in the distal convoluted tubule and collecting duct of the nephron. Leaky epithelia have higher paracellular permeability; for example, TJs in the kidney proximal tubule. TJs can be rapidly formed and disassembled. Under various physiological conditions, material transport across TJs occurs in a regulated fashion. The TJs undergo dynamic modulation by a number of molecules. Insulin, hepatocyte growth factor (HGF), epidermal growth factor (EGF), protamine sulfate, D-glucose, Ras homolog gene family, member A (RhoA), ras-related C3 botulinum toxin substrate 1 (Rac1), $Ca^{2+}$, and many other factors have been implicated in the regulation of the assembly and barrier function of TJs [4-10]. The barrier function of TJs can be measured by transepithelial electrical resistance (TER) or the paracellular flux of ions or small molecules.

There are two major components of TJs: transmembrane components and scaffolding components (Figure 1A) [3]. Three main types of structural transmembrane components are enriched at TJs: the IgG-like family of junctional adhesion molecules (JAMs), the occludin family, and the claudin family. Only recently, proteins MARVEL-D3 (MAL and related proteins for vesicle trafficking and membrane link domain containing-3) and MARVEL-D2 (tricellulin) were identified as being structurally similar to occludin [11]. MARVEL-D3 is an alternatively spliced protein that localizes with occludin, while tricellulin is expressed in regions where three cells make contact [3]. JAMs (~45kDa) are members of the immunoglobulin gene superfamily, which contains single transmembrane domain. The three most common members of the JAMs family are JAM-A, JAM-B, and JAM-C. JAM-A deficient mice are viable but show irregularly-shaped corneal epithelium compared to the wild-type mice with normal cobblestone shape of corneal epithelium [12]. JAM-B regulates the maintenance of hematopoietic stem cells in the bone marrow. Deletion of JAM-B in mice leads to a decreased pool of quiescent hematopoietic stem cells, which is due to alterations of bone marrow stromal compartments [13]. JAM-C controls homeostatic chemokine secretion in lymph node fibroblastic reticular cells, and JAM-C deficient mice showed decreased chemokine secretion [14]. In addition, loss of integrity of the myelin sheath and defective nerve conduction were also observed in JAM-C deficient mice [15].

Occludin (~65kDa) has four transmembrane domains and two extracellular loops that are similar in size with N- and C- termini in the cytoplasm. Occludin knockout pups are viable but do not have a significant phenotype. However, by 2-6 weeks of age, knockout mice show atrophy of the fundic mucosa and develop gastritis [16].

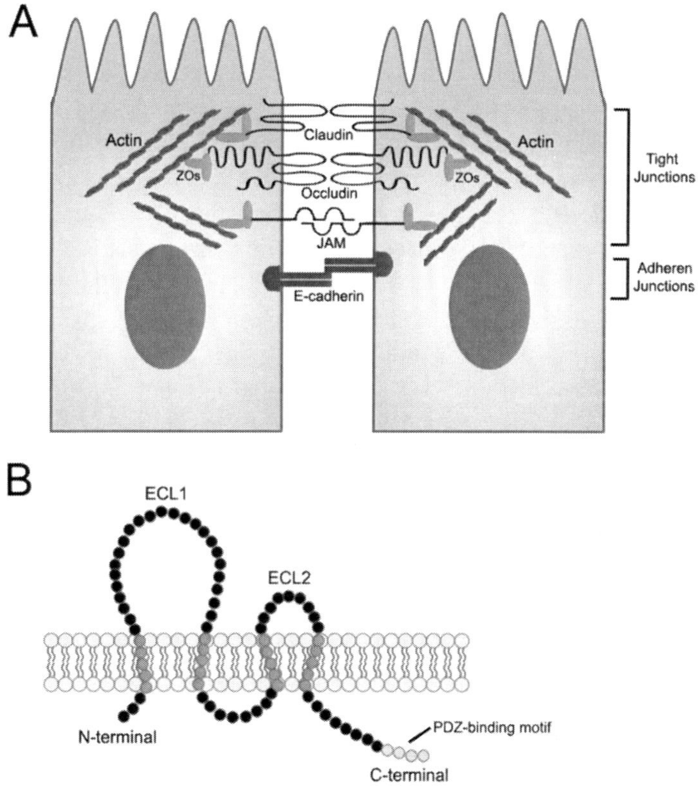


Figure 1. Models of tight junction and claudin protein. A. Tight junctions contain two major components: transmembrane and scaffolding components. Three main types of structural transmembrane proteins are enriched at tight junctions: claudins, occludin, and the IgG-like family of junctional adhesion molecules (JAMs). The association and incorporation of occludin, claudins, and JAMs into tight junctions require local clustering of scaffolding proteins such as ZO-1, ZO-2, and ZO-3 proteins (ZOs). Extracellular domains of transmembrane proteins contributed from two adjacent epithelial cells interact with each other to form tight junction structure. B. A membrane-folding model of claudin structure. Each claudin protein contains two extracellular loops and one intracellular loop with N- and C-termini in the cytoplasm. Claudins contain a PDZ-binding motif, which binds to ZOs, at intracellular C-terminal positions -3, -2, -1 and 0.

Claudins (20~27 kDa) are a family of proteins with similar topology as occludin. In this chapter, we will mainly focus on claudin family proteins in human lung cancer. The incorporation and association of occludin, claudins, and JAMs into TJ strands require local clustering of scaffolding proteins. An important group of these proteins includes the ZO proteins, such as ZO-1, ZO-2 and ZO-3, cingulin, the membrane-associated guanylate kinase inverted (MAGI) [17], as well as partitioning-defective proteins PAR-3 and PAR-6 [18], the multi-PDZ domain protein 1 (MUPP1) [19], and c-Yes [20]. These peripheral cytoplasmic plaque proteins anchor the TJ integral membrane proteins to cytoplasmic and cytoskeletal elements. The interlamellar strands of oligodendrocyte myelin sheaths [21] and filtration slits in renal glomerular epithelial cells [6] are considered as variants of TJs where claudin-11 and ZO-1 are expressed, respectively.

While the barrier and fence functions of TJs have been well-appreciated, functions of TJs in the initiation and progression of cancers are only just beginning to be recognized. Deficient expression of TJ proteins are known to increase epithelial proliferation in gastric and intestinal epithelium [16, 22]. Down-regulation of claudins may contribute to increased paracellular permeability, allowing more nutrients and growth factors to cancerous cells. In cases of up-regulation of claudin expression, the barrier function of the cancerous epithelia could also be altered as they display a disorganized arrangement of TJ strands with increased permeability to paracellular tracers [23]. This defective form of TJs can also enable the additional source of nutrients and other growth factors to be obtained from the luminal fluid and help the tumor grow aggressively.

Changes in expression of claudins not only affect the cell proliferation but also the invasive and migratory properties of cancer cells. During metastasis, several important steps occur including epithelial-mesenchymal transition (EMT). By definition, the term EMT applies only to epithelial-derived cancers. During this process, epithelial cells down-regulate cell-cell adhesion structures, alter their polarity, reorganize their cytoskeleton, and become isolated and motile [24]. Following EMT, cancer cells detach from the neighboring cells, degrade and travel through the extracellular matrix that imposes a barrier to cancer dissemination, and penetrate the walls of the lymphatic and/or blood vessels, known as intravasation, through which they are able to circulate through the bloodstream. Finally, metastatic cells exit the bloodstream by a process known as extravasation and reach other sites in the body. TJs have been shown to be involved in this cancer metastatic process. As TJ proteins are important structures for maintaining the cell-cell adhesion, altered expression of these proteins can cause the disruption of cell-cell adhesion, which is an initial step for cancer cell invasion. Expressional changes in junctional complex proteins are responsible for this step. Altered TJ protein expression has been found in a wide variety of human malignancies, including ovarian, pancreatic, liver, and prostate cancers [25].

In this chapter, we will mainly focus on claudin family proteins and their structure, function, and expressional changes in lung cancer.

## Claudin Family Proteins

Claudin proteins were first discovered in 1999 [26]. Since then, at least 24 members of the claudin family have been identified. Claudins are the major structural and functional components of TJs (Figure 1B). They are transmembrane proteins that span the cell membrane four times with molecular masses of ~20 kDa, contain two extracellular domains (~53 amino acids) and one intracellular loop (~24 amino acids), and have the N- and C-termini oriented toward the cytoplasm [27]. According to the alignment analysis of their full-length sequences, claudins can be divided into two groups: the classic claudins, such as claudin-1, -2, -3, -4, -5, and -7, and non-classic claudins, such as claudin-11, -12, -13, and -16. Classic claudins exhibit a much stronger consensus sequence (sequence homology) than non-classic claudins.

The first extracellular loop of claudins has a common motif, GLWXXCC (X indicates any amino acid), which is also found in some non-claudin molecules. The two conserved cysteine residues are involved in the barrier function [28]. Negative and positive charges of the first extracellular loop contribute to TJ permeability [29]. The function of the second extracellular loop has not been studied to a large extent. Only in claudin-3 and -4 does the second extracellular loop contain a clostridium perfingens endotoxin (CPE) binding domain. This endotoxin is secreted by *Clostridium. C. perfingens* and causes the degradation and redistribution of TJ components, such as claudin-4, ZO-1, and occludin [30-31]. Mutations in the first or second extracellular loop of claudin-16 result in familial hypomagnesaemia, hypercalciuria, and nephrocalcinosis (FHHNC disorder) [32]. A mutation in the first extracellular loop of claudin-19 causes hypomagnesaemia [28]. Claudins also have a PDZ-binding motif (PDZ is an acronym combining the first letters of three proteins: Post synaptic density protein, Drosophila disc large tumor suppressor, and ZO-1, which were first discovered to share the domain) at their intracellular C-terminal positions -3, -2, -1, and 0. They bind to PDZ domain-containing peripheral membrane proteins such as ZO-1, ZO-2, ZO-3, MUPP1, and protein associated with Lin seven 1 (PALS1) associated TJ proteins [26], which then further interact with the cytoplasmic and cytoskeleton proteins. Intramembranous domains of claudin proteins also play an important role. For example, mutations in the first transmembrane domain of claudin-19 are associated with renal magnesium wasting, renal failure, and severe ocular involvement [33]. Mutations in either one of the four transmembrane domains of claudin-16 result in the FHHNC disorder [32].

Claudins comprise a multigene family; two or more different claudins in adjacent cells can interact heterotypically through the extracellular loops. However, this interaction is not universal, but rather limited to specific claudin combinations. NIH3T3 mouse fibroblasts are often used to study claudin compatibility since they do not express endogenous claudins. Transfection of distinct claudins into fibroblast cells establishes the random localized TJ-like strand morphology [34]. Studies show that claudin-1 heterotypically binds to claudin-3 but not claudin-2 or -5, and claudin-2 and -5 heterotypically bind to claudin-3. Transfecting claudin-1 or -3 into 3T3 cells neither increased the TER nor decreased the permeability of dextran. Cotransfecting claudin-1 and -3 significantly increased TER as well as decreased the permeability of dextran when compared to the wild type. Claudin-1 and -3 indeed were colocalized and formed a heterodimer in both 3T3 and lung carcinoma NCI-H1299 cells [34-35]. Point mutations and/or chimeric construction of claudin proteins show that the extracellular domains control the heterotypic claudin compatibility [36]. Claudins have different expression patterns in different organs [37]. Claudin-1, -2, -3, -4, -7, -8, -10 are expressed in kidneys, while claudin-5, -6, -9, -12 are not [38]. Claudin-1 has been found to be expressed in human liver, pancreas, colon, placenta, prostate, and skin, while claudin-7 is expressed in lung, kidney, ovary, prostate, and colon [26].

Claudins regulate the paracellular permeability of ions and small molecules, which are tissue-, size-, and charge-specific. Most of the research has been performed in cell lines. For example, claudin-2 is typically present in leaky epithelia, such as the proximal renal tubule and human ovarian surface epithelium, and is found to increase paracellular cation $Na^+$ and $K^+$ permeability in Madin-Darbey canine kidney C7 (MDCK-C7) cells [39]. Overexpression of claudin-7 increases paracellular $Na^+$ but decreases $Cl^-$ permeability in LLC-Pig Kidney 1 cells [40]. Several claudin gene-deficient mouse models are currently available, including models deficient in claudin-1, -5, -7, -11, -14, -15, -16, and -19. Claudin-5 knockout mice died shortly after birth, showing the size-selective loosening of the blood-brain barrier [41]. Claudin-7 deficient mice exhibited growth retardation, salt wasting, mucosal disruption in intestines, and died within 12 days after birth [22, 42]. Claudin-15 null mice show a two-fold enlargement of the upper small intestines in comparison to wild type mice [43]. Claudin-11 knockout mice show deafness due to the absence of basal cell paracellular diffusion barrier, male sterility due to defective blood-testis barrier, and neurological abnormalities due to absent myelin TJ in oligodendrocytes that results in slowed conduction velocities in the central nervous system [21, 44]. Claudin-19 knockout mice display peripheral nervous system deficits due to the absence of TJs from Schwann cells of peripheral myelinated axons [45].

## Post-Translational Modifications of Tight Junction Proteins

The assembly and barrier function of TJs can be regulated through the phosphorylation of TJ proteins by kinases, such as protein kinase C (PKC), extracellular signal-regulated kinase (ERK)/mitogen-activated protein kinase (MAPK), and c-Yes [20, 46]. Growth factor stimulation leads to increased phosphorylation [47]. Different types of stimulation applied to different cell types have contributed to the discovery of various phosphorylated residues in claudins. Hyper-phosphorylation of occludin at the C-terminus is associated with its localization at TJs [48-49]. During the disruption of TJs by various factors, occludin undergoes de-phosphorylation on Ser/Thr residues and elevated phosphorylation on Tyr residues; phosphorylation of Tyr residues attenuates its interaction with ZO-1 [20, 50-51]. Phosphorylation of occludin at Thr403 and Thr404 residues by PKCη enhances both occludin trafficking to the TJs and paracellular barrier function in human colon cancer cell line Caco-2 and MDCK cells [52]. Tyr398 and Tyr402 phosphorylation by c-Src reduces occludin localization to the TJs and interferes with its interaction with ZO-1 in MDCK cells [53]. Increased tyrosine phosphorylation of occludin and ZO-1 is associated with TJ barrier dysfunction during oxidative stress in Caco-2 cells [54]. Occludin Ser/Thr de-phosphorylation following *Pseudomonas aeruginosa* infection increased the paracellular permeability in both intestinal epithelium and Caco-2 cells [55]. Increases in tyrosine phosphorylation of occludin play an important role in its redistribution and disruption of TJs, which may lead to increased macromolecular permeability in blood-brain barrier after cerebral ischemia [56]. Cigarette smoke exposure increased macromolecular permeability, increased tyrosine phosphorylation of occludin, and decreased occludin association with ZO-1 in the airway epithelial cell line, Calu-3 [57]. However, other studies have shown that tyrosine phosphorylation and serine de-phosphorylation can be positively and temporally correlated with TJ assembly and function.

Tsukamoto and Nigam show that tyrosine phosphorylation of occludin and possibly other proteins are necessary for TJ reassembly during adenosine triphosphate repletion [58]. Inhibition of MAPK pathway increases both protein half-life and tyrosine phosphorylation of occludin [46]. PKCβ directly phosphorylates occludin at Ser490 residue and leads to the ubiquitination of occludin, disruption of its interaction with ZO-1, and increased blood-retinal barrier permeability [59-60]. Casein kinase II phosphorylates occludin at Ser408 residue and decreases TER by increasing paracellular cation flux [61]. In addition, kinases, such as p160 Rho-associated protein kinase (ROCK), can also phosphorylate occludin and affect the barrier function of TJs [62].

The sealing function of claudins at TJs can be mediated through phosphorylation or palmitoylation events. Claudins undergo post-translational modification in which the C-termini can be phosphorylated (Figure 2). For example, Thr203 residue of claudin-1 can be phosphorylated by MAPK, which is required to promote the barrier function of TJs [63]; phosphorylation of claudin-3 at Thr192 residue by cAMP-dependent protein kinase (PKA) disrupts TJ barrier function in ovarian cancer cells [64]; PKCε colocalizes with claudin-4 at the TJs and phosphorylates claudin-4 at Thr189 and Ser194 residues, which alter claudin-4 localization and disrupt the barrier function of TJs [65]. EphA2 associates with claudin-4 via their extracellular domains and leads to phosphorylation of the C-terminus of claudin-4 at Tyr208 residue and increases the paracellular permeability [66]; cAMP regulates the barrier function of TJs in endothelial cells by phosphorylating claudin-5 on the Thr207 residue [67]; WNK4 phosphorylates Ser206 residue of claudin-7 and promotes paracellular $Cl^-$ permeability [68]. Palmitoylation of claudin-14 at Cys107 and Cys185 residues in the second and/or fourth transmembrane domains is required for its efficient TJ localization [69]. Tyrosine phosphorylation of claudin-1 is decreased by two-folds after alcohol/ethanol intoxication and burn injury [70]. Activation of PKC by its activator 12-O-tetradecanoylphorbol 13-acetate (TPA) increases the serine phosphorylation of claudin-4, alters the localization of claudin-4, and changes the TJ barrier function in pancreatic cancer HPAC cells [71].

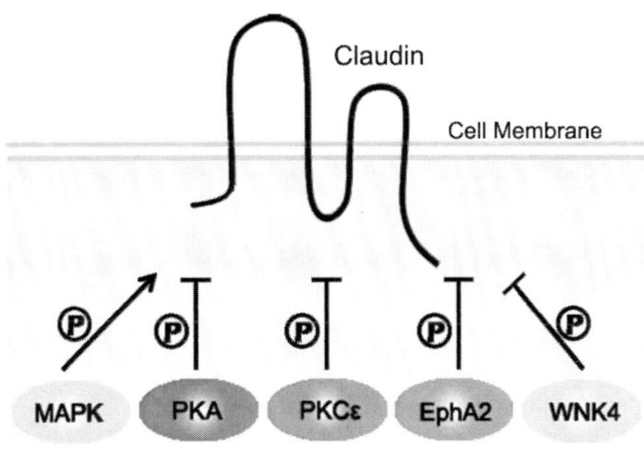


Figure 2. Schematic diagram showing that phosphorylation of claudins by protein kinases can affect the barrier function of tight junctions. For example, phosphorylation of claudin-1 by MAPK promotes the barrier function of tight junctions. PKA, PKCε, EphA2, and WNK4 phosphorylate claudins and attenuate the tight junction barrier function as measured by transepithelial electric resistance (TER).

Mutation in claudin-14 at Gly232 residue affects its phosphorylation and results in autosomal recessive non-syndromic hearing loss [72]. A number of molecules, such as acetaldehyde, can induce the tyrosine phosphorylation of claudin-3 in Caco-2 cells. EGF attenuates this tyrosine phosphorylation, but not through the ERK/MAPK pathway [73]. Ischemia and tissue plasminogen activator treatment induces phosphorylation of claudin-5 and enhances the paracellular permeability of blood-brain barrier in rats [74]. Alternate phosphorylation and O-β-GlcNAc modification on Ser192, Ser205, Ser206, and Thr191 lead to the disassembly of claudin-1 at TJs during hepatitis C virus entry into the host cells [75-76]. Phosphorylation of claudin-1 by PKC and PKA translocates claudin-1 from nucleus to cytoplasm and increases the motility of G361 melanoma cells [77]. One of the PKC isoforms, PKC-θ, phosphorylates claudin-1 and claudin-2 at serine and threonine sites, which is required for normal claudin assembly and the integrity of the intestinal epithelial barrier in Caco-2 cells [78]. Disease-causing mutant WNK4 (D564A) increases paracellular $Cl^-$ permeability and phosphorylates claudin-1, -2, -3 and -4 in COS-7 cells and MDCK II cells [79]. $Mg^{2+}$ deprivation inhibits the localization of claudin-16 at TJs and decreases the MEK/ERK-dependent phosphothreonine levels of claudin-16 [80]. Post-translational modifications can be predicted by certain programs. Netphos 2.0 and Disphos 1.3 programs can be used to predict potential phosphorylation sites, while YinOYang 1.2 and OGPET can be used to predict possible O-glycosylation sites. CSS-Palm 2.0 can be used to predict potential palmitoylation sites [76, 81].

## Tight Junction Proteins and Lung Cancer

In human airways, TJs serve to separate the internal and external environment of the lungs. The airway TJs are moderately leaky with relatively low TER of ~100 $\Omega$*cm$^2$ [82]. Lungs are exposed to pathogens and exogenous compounds, which can influence the normal function of bronchial airways and alveolar cells. TJs in airway epithelial cells create a physicochemical defense barrier against inhaled pathogens or noxious agent intrusions into the interstitial compartment. The airway epithelium can also be frequently injured from permanent contact with the external environment. Cytotoxicity and inflammation can disrupt this paracellular barrier. TJs are also key regulators of ion and solute homeostasis controlling airway surface liquid height and ionic composition necessary for lung defense [83]. Several claudins, such as claudin-1, -2, -3, -4, -5, and -7, are detected in normal human airway epithelial cells, whereas other claudins, including claudin-6, -9, -10, -11, -15, and -16, are not detected in the lung [34, 84-86].

Tobioka *et al.* have shown that in normal lung tissues, occludin is localized at the apicoluminal borders of the bronchial or bronchiolar epithelial and bronchial glands as a dot or short line, as well as the intercellular borders of alveolar epithelia. In all adenocarcinomas (ADCs), occludin shows an expression pattern identical to those of the normal bronchial and alveolar epithelia. However, it has negative reactivity in all cases of squamous cell carcinoma (SCC), large cell carcinoma (LCC), and small cell lung cancer (SCLC). Thus, occludin can serve as an immunohistochemical indicator of the glandular differentiation in human lung cancer [87]. Occludin mRNA is detected in normal human lung tissues [88]; however, mRNA levels are significantly decreased in SCCs [89].

Moldvay *et al.* performed immunohistochemical staining on claudin-1, -2, -3, -4, and -7 proteins using 104 human lung cancer tissue samples including 46 ADCs, 30 SCCs, 15 SCLCs, 8 typical and 5 atypical carcinoids. Adjacent normal lung cancer tissues were used as controls. Claudin-1 was strongly stained at the cell membranes of the bronchial cells at the basolateral surface, while no staining of claudin-1 was observed in pneumocytes, cylindrical cells, fibroblasts, endothelial cells, or lymphocytes of peripheral parenchyma [90]. Claudin-1 showed basolateral staining and circular cell membrane staining in ADCs, as well as circular cell membrane staining in SCCs. Conversely, Paschoud *et al.* have performed immunohistochemical staining on 90 lung carcinomas containing 41 ADCs and 49 SCCs, and showed no claudin-1 expression in ADCs [89]. Its expression was weaker in SCLCs than in the adjacent normal epithelial tissues [90]. Claudin-2 is predominantly localized in the cytoplasm of the bronchial cells at the apical surface [90]. Claudin-2 is present in a cytoplasmic, granular manner in ADCs, and its expression is often stronger at the border of the tumor islands in SCCs. Expression of claudin-2 was absent in all SCLC samples [90]. Claudin-3 is localized continuously along the cell membranes in normal bronchial basal cells and cylindrical cells [91]. Claudin-3 staining tends to move to the apical membrane in ADCs, and its expression is barely detected in SCCs but shows strong staining in SCLC samples. Like claudin-3, claudin-4 is also localized continuously along the cell membranes of normal bronchial epithelial cells and the lateral membrane of cylindrical cells and pneumocytes, whereas no staining of claudin-4 is detected in endothelial cells, lymphocytes, or fibroblasts [89]. Most ADCs show strong basal surface staining of claudin-4 [91]; in contrast to claudin-2 expression, claudin-4 is often found in the central part of the tumor cell islands in SCCs. No significant difference of claudin-4 staining is observed in SCLC samples when compared to the adjacent normal epithelial tissues. Claudin-5 is detected in the lateral membranes of cylindrical cells, endothelial cells, and pneumocytes, while it is not detected in the basal cells of normal human lung tissues [89]. Claudin-5 shows strong staining in ADCs but not in SCCs [89, 91]. Claudin-7 stains the cell membrane strongly and homogenously and shows no predominance concerning cellular polarity. There is controversy over claudin-7 expression in lung cancers. To investigate whether claudin-7 is dysregulated in lung cancer, we performed tissue microarray analyses using claudin-7 immunohistochemical staining method on 36 cases of different lung cancer types in comparison to normal lung tissues. After we examined the tissue microarray platform of 96 cores, including all the common types of lung cancer (36 cases) and normal and inflammatory lung tissues (12 cases) in duplicate, our data showed that while claudin-7 was distributed to cell-cell junction area in normal lung epithelia, its expression was altered in lung tumors. It was discontinuous in lung carcinoma specimens or completely absent in SCCs [35]. Using immunohistochemical staining on 101 cases of lung squamous cell carcinoma and adenocarcinoma samples and Western blot on 30 specimens of fresh lung cancer, Li *et al.* found that claudin-7 was remarkably decreased in SCCs and ADCs compared with normal lung tissues, and its expression level was closely correlated with differentiation grade and lymphatic metastasis [92].

However, Moldvay *et al.* showed that there was no significant difference of claudin-7 staining between SCLC samples and the adjacent normal epithelial tissues, only one case out of 15 SCLC samples was negative for claudin-7 [90]. Merikallio *et al.* have also found that claudin-7 expression was strong in both ADCs and SCCs but significantly lower in LCCs when compared to SCCs [93]. Claudin-18 is present in both type I and type II alveolar pneumocytes, and shows intensive membrane staining in lung ADCs. Patients displaying claudin-18 expression in their tumors have a better survival rate [94].

RT-PCR results reveal elevated claudin-1 mRNA expression in 82.1% (23 out of 28 cases) of the lung SCCs [95] and decreased claudin-1 mRNA expression in ADCs [89]. The protein level of claudin-1 is also high in SCCs and low in ADCs [89]. Chao *et al.* have shown that claudin-1 is a cancer invasion and metastasis suppressor, and that low claudin-1 mRNA and protein expressions are correlated with poor overall survival in lung ADCs [96]. Hewitt et al. performed in silico analysis of claudin expression and confirmed that claudin-3 and -4 are elevated in ADCs [97]. However, Paschoud *et al.* showed significant decrease in mRNA levels of claudin-3 and -4 in ADCs when normal bronchial cells are used as a negative control instead of parenchyma cells [89].

The mRNA level of claudin-5 increases in both ADCs and SCCs, though antibody staining does not show claudin-5 in SCCs. Claudin-7 is normally expressed in human bronchial cells, type I and type II alveolar cells by RT-PCR and Western blot [98]. The mRNA level of claudin-7 is decreased in both SCCs and ADCs when compared to the normal bronchial cells [89]. However, Hewitt *et al.* have shown that claudin-7 is elevated in ADCs by in silico analysis [97]. Some of these contradictory results could be due to the different stages or grades of the cancers.

Lung cancer cells can spread from the primary site to other parts of the body, a process known as metastasis. Common metastasis sites are heart, trachea, esophagus, kidneys, bone, and brain [99-100]. In human lung adenocarcinoma cell line A549, the expression levels of claudin-1, -2, -6, and -9 are significantly increased with claudin-2 expression 160-fold higher than in normal lung tissue [101].

Knockdown of claudin-2 decreases the cell migration by down-regulating the mRNA level and enzymatic activity of matrix metalloproteinase (MMP)-9 [101]. In human lung adenocarcinoma cell line HCC827 cells, knockdown of claudin-7 increases the mRNA and protein levels of MMP-3 [22]. MMPs, a group of zinc-dependent endopeptidases, are capable of degrading extracellular matrix proteins, such as collagens, laminins, and fibronectins. In addition, during the process of intravasation and extravasation processes, the cancer cells must disrupt the cell-cell junctions that serve as a barrier for the cancer cells metastases and transverse through the paracellular pathway of the endothelial cells. Elimination and/or reduction of TJ barriers in cancer cells are essential for allowing metastatic cells to break in and out of blood vessels [102-103].

For example, when small cell lung cancer cell line NCI-H209 was co-cultured with human brain microvascular endothelial cells (HBMECs), the continuous membrane staining of ZO-1, occludin, and claudin-5 in HBMECs gradually became discontinuous, segmented, and dotted while the NCI-H209 cells transmigrated through the cell layer of HBMECs [104].

The most common cause of lung cancer is long-term exposure to cigarette smoking. Cigarette smoking increases the permeability of lung epithelium and permits more toxins and pathogens to travel from the air spaces to the interstitium and blood stream. Studies have been performed to investigate the effect of cigarette smoke on expressional changes of claudins. Bronchial cell line BEAS-2B and two carcinoma cell lines SK-LU-1 and SK-MES-1 were treated with tobacco smoke for 24 hours; initial increases of claudin-2, -3, -4, and -7 in BEAS-2B and SK-LU-1 were followed by a decline in the mRNA levels of those claudins. SK-MES-1 did not display any changes of claudins. Intense claudin-1, -4 and -7 signals are found more often in SCC samples of heavy smokers. The increased claudin-2 expression in ADCs is associated with fewer pack-years [93].

Nicotine, the major addictive component of tobacco smoke, reduces the expression of ZO-1 and facilitates EMT-like changes in mouse models of lung cancer [105]. Nicotine also induces cell proliferation as well as the migratory and invasive behavior of bronchioalveolar lung cancer cells A549 [106]. Claudin-18 is more commonly found in nonsmokers, and patient pack-years are significantly lower in patients with claudin-18-positive tumors, which underlines its role as an indicator of a tobacco unrelated carcinogenic pathway in lung carcinogenesis [94].

## Crosstalk of Claudins and Occludin with Other Signaling Pathways in Lung Cancer

MAPK cascades are key signaling pathways involved in the regulation of normal cell proliferation, survival, and differentiation. Aberrant regulation of MAPK cascades contributes to cancer and other human diseases. ERK/MAPK is the most extensively studied subfamily of MAPKs. It is regulated by a wide variety of growth factors and mitogens, and is often over-activated in lung cancers [107]. First, the receptor-linked tyrosine kinases such as epidermal growth factor receptor (EGFR) are activated by extracellular ligands, such as EGF. The binding of EGF to EGFR activates the tyrosine kinase activity of the cytoplasmic domain of the receptor. After EGFR becomes phosphorylated on tyrosine residues, it activates Ras-Raf-mitogen-activated protein kinase kinase (MEK)-ERK, in which Ras serves as a key downstream effector of EGFR [108]. Currently, there are about 160 ERK substrates already identified that function as kinases, phosphatases, proteinases, transcription factors, and cytoskeletal proteins [109]. EGFR is overexpressed in 40-80% of the lung cancer and mutated in 10% of NSCLC (30% of mutation in East Asians versus 8% in non-Asians) [110]. Ras is found to be mutated in 30% of the NSCLC [108]. The interactions between MAPK pathway and TJ proteins have been previously reported [111-112]. For example, TJ membrane protein occludin participates in the activation of the MAPK signaling pathway [113]. In the hepatic cell line derived from occludin-deficient mice, MAPK activation is down-regulated, which triggers apoptosis and increases claudin-2 expression. However, when occludin is transfected into these occludin-deficient cells, MAPK becomes activated and the increases in claudin-2 expression and apoptosis are diminished [113]. Chen *et al.* have found that inhibition of the MEK pathway restores the TJ formation and claudin-1 and E-cadherin localization in Ras-transformed MDCK cells [46]. Fujibe *et al.* reported that Thr203 of claudin-1 is a putative phosphorylation site of MAPK, which is required to promote the barrier function of TJs [63]. EGF treatment increases claudin-2 expression by 46% and accelerates claudin-2-induced colonization of NSCLC cells A549 through ERK/MAPK pathway [114]. In pneumocytes, EGF increases the expression of claudin-4 and -7 as well as decreases the expression of claudin-3 and -5 [115].

Binding of hepatocyte growth factor (HGF) to its receptor c-Met activates the tyrosine kinase domain, resulting in autophosphorylation of several tyrosine residues in its cytoplasmic domain. The phosphorylation of each tyrosine residue initiates distinct signal transduction cascades involving ERK/MAPK pathway. MAPK activation is required for cell-

cell dissociation and cell movement induced by HGF [116]. The c-Met gene amplification and/or overexpression have been reported in a wide variety of cancer types including lung, stomach, liver, prostate, ovarian, colon, and pancreatic cancers. HGF is normally secreted by fibroblasts and smooth muscle cells, but it can also be produced by tumor cells with variable expression observed in 45% of lung cancer tumors [117-118]. Data suggest that the HGF-Met loop is one of the factors that may promote metastasis in early-stage lung cancer [119]. Co-expression of Met and HGF promotes systemic metastasis in NCI-H460, a human NSCLC cell line [119]. We have found that transfection of claudin-7 into NCI-H1299 human lung carcinoma cells reduces migration and invasion ability under HGF treatment when compared to the control cells. These effects are mediated through the ERK/MAPK signaling pathway. It is possible that claudin-7 may serve as an inhibitor of the upstream elements of ERK/MAPK pathway, thus down-regulating the ERK1/2 activity and reducing cell motility [35].

Other signaling pathways, such as PI3K/Akt pathway, can also interact with TJ proteins. It has been reported that in the hepatic cell lines derived from occludin-deficient mice, the activation of MAPK and Akt is decreased and cell apoptosis is increased. Ectopic expression of occludin in these hepatic cells increases Akt activity and inhibits apoptosis, which suggests that lack of occludin renders hepatocytes sensitive to proapoptotic stimuli due to a decrease in Akt activity [113]. Phosphorylation of glycogen synthase kinase-3β (GSK-3β) and Akt contributes to the increased claudin-2 expression and its cell membrane distribution in A549 cells under treatment of Der p2 (DP2), a major allergen derived from house dust mite *Dermatophagoides pteronyssinus* [120]. As discussed previously, claudin expression can regulate the tumor invasion process by altering MMPs activity in human lung cancer cells. In human lung adenocarcinoma cell line A549, the expression levels of claudin-1, -2, -6, and -9 are significantly higher, and claudin-2 expression is 160-fold higher than in normal lung tissue. Knockdown of claudin-2 decreases the cell migration by down-regulating mRNA levels and the enzymatic activity of MMP-9. In human lung adenocarcinoma cell line HCC827 cells, knockdown of claudin-7 increases the mRNA and protein levels of MMP-3 [22]. Increased levels of the proinflammatory cytokines interleukin-8 (IL-8), tumor necrosis factor α (TNF- α), and interferon γ (IFN- γ) induce alterations in TJ ion selectivity in primary human airway epithelial cells [121]. Claudin-5 is involved in angiopoietin-like 4 (ANGPTL4) modulated vascular junction integrity and triggered lung metastasis. ANGPTL4 instigates the disruption of endothelial continuity by weakening the intercellular VE-cadherin and claudin-5 clusters [122]. The functions of TJs in epithelial cells can also be modulated by signal transduction pathways that are triggered by exogenous agents, such as bacterial toxins and dietary constituents, or by endogenous factors, such as cytokines and growth factors. Classic secondary messengers, including calcium, calmodulin, cAMP, phospholipase C, nitric oxide, and G-proteins, have been implicated in regulating the assembly and permeability of TJs [37]. It has been shown that aspirin can induce gastric epithelial barrier dysfunction by activating p38 MAPK via claudin-7 [123].

## Claudins as Therapeutic Targets

Accurate staging of lung cancer can provide important information for designing treatment protocols, evaluating treatment outcomes, and determining prognosis. Lack of sufficient lung cancer subclassification information could potentially expose patients to treatments with unnecessary risks. Robust predictive markers will allow the successful implementation of targeted agents. Nowadays, oncologists generally differentiate subtypes of lung cancer and select appropriate therapeutic treatments based on two main groups, NSCLC and SCLC. The combination regimen of platinum and etoposide is the first-line approach in SCLCs; however, this is not the case for NSCLC. SCC patients have a survival advantage when they receive a combined treatment of cisplatin and gemcitabine; ADC patients with low thymidylate synthase (a main cellular target of pemetrexed) or EGFR mutations have a better response to pemetrexed or erlotinib treatments, respectively [124]. Therefore, it is important to distinguish SCC from ADC. Due to the high specificity of claudin expression patterns in different lung cancer subtypes, it has been suggested that claudins may represent useful molecular markers. Based on the immunohistochemical staining results, claudin-3, -4, and -7 can be used to distinguish ADCs from SCCs because of the different staining patterns in these two types of lung cancers. Claudin-2 can be used to distinguish SCLCs from ADCs. Claudin-2, -3, and -4 can be used to distinguish SCCs from SCLCs. Claudin-1 positivity predicted a better survival in ADCs and SCCs, but claudin-4 positivity predicts a better survival only in ADCs. Additionally, claudin-7 positivity predicts a better survival in SCCs [93], while only claudin-5 is found to be associated with high clinical stage in SCC [91]. Increased protein expression of vimentin combined with the loss of E-cadherin, claudin-4, and -7 is associated with gefitinib resistance in NSCLC cell lines [125].

The altered expression of various claudin proteins in cancer and their membrane localization (containing two extracellular domains that serve as potential target sites) make these proteins attractive targets for cancer therapy.

The differential expression and localization of claudins between tumor and normal cells also make them attractive candidates for biomarkers. For those claudins with altered expression in cancers, down-regulating or up-regulating the expression of specific claudins could be a potential way to facilitate lung cancer treatment. Since claudins are important proteins involved in various pathological diseases, a number of studies are investigating the transcription factors that can regulate TJ protein expression. Snail, a zinc-finger transcription factor, serves as a transcriptional repressor inducing EMT with the repression of claudin-3, -4, and -7 mRNA and protein [126]. In the case of claudin-1, the inhibition exerted by snail is only at the protein level [127]. Cdx2, an intestine specific homeobox protein, exerts a potent activation of claudin-2 transcription in Caco-2 cells [128]. Thyroid transcription factor-1 (TTF-1), a homeodomain transcription factor, is only expressed in lung, thyroid, and parts of the brain, and regulates the expression of claudin-18 in these tissues [129-130]. Carcinogenic compounds from tobacco smoke influence claudin synthesis by up-regulating transcription factors like twist, snail, or ZEB1 [93]. Our recent work revealing the role of claudin-7 in suppressing ERK/MAPK signaling pathway in human lung carcinoma cell line NCI-H1299 implies a new way to target lung cancer by regulating both the transcription factors of claudin-7 and ERK/MAPK signaling pathway.

Anti-claudin antibodies and cytolytic enterotoxin from *Clostridium perfringens* are emerging agents in the treatment of cancers. For claudins increased in cancers, such as claudin-3 and -4, antibodies targeting the extracellular domains of claudin-3 and -4 are generated [131]. These antibodies are able to bind to the surface of non-permeabilized breast and colon cancer cells, and tumor cells can be eliminated by attaching radionuclides or toxins to these antibodies, or stimulating immune responses [132]. Claudin-3 and -4 serve as receptors for CPE, which is capable of inducing cytolysis of mammalian cells. CPE binds to the second extracellular domain of claudin-3 or -4, triggers the formation of a large multi-protein membrane-pore complex, disrupts cellular osmotic equilibrium, and causes cell lysis [133]. CPE may either directly treat the tumors or deliver radionuclides or toxins to tumors with high claudin-3 and -4 expression [30]. Breast, ovarian, and prostate cancer cells expressing high levels of claudin-3 and -4 are sensitive to CPE-mediated cytolysis [134-136]. As the whole CPE has strong cytotoxicity, the C-terminal of CPE may therefore serve as a binding domain for claudin-3 or -4, and could be used for claudin-targeted cancer therapy. Fusion of C-terminal fragment of CPE to protein synthesis inhibitory factor (PSIF) derived from Pseudomonas exotoxin has successfully suppressed the claudin-4 expressing lung tumor metastasis in mice [137]. High levels of claudin-3 in SCLCs may provide an opportunity for therapeutic targeting. Since claudin-3 and -4 are widely expressed in kidneys and intestines, systemic cancer treatment should be used with caution. Nevertheless, it has been shown that claudin-3 and -4 specific CPE fragment can be delivered locally to lung cancer tissues [25]. Vaccine-induced antibodies are emerging as promising therapeutics in oncology. Highly specific auto-antibodies against claudin-18 isoform 2 induced by a chimeric hepatitis B virus core antigen (HBcAg) virus-like particle vaccine kill tumor cells and inhibit the growth of lung metastases [138]. Besides antibody-based treatment, hydroxycamptothecin-loaded $Fe_3O_4$ nanoparticles induce human HCC827 lung cancer cell apoptosis and disrupt TJs by internalizing the claudin-1, -3, -4, and -7 proteins and decreasing their protein expression [139]. HangAmDan-B, an anti-invasive agent extracted from eight Korean medical animals and plants, can inhibit the cell migration and invasion of a NSCLC cell line NCI-H460 and tighten the TJs through down-regulating claudin-1, -2, -3, and -4 at both transcriptional and translational levels [140].

## Conclusion

In the future, claudins may have a role as both a biomarker to distinguish different subtypes of lung cancers and facilitate better diagnosis and as a target for treatment. However, given the controversy over changes in expression of some claudins in lung cancers, more studies are required to elucidate the expressional patterns of claudins in different subtypes and different stages of cancers versus normal tissues.

Claudin-targeted therapy may have higher specificity towards tumor cells than the traditional chemo- and radio-therapies. Since claudins are widely expressed in human organs, future targeted therapy needs to be further validated and applied practically and safely in a clinical setting.

## Acknowledgments

This work was supported by National Institute of Health grants ES016888 and HL085752.

# References


[1] Farquhar MG, Palade GE. Junctional complexes in various epithelia. *J. Cell Biol.* 1963;17:375-412.

[2] Tsukita S, Furuse M, Itoh M. Multifunctional strands in tight junctions. *Nat. Rev. Mol. Cell Biol.* 2001;2:285-93.

[3] Niessen CM. Tight junctions/adherens junctions: basic structure and function. *J. Invest Dermatol.* 2007;127:2525-32.

[4] Balda MS, Gonzalez-Mariscal L, Contreras RG, et al. Assembly and sealing of tight junctions: possible participation of G-proteins, phospholipase C, protein kinase C and calmodulin. *J. Membr. Biol.* 1991;122:193-202.

[5] McRoberts JA, Aranda R, Riley N, et al. Insulin regulates the paracellular permeability of cultured intestinal epithelial cell monolayers. *J. Clin. Invest.* 1990;85:1127-34.

[6] Kurihara H, Anderson JM, Farquhar MG. Increased Tyr phosphorylation of ZO-1 during modification of tight junctions between glomerular foot processes. *Am. J. Physiol.* 1995;268:F514-24.

[7] Fine KD, Santa Ana CA, Porter JL, et al. Effect of D-glucose on intestinal permeability and its passive absorption in human small intestine in vivo. *Gastroenterology.* 1993;105:1117-25.

[8] Nusrat A, Parkos CA, Bacarra AE, et al. Hepatocyte growth factor/scatter factor effects on epithelia. Regulation of intercellular junctions in transformed and nontransformed cell lines, basolateral polarization of c-met receptor in transformed and natural intestinal epithelia, and induction of rapid wound repair in a transformed model epithelium. *J. Clin. Invest.* 1994;93:2056-65.

[9] Jou TS, Schneeberger EE, Nelson WJ. Structural and functional regulation of tight junctions by RhoA and Rac1 small GTPases. *J. Cell Biol.* 1998;142:101-15.

[10] Borok Z, Hami A, Danto SI, et al. Effects of EGF on alveolar epithelial junctional permeability and active sodium transport. *Am. J. Physiol.* 1996;270:L559-65.

[11] Cummins PM. Occludin: one protein, many forms. *Mol. Cell Biol.* 2012;32:242-50.

[12] Kang LI, Wang Y, Suckow AT, et al. Deletion of JAM-A causes morphological defects in the corneal epithelium. *Int. J. Biochem. Cell Biol.* 2007;39:576-85.

[13] Arcangeli ML, Frontera V, Bardin F, et al. JAM-B regulates maintenance of hematopoietic stem cells in the bone marrow. *Blood.* 2011;118:4609-19.

[14] Frontera V, Arcangeli ML, Zimmerli C, et al. Cutting edge: JAM-C controls homeostatic chemokine secretion in lymph node fibroblastic reticular cells expressing thrombomodulin. *J. Immunol.* 2011;187:603-7.

[15] Scheiermann C, Meda P, Aurrand-Lions M, et al. Expression and function of junctional adhesion molecule-C in myelinated peripheral nerves. *Science.* 2007;318:1472-5.

[16] Saitou M, Furuse M, Sasaki H, et al. Complex phenotype of mice lacking occludin, a component of tight junction strands. *Mol. Biol. Cell.* 2000;11:4131-42.

[17] Shin K, Fogg VC, Margolis B. Tight junctions and cell polarity. *Annu. Rev. Cell Dev. Biol.* 2006;22:207-35.

[18] Gonzalez-Mariscal L, Betanzos A, Nava P, et al. Tight junction proteins. *Prog. Biophys. Mol. Biol.* 2003;81:1-44.

[19] Furuse M, Tsukita S. Claudins in occluding junctions of humans and flies. *Trends Cell Biol.* 2006;16:181-8.
[20] Chen YH, Lu Q, Goodenough DA, et al. Nonreceptor tyrosine kinase c-Yes interacts with occludin during tight junction formation in canine kidney epithelial cells. *Mol. Biol. Cell.* 2002;13:1227-37.
[21] Kitajiri S, Miyamoto T, Mineharu A, et al. Compartmentalization established by claudin-11-based tight junctions in stria vascularis is required for hearing through generation of endocochlear potential. *J. Cell Sci.* 2004;117:5087-96.
[22] Ding L, Lu Z, Foreman O, et al. Inflammation and disruption of the mucosal architecture in claudin-7-deficient mice. *Gastroenterology.* 2012;142:305-15.
[23] Gonzalez-Mariscal L, Lechuga S, Garay E. Role of tight junctions in cell proliferation and cancer. *Prog. Histochem. Cytochem.* 2007;42:1-57.
[24] Klymkowsky MW, Savagner P. Epithelial-mesenchymal transition: a cancer researcher's conceptual friend and foe. *Am. J. Pathol.* 2009;174:1588-93.
[25] Morin PJ. Claudin proteins in human cancer: promising new targets for diagnosis and therapy. *Cancer Res.* 2005;65:9603-6.
[26] Morita K, Furuse M, Fujimoto K, et al. Claudin multigene family encoding four-transmembrane domain protein components of tight junction strands. *Proc. Natl. Acad. Sci. USA.* 1999;96:511-6.
[27] Van Itallie CM, Anderson JM. The molecular physiology of tight junction pores. *Physiology* (Bethesda). 2004;19:331-8.
[28] Krause G, Winkler L, Mueller SL, et al. Structure and function of claudins. *Biochim. Biophys. Acta.* 2008;1778:631-45.
[29] Alexandre MD, Jeansonne BG, Renegar RH, et al. The first extracellular domain of claudin-7 affects paracellular Cl- permeability. *Biochem. Biophys. Res. Commun.* 2007;357:87-91.
[30] Kominsky SL. Claudins: emerging targets for cancer therapy. *Expert Rev. Mol. Med.* 2006;8:1-11.
[31] Takahashi A, Kondoh M, Suzuki H, et al. Claudin as a target for drug development. *Curr. Med. Chem.* 2011;18:1861-5.
[32] Kausalya PJ, Amasheh S, Gunzel D, et al. Disease-associated mutations affect intracellular traffic and paracellular Mg2+ transport function of Claudin-16. *J. Clin. Invest.* 2006;116:878-91.
[33] Konrad M, Schaller A, Seelow D, et al. Mutations in the tight-junction gene claudin 19 (CLDN19) are associated with renal magnesium wasting, renal failure, and severe ocular involvement. *Am. J. Hum. Genet.* 2006;79:949-57.
[34] Coyne CB, Gambling TM, Boucher RC, et al. Role of claudin interactions in airway tight junctional permeability. *Am. J. Physiol. Lung Cell Mol Physiol.* 2003;285:L1166-78.
[35] Lu Z, Ding L, Hong H, et al. Claudin-7 inhibits human lung cancer cell migration and invasion through ERK/MAPK signaling pathway. *Exp. Cell Res.* 2011;317:1935-46.
[36] Daugherty BL, Ward C, Smith T, et al. Regulation of heterotypic claudin compatibility. *J. Biol. Chem.* 2007;282:30005-13.
[37] Heiskala M, Peterson PA, Yang Y. The roles of claudin superfamily proteins in paracellular transport. *Traffic.* 2001;2:93-8.

[38] Li J, Ananthapanyasut W, Yu AS. Claudins in renal physiology and disease. *Pediatr Nephrol.* 2011;26:2133-42.

[39] Amasheh S, Meiri N, Gitter AH, et al. Claudin-2 expression induces cation-selective channels in tight junctions of epithelial cells. *J. Cell Sci.* 2002;115:4969-76.

[40] Alexandre MD, Lu Q, Chen YH. Overexpression of claudin-7 decreases the paracellular Cl- conductance and increases the paracellular Na+ conductance in LLC-PK1 cells. *J. Cell Sci.* 2005;118:2683-93.

[41] Nitta T, Hata M, Gotoh S, et al. Size-selective loosening of the blood-brain barrier in claudin-5-deficient mice. *J. Cell Biol.* 2003;161:653-60.

[42] Tatum R, Zhang Y, Salleng K, et al. Renal salt wasting and chronic dehydration in claudin-7-deficient mice. *Am. J. Physiol. Renal. Physiol.* 2010;298:F24-34.

[43] Tamura A, Kitano Y, Hata M, et al. Megaintestine in claudin-15-deficient mice. *Gastroenterology.* 2008;134:523-34.

[44] Gow A, Davies C, Southwood CM, et al. Deafness in Claudin 11-null mice reveals the critical contribution of basal cell tight junctions to stria vascularis function. *J. Neurosci.* 2004;24:7051-62.

[45] Miyamoto T, Morita K, Takemoto D, et al. Tight junctions in Schwann cells of peripheral myelinated axons: a lesson from claudin-19-deficient mice. *J. Cell Biol.* 2005;169:527-38.

[46] Chen Y, Lu Q, Schneeberger EE, et al. Restoration of tight junction structure and barrier function by down-regulation of the mitogen-activated protein kinase pathway in ras-transformed Madin-Darby canine kidney cells. *Mol. Biol. Cell.* 2000;11:849-62.

[47] Harhaj NS, Felinski EA, Wolpert EB, et al. VEGF activation of protein kinase C stimulates occludin phosphorylation and contributes to endothelial permeability. *Invest Ophthalmol. Vis. Sci.* 2006;47:5106-15.

[48] Sakakibara A, Furuse M, Saitou M, et al. Possible involvement of phosphorylation of occludin in tight junction formation. *J. Cell Biol.* 1997;137:1393-401.

[49] Wong V. Phosphorylation of occludin correlates with occludin localization and function at the tight junction. *Am. J. Physiol.* 1997;273:C1859-67.

[50] Clarke H, Soler AP, Mullin JM. Protein kinase C activation leads to dephosphorylation of occludin and tight junction permeability increase in LLC-PK1 epithelial cell sheets. *J. Cell Sci.* 2000;113 ( Pt 18):3187-96.

[51] Rao R. Occludin phosphorylation in regulation of epithelial tight junctions. *Ann. N. Y. Acad. Sci.* 2009;1165:62-8.

[52] Suzuki T, Elias BC, Seth A, et al. PKC eta regulates occludin phosphorylation and epithelial tight junction integrity. *Proc. Natl. Acad. Sci. USA.* 2009;106:61-6.

[53] Elias BC, Suzuki T, Seth A, et al. Phosphorylation of Tyr-398 and Tyr-402 in occludin prevents its interaction with ZO-1 and destabilizes its assembly at the tight junctions. *J. Biol. Chem.* 2009;284:1559-69.

[54] Sheth P, Basuroy S, Li C, et al. Role of phosphatidylinositol 3-kinase in oxidative stress-induced disruption of tight junctions. *J. Biol. Chem.* 2003;278:49239-45.

[55] Vikstrom E, Bui L, Konradsson P, et al. The junctional integrity of epithelial cells is modulated by Pseudomonas aeruginosa quorum sensing molecule through phosphorylation-dependent mechanisms. *Exp. Cell Res.* 2009;315:313-26.

[56] Kago T, Takagi N, Date I, et al. Cerebral ischemia enhances tyrosine phosphorylation of occludin in brain capillaries. *Biochem. Biophys. Res. Commun.* 2006;339:1197-203.

[57] Olivera D, Knall C, Boggs S, et al. Cytoskeletal modulation and tyrosine phosphorylation of tight junction proteins are associated with mainstream cigarette smoke-induced permeability of airway epithelium. *Exp. Toxicol. Pathol.* 2010;62:133-43.

[58] Tsukamoto T, Nigam SK. Role of tyrosine phosphorylation in the reassembly of occludin and other tight junction proteins. *Am. J. Physiol.* 1999;276:F737-50.

[59] Murakami T, Felinski EA, Antonetti DA. Occludin phosphorylation and ubiquitination regulate tight junction trafficking and vascular endothelial growth factor-induced permeability. *J. Biol. Chem.* 2009;284:21036-46.

[60] Murakami T, Frey T, Lin C, et al. Protein kinase cbeta phosphorylates occludin regulating tight junction trafficking in vascular endothelial growth factor-induced permeability in vivo. *Diabetes.* 2012;61:1573-83.

[61] Raleigh DR, Boe DM, Yu D, et al. Occludin S408 phosphorylation regulates tight junction protein interactions and barrier function. *J. Cell Biol.* 2011;193:565-82.

[62] Hirase T, Kawashima S, Wong EY, et al. Regulation of tight junction permeability and occludin phosphorylation by Rhoa-p160ROCK-dependent and -independent mechanisms. *J. Biol. Chem.* 2001;276:10423-31.

[63] Fujibe M, Chiba H, Kojima T, et al. Thr203 of claudin-1, a putative phosphorylation site for MAP kinase, is required to promote the barrier function of tight junctions. *Exp. Cell Res.* 2004;295:36-47.

[64] D'Souza T, Agarwal R, Morin PJ. Phosphorylation of claudin-3 at threonine 192 by cAMP-dependent protein kinase regulates tight junction barrier function in ovarian cancer cells. *The Journal of biological chemistry.* 2005;280:26233-40.

[65] D'Souza T, Indig FE, Morin PJ. Phosphorylation of claudin-4 by PKCepsilon regulates tight junction barrier function in ovarian cancer cells. *Exp. Cell Res.* 2007;313:3364-75.

[66] Tanaka M, Kamata R, Sakai R. EphA2 phosphorylates the cytoplasmic tail of Claudin-4 and mediates paracellular permeability. *J. Biol. Chem.* 2005;280:42375-82.

[67] Soma T, Chiba H, Kato-Mori Y, et al. Thr(207) of claudin-5 is involved in size-selective loosening of the endothelial barrier by cyclic AMP. *Exp. Cell Res.* 2004;300:202-12.

[68] Tatum R, Zhang Y, Lu Q, et al. WNK4 phosphorylates ser(206) of claudin-7 and promotes paracellular Cl(-) permeability. *FEBS Lett.* 2007;581:3887-91.

[69] Van Itallie CM, Gambling TM, Carson JL, et al. Palmitoylation of claudins is required for efficient tight-junction localization. *J. Cell Sci.* 2005;118:1427-36.

[70] Li X, Akhtar S, Choudhry MA. Alteration in intestine tight junction protein phosphorylation and apoptosis is associated with increase in IL-18 levels following alcohol intoxication and burn injury. *Biochim. Biophys. Acta.* 2012;1822:196-203.

[71] Kyuno D, Kojima T, Ito T, et al. Protein kinase Calpha inhibitor enhances the sensitivity of human pancreatic cancer HPAC cells to Clostridium perfringens enterotoxin via claudin-4. *Cell Tissue Res.* 2011;346:369-81.

[72] Lee K, Ansar M, Andrade PB, et al. Novel CLDN14 mutations in Pakistani families with autosomal recessive non-syndromic hearing loss. *Am. J. Med. Genet A.* 2012;158A:315-21.

[73] Samak G, Aggarwal S, Rao RK. ERK is involved in EGF-mediated protection of tight junctions, but not adherens junctions, in acetaldehyde-treated Caco-2 cell monolayers. *Am. J. Physiol. Gastrointest Liver Physiol.* 2011;301:G50-9.

[74] Kaur J, Tuor UI, Zhao Z, et al. Quantitative MRI reveals the elderly ischemic brain is susceptible to increased early blood-brain barrier permeability following tissue plasminogen activator related to claudin 5 and occludin disassembly. *J. Cereb. Blood Flow Metab.* 2011;31:1874-85.
[75] Evans MJ, von Hahn T, Tscherne DM, et al. Claudin-1 is a hepatitis C virus co-receptor required for a late step in entry. *Nature*. 2007;446:801-5.
[76] Ahmad W, Shabbiri K, Ijaz B, et al. Claudin-1 required for HCV virus entry has high potential for phosphorylation and O-glycosylation. *Virol J.* 2011;8:229.
[77] French AD, Fiori JL, Camilli TC, et al. PKC and PKA phosphorylation affect the subcellular localization of claudin-1 in melanoma cells. *Int. J. Med. Sci.* 2009;6:93-101.
[78] Banan A, Zhang LJ, Shaikh M, et al. theta Isoform of protein kinase C alters barrier function in intestinal epithelium through modulation of distinct claudin isotypes: a novel mechanism for regulation of permeability. *J. Pharmacol. Exp. Ther.* 2005;313:962-82.
[79] Yamauchi K, Rai T, Kobayashi K, et al. Disease-causing mutant WNK4 increases paracellular chloride permeability and phosphorylates claudins. *Proc. Natl. Acad. Sci. USA*. 2004;101:4690-4.
[80] Ikari A, Kinjo K, Atomi K, et al. Extracellular Mg(2+) regulates the tight junctional localization of claudin-16 mediated by ERK-dependent phosphorylation. *Biochim. Biophys. Acta*. 2010;1798:415-21.
[81] Butt AM, Khan IB, Hussain M, et al. Role of post translational modifications and novel crosstalk between phosphorylation and O-beta-GlcNAc modifications in human claudin-1, -3 and -4. *Mol. Biol. Rep.* 2012;39:1359-69.
[82] Knowles M, Murray G, Shallal J, et al. Bioelectric properties and ion flow across excised human bronchi. *J. Appl. Physiol.* 1984;56:868-77.
[83] Berube K, Prytherch Z, Job C, et al. Human primary bronchial lung cell constructs: the new respiratory models. *Toxicology*. 2010;278:311-8.
[84] Daugherty BL, Mateescu M, Patel AS, et al. Developmental regulation of claudin localization by fetal alveolar epithelial cells. *Am. J. Physiol. Lung Cell Mol. Physiol.* 2004;287:L1266-73.
[85] Kaarteenaho-Wiik R, Soini Y. Claudin-1, -2, -3, -4, -5, and -7 in usual interstitial pneumonia and sarcoidosis. *J. Histochem. Cytochem.* 2009;57:187-95.
[86] Kaarteenaho R, Merikallio H, Lehtonen S, et al. Divergent expression of claudin -1, -3, -4, -5 and -7 in developing human lung. *Respir Res.* 2010;11:59.
[87] Tobioka H, Tokunaga Y, Isomura H, et al. Expression of occludin, a tight-junction-associated protein, in human lung carcinomas. *Virchows Arch.* 2004;445:472-6.
[88] Saitou M, Ando-Akatsuka Y, Itoh M, et al. Mammalian occludin in epithelial cells: its expression and subcellular distribution. *Eur. J. Cell Biol.* 1997;73:222-31.
[89] Paschoud S, Bongiovanni M, Pache JC, et al. Claudin-1 and claudin-5 expression patterns differentiate lung squamous cell carcinomas from adenocarcinomas. *Mod. Pathol.* 2007;20:947-54.
[90] Moldvay J, Jackel M, Paska C, et al. Distinct claudin expression profile in histologic subtypes of lung cancer. *Lung Cancer*. 2007;57:159-67.
[91] Jung JH, Jung CK, Choi HJ, et al. Diagnostic utility of expression of claudins in non-small cell lung cancer: different expression profiles in squamous cell carcinomas and adenocarcinomas. *Pathol. Res. Pract.* 2009;205:409-16.

[92] Li R, Zhang D, Cai C, et al. [The clinical significance of Claudin-7 and slug expression in lung squamous cell carcinoma and adenocarcinoma]. *Zhongguo Fei Ai Za Zhi.* 2011;14:492-6.
[93] Merikallio H, Kaarteenaho R, Paakko P, et al. Impact of smoking on the expression of claudins in lung carcinoma. *European journal of cancer.* 2011;47:620-30.
[94] Merikallio H, Paakko P, Harju T, et al. Claudins 10 and 18 are predominantly expressed in lung adenocarcinomas and in tumors of nonsmokers. *Int. J. Clin. Exp Pathol.* 2011;4:667-73.
[95] Liu Y, Sun W, Zhang K, et al. Identification of genes differentially expressed in human primary lung squamous cell carcinoma. *Lung Cancer.* 2007;56:307-17.
[96] Chao YC, Pan SH, Yang SC, et al. Claudin-1 is a metastasis suppressor and correlates with clinical outcome in lung adenocarcinoma. *Am. J. Respir Crit. Care Med.* 2009;179:123-33.
[97] Hewitt KJ, Agarwal R, Morin PJ. The claudin gene family: expression in normal and neoplastic tissues. *BMC Cancer.* 2006;6:186.
[98] Soini Y. Claudins in lung diseases. Respir Res. 2011;12:70.
[99] Greene FL. The American Joint Committee on Cancer: updating the strategies in cancer staging. *Bull Am. Coll Surg.* 2002;87:13-5.
[100] Jones KD. An update on lung cancer staging. *Adv. Anat. Pathol.* 2010;17:33-7.
[101] Ikari A, Sato T, Takiguchi A, et al. Claudin-2 knockdown decreases matrix metalloproteinase-9 activity and cell migration via suppression of nuclear Sp1 in A549 cells. *Life Sci.* 2011;88:628-33.
[102] Martin TA, Watkins G, Mansel RE, et al. Hepatocyte growth factor disrupts tight junctions in human breast cancer cells. *Cell Biol. Int.* 2004;28:361-71.
[103] Tan X, Tamori Y, Egami H, et al. Analysis of invasion-metastasis mechanism in pancreatic cancer: involvement of tight junction transmembrane protein occludin and MEK/ERK signal transduction pathway in cancer cell dissociation. *Oncol. Rep.* 2004;11:993-8.
[104] Li B, Zhao WD, Tan ZM, et al. Involvement of Rho/ROCK signalling in small cell lung cancer migration through human brain microvascular endothelial cells. *FEBS Lett.* 2006;580:4252-60.
[105] Davis R, Rizwani W, Banerjee S, et al. Nicotine promotes tumor growth and metastasis in mouse models of lung cancer. *PLoS One.* 2009;4:e7524.
[106] Dasgupta P, Rizwani W, Pillai S, et al. Nicotine induces cell proliferation, invasion and epithelial-mesenchymal transition in a variety of human cancer cell lines. *Int. J. Cancer.* 2009;124:36-45.
[107] Johnson GL, Lapadat R. Mitogen-activated protein kinase pathways mediated by ERK, JNK, and p38 protein kinases. *Science.* 2002;298:1911-2.
[108] Roberts PJ, Der CJ. Targeting the Raf-MEK-ERK mitogen-activated protein kinase cascade for the treatment of cancer. *Oncogene.* 2007;26:3291-310.
[109] Yoon S, Seger R. The extracellular signal-regulated kinase: multiple substrates regulate diverse cellular functions. *Growth Factors.* 2006;24:21-44.
[110] Bell DW, Brannigan BW, Matsuo K, et al. Increased prevalence of EGFR-mutant lung cancer in women and in East Asian populations: analysis of estrogen-related polymorphisms. *Clin. Cancer Res.* 2008;14:4079-84.

[111] Lan M, Kojima T, Osanai M, et al. Oncogenic Raf-1 regulates epithelial to mesenchymal transition via distinct signal transduction pathways in an immortalized mouse hepatic cell line. *Carcinogenesis.* 2004;25:2385-95.
[112] Lipschutz JH, Li S, Arisco A, et al. Extracellular signal-regulated kinases 1/2 control claudin-2 expression in Madin-Darby canine kidney strain I and II cells. *J. Biol. Chem.* 2005;280:3780-8.
[113] Murata M, Kojima T, Yamamoto T, et al. Down-regulation of survival signaling through MAPK and Akt in occludin-deficient mouse hepatocytes in vitro. *Exp. Cell Res.* 2005;310:140-51.
[114] Peter Y, Comellas A, Levantini E, et al. Epidermal growth factor receptor and claudin-2 participate in A549 permeability and remodeling: implications for non-small cell lung cancer tumor colonization. *Mol. Carcinog.* 2009;48:488-97.
[115] Chen SP, Zhou B, Willis BC, et al. Effects of transdifferentiation and EGF on claudin isoform expression in alveolar epithelial cells. *J. Appl. Physiol.* 2005;98:322-8.
[116] Potempa S, Ridley AJ. Activation of both MAP kinase and phosphatidylinositide 3-kinase by Ras is required for hepatocyte growth factor/scatter factor-induced adherens junction disassembly. *Mol. Biol. Cell.* 1998;9:2185-200.
[117] Ma PC, Tretiakova MS, MacKinnon AC, et al. Expression and mutational analysis of MET in human solid cancers. *Genes Chromosomes Cancer.* 2008;47:1025-37.
[118] Lawrence RE, Salgia R. MET molecular mechanisms and therapies in lung cancer. *Cell Adh Migr.* 2010;4:146-52.
[119] Navab R, Liu J, Seiden-Long I, et al. Co-overexpression of Met and hepatocyte growth factor promotes systemic metastasis in NCI-H460 non-small cell lung carcinoma cells. *Neoplasia.* 2009;11:1292-300.
[120] Wang WC, Tsai JJ, Kuo CY, et al. Non-proteolytic house dust mite allergen, Der p 2, upregulated expression of tight junction molecule claudin-2 associated with Akt/GSK-3beta/beta-catenin signaling pathway. *J. Cell Biochem.* 2011;112:1544-51.
[121] Coyne CB, Vanhook MK, Gambling TM, et al. Regulation of airway tight junctions by proinflammatory cytokines. *Mol. Biol. Cell.* 2002;13:3218-34.
[122] Huang RL, Teo Z, Chong HC, et al. ANGPTL4 modulates vascular junction integrity by integrin signaling and disruption of intercellular VE-cadherin and claudin-5 clusters. *Blood.* 2011;118:3990-4002.
[123] Oshima T, Miwa H, Joh T. Aspirin induces gastric epithelial barrier dysfunction by activating p38 MAPK via claudin-7. *Am. J. Physiol. Cell Physiol.* 2008;295:C800-6.
[124] Selvaggi G, Scagliotti GV. Histologic subtype in NSCLC: does it matter? *Oncology* (Williston Park). 2009;23:1133-40.
[125] Frederick BA, Helfrich BA, Coldren CD, et al. Epithelial to mesenchymal transition predicts gefitinib resistance in cell lines of head and neck squamous cell carcinoma and non-small cell lung carcinoma. *Molecular cancer therapeutics.* 2007;6:1683-91.
[126] Ikenouchi J, Matsuda M, Furuse M, et al. Regulation of tight junctions during the epithelium-mesenchyme transition: direct repression of the gene expression of claudins/occludin by Snail. *J. Cell Sci.* 2003;116:1959-67.
[127] Ohkubo T, Ozawa M. The transcription factor Snail downregulates the tight junction components independently of E-cadherin downregulation. *J. Cell Sci.* 2004;117:1675-85.

[128] Sakaguchi T, Gu X, Golden HM, et al. Cloning of the human claudin-2 5'-flanking region revealed a TATA-less promoter with conserved binding sites in mouse and human for caudal-related homeodomain proteins and hepatocyte nuclear factor-1alpha. *J. Biol. Chem.* 2002;277:21361-70.

[129] Kimura S. Thyroid-specific enhancer-binding protein Role in thyroid function and organogenesis. *Trends Endocrinol. Metab.* 1996;7:247-52.

[130] Niimi T, Nagashima K, Ward JM, et al. claudin-18, a novel downstream target gene for the T/EBP/NKX2.1 homeodomain transcription factor, encodes lung- and stomach-specific isoforms through alternative splicing. *Molecular and cellular biology.* 2001;21:7380-90.

[131] Offner S, Hekele A, Teichmann U, et al. Epithelial tight junction proteins as potential antibody targets for pancarcinoma therapy. *Cancer Immunol Immunother.* 2005;54:431-45.

[132] Carter P. Improving the efficacy of antibody-based cancer therapies. *Nature reviews Cancer.* 2001;1:118-29.

[133] McClane BA. The complex interactions between Clostridium perfringens enterotoxin and epithelial tight junctions. *Toxicon.* 2001;39:1781-91.

[134] Long H, Crean CD, Lee WH, et al. Expression of Clostridium perfringens enterotoxin receptors claudin-3 and claudin-4 in prostate cancer epithelium. *Cancer Res.* 2001;61:7878-81.

[135] Kominsky SL, Vali M, Korz D, et al. Clostridium perfringens enterotoxin elicits rapid and specific cytolysis of breast carcinoma cells mediated through tight junction proteins claudin 3 and 4. *Am. J. Pathol.* 2004;164:1627-33.

[136] Santin AD, Cane S, Bellone S, et al. Treatment of chemotherapy-resistant human ovarian cancer xenografts in C.B-17/SCID mice by intraperitoneal administration of Clostridium perfringens enterotoxin. *Cancer Res.* 2005;65:4334-42.

[137] Saeki R, Kondoh M, Kakutani H, et al. A claudin-targeting molecule as an inhibitor of tumor metastasis. *J. Pharmacol. Exp. Ther.* 2010;334:576-82.

[138] Klamp T, Schumacher J, Huber G, et al. Highly specific auto-antibodies against claudin-18 isoform 2 induced by a chimeric HBcAg virus-like particle vaccine kill tumor cells and inhibit the growth of lung metastases. *Cancer Res.* 2011;71:516-27.

[139] Zhang G, Ding L, Renegar R, et al. Hydroxycamptothecin-loaded Fe3O4 nanoparticles induce human lung cancer cell apoptosis through caspase-8 pathway activation and disrupt tight junctions. *Cancer Sci.* 2011;102:1216-22.

[140] Choi YJ, Shin DY, Lee YW, et al. Inhibition of cell motility and invasion by HangAmDan-B in NCI-H460 human non-small cell lung cancer cells. *Oncol. Rep.* 2011;26:1601-8.

In: Lung Cancer: A Comprehensive Overview
Editor: Kathy Gately
ISBN: 978-1-62618-447-3


*Chapter XIII*

# The Role of the Arachidonic Acid Pathway in NSCLC Development and Progression: Novel Approaches for Therapeutic Intervention

***Mary-Clare Cathcart*, Ken O' Byrne and Graham P. Pidgeon***
Department of Surgery, Trinity College Dublin, Ireland

## Abstract

Arachidonic acid metabolism through cyclooxygenase (COX), lipoxygenase (LOX) and cytochrome P-450 epoxygenase (EPOX) pathways is responsible for the formation of biologically active eicosanoids, including prostanoids, leukotrienes, hydroxyeicosatetraenoic acid, epoxyeicosatrienoic acid and hydroperoxyeicosatetraenoic acids. Altered eicosanoid expression levels are commonly obsereved during tumour development and progression of a range of malignancies, including non-small cell lung cancer (NSCLC). Arachidonic acid-derived eicosanoids affect a range of biological phenomena to modulate tumour processes such as cell growth, survival, angiogenesis, cell adhesion, invasion and migration and metastatic potential. Numerous studies have demonstrated that eicosanoids modulate NSCLC development and progression, while targeting these pathways has generally been shown to inhibit tumour growth/progression. Modulation of these arachidonic acid-derived pathways for the prevention and/or treatment of NSCLC has been the subject of significant interest over the past number of years, with a number of clinical trials examining the potential of COX and LOX inhibitors in combination with traditional and novel molecular approaches. However, results from these trials have been largely disappointing. Furthermore, enthusiasm for the use of selective COX-2 inhibitors for cancer prevention/treatment waned, due to their association with adverse cardiovascular events in chemoprevention trials.

While COX and LOX targeting may both retain promise for NSCLC prevention and/or treatment, there is an urgent need to understand the downstream signalling

* Email: CATHCARM@tcd.ie.

mechanisms through which these and other arachidonic acid-derived signalling pathways mediate their effects on tumourigenesis. This will allow for development of safer and potentially more effective strategies for NSCLC prevention and/or treatment. Chemoprevention studies with $PGI_2$ analogues have demonstrated considerable promise, while binding to/signalling through $PGE_2$ receptors have also been the subject of interest for NSCLC treatment. In this chapter, the role of the eicosanoid signalling pathways in non-small cell lung cancer will be discussed. In particular, the effect of the eicosanoids on tumour cell proliferation, their roles in induction of cell death, effects on angiogenesis, migration, invasion and their regulation of the immune response will be assessed, with signal transduction pathways involved in these processes also discussed. Finally, novel approaches targeting these arachidonic acid-derived eicosanoids (using pharmacological or natural agents) for chemoprevention and/or treatment of NSCLC will be outlined. Elucidating the molecular mechanisms underlying the effects of specific or general arachidonic acid pathway modulators may lead to the design of biologically and pharmacologically targeted therapeutic strategies for NSCLC prevention/treatment, which may be used alone or in combination with conventional therapies.

## Introduction

The arachidonic acid signalling pathway plays a crucial role in chronic inflammation and cancer. This functional relationship between polyunsaturated fatty acid metabolism, inflammation and carcinogenesis has been examined in numerous molecular studies, revealing potential novel targets for chemoprevention and/or treatment of a number of cancers [1, 2]. Multiple lines of evidence have shown that activation of downstream COX and LOX pathways during chronic inflammation and carcinogenesis leads to altered arachidonic acid metabolism, which may promote carcinogenesis. A number of studies have recently demonstrated the importance of arachidonic acid derived eicosanoids in the development of a number of cancers, including NSCLC [3].

The arachidonic acid (AA) pathway is responsible for the generation of a wide variety of bioactive metabolites. These metabolites, otherwise known as eicosanoids, have been shown to be involved in many different pathologies, including inflammation and cancer [4]. The various eicosanoids generated by AA metabolism can regulate cellular proliferation, apoptosis, differentiation and senescence. Eicosanoids are a group of diverse biological molecules, which include prostanoids (synthesized *via* the 'cyclooxygenase' pathway), leukotrienes and hydroxy eicosatetraenoic acids (HETEs) (synthesized *via* the 'lipoxygenase' pathway), and the epoxides (synthesized *via* the cyctochrome P-450 pathway) [4, 5]. Evidence from laboratory and epidemiological studies suggests that aberrant arachidonic acid metabolism *via* COX and LOX pathways can promote carcinogenesis. The development of cancer in both humans and experimental animals is consistently linked to an imbalance in COX signalling [1, 6]. Both non-steroidal anti-inflammatory drugs (NSAIDs) and selective cyclooxygenase-2 inhibitors (which reduce prostanoid formation *via* COX inhibition) have been associated with a reduced risk of cancer development, including NSCLC. There has been a significant interest in COX-2 and its role carcinogenesis over the past number of years, with a number of clinical trials examining selective COX-2 inhibition as a potential therapeutic strategy [7-10]. However, the association of both NSAIDs and selective COX-2 inhibitors with a heightened cardiovascular risk has dampened enthusiasm for this class of drugs as anti-cancer agents [11-15]. Targeting downstream effectors of cyclooxygenase (COX) signalling has the advantage of avoiding the adverse effects associated with COX-inhibition, with the potential to maintain/enhance anti-tumour reactivity. While the effects of COX expression in cancer are thought to be related to the expression pattern of downstream prostanoids, the relationship of prostanoid profile to tumour development and progression has not been fully investigated [16].

Lipoxygenase (LOX) signalling pathways have also been implicated in tumour development/progression. Both 5-LOX and 12-LOX have been strongly implicated in carcinogenesis. While 15-LOX-2 is generally anti-carcinogenic, the role of 15-LOX-1 is unclear [17]. The cytochrome P-450 (CYP) pathway has also more recently been implicated in carcinogenesis, although to a lesser extent. CYP enzymes convert arachidonic acid into hydroxyeicosatetraenoic acids (HETEs) or epoxyeicosatetraenoic acids, which are thought to play a role in tumour growth. The role of CYP-derived prostanoids in tumourigenesis has not been well investigated however, suggesting that further studies into this arachidonic acid pathway are warranted [18]. A clearer understanding of the individual roles of the arachidonic acid-derived eicosanoids and their contributions to tumour development/progression will allow development of safer novel therapeutic agents for chemoprevention and/or treatment.

In this chapter we discuss the current state of knowledge regarding the contributions of the arachidonic acid-derived eicosanoids and the signalling pathways activated by these eicosanoids in NSCLC development and progression. With reference to the hallmarks of cancer [19, 20], we detail their involvement in underlying mechanisms of tumour development and progression, from tumour cell growth/survival and immune surveillance, to their involvement in the metastatic spread of tumours by influencing angiogenesis and migration. A number of pharmacological and natural agents have been recently been shown to affect eicosanoid signalling. With reference to these agents, we assess a role for AA-derived eicosanoids as potential targets for chemoprevention and/or treatment of NSCLC, which may be used alone, or in combination with other agents/conventional therapies.

# 1. Arachidonic Acid Metabolism: Generation and Classification of Eicosanoids

The eicosanoids are derived from 20-carbon (termed 'eicosa') essential fatty acids containing three, four or five double bonds [21]. The omega-6 family of eicosanoids consists of the well-known prostanoids, leukotrienes, and epoxygenases [22], while the newer, omega-3 family of eicosanoids includes the EPA and DHA-derived resolvins and protectins [23]. Eicosanoids are a group of diverse biological molecules derived from arachidonic acid, which include prostanoids (synthesized *via* the 'cyclooxygenase' pathway), leukotrienes and hydroxy eicosatetraenoic acids (HETEs) (synthesized via the 'lipoxygenase' pathway), and the epoxides (synthesized by a cytochrome *P*-450 'epoxygenase' pathway) [5]. Once it is released, arachidonic acid is rapidly metabolised by microsomal enzymes to produce eicosanoids. It is metabolised by cyclooxygenase to form prostaglandins and thromboxanes, by lipoxygenase to form leukotrienes, hydroxy eicosatetraenoic acids (HETEs) and lipoxins, and by cytochrome *P*-450 to generate dihydroxy acids and epoxyeicosantrenoic acids (EETs). The pathways involved in arachidonic acid metabolism are summarised in Figure 1.

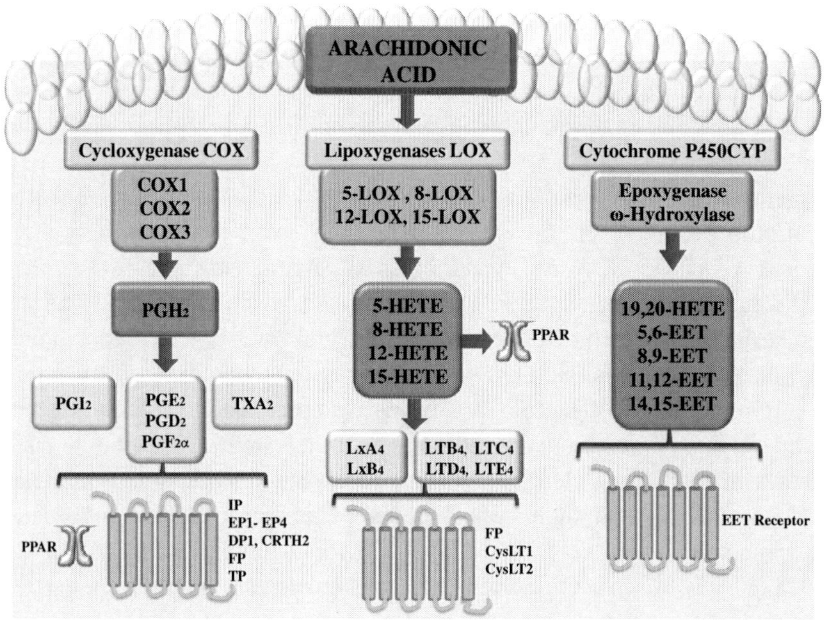


Figure 1. Generation of the eicosanoids *via* arachidonic acid metabolism. Arachidonic acid is metabolised to eicosanoids by one of three major pathways: the cyclooxygenase (COX), the lipoxygenase (LOX) and the cytochrome P-450 epoxygenase pathway (EPOX). In the COX pathway, COX enzymes convert arachidonic acid to prostaglandin $G_2$ ($PGG_2$), which is then reduced to an intermediate $PGH_2$ by the peroxidase activity of COX. $PGH_2$ is then further converted to prostanoids, including prostaglandins (PGs) and thromboxanes (TXs) by the action of cell specific synthases and isomerases. The LOX isoforms convert arachidonic acid into biologically active metabolites such as leukotrienes and hydroxyeicosatetraenoic acids (HETEs), while cytochrome *P*-450 metabolizes arachidonic acid into epoxyeicosatrienoic acids (EETs), HETEs and hydroperoxyeicosatetraenoic acids (HPETEs). Reproduced by permission from Tumor Angiogenesis Regulators, 2013 (Eds. Ruben R. Gonzalez-Perez and Bo R. Rueda), CRC Press, Boca Raton, FL.

The cyclooxygenase or prostaglandin H synthase (PGHS), enzymes catalyse the conversion of arachidonic acid to $PGH_2$ [24]. This rate-limiting step in the formation of prostaglandins is irreversible. Two isoforms of COX have been identified, COX-1 and COX-2 [25, 26]. COX-1 is constitutively expressed in most tissue types. COX-1 is the only isoform expressed within platelets [27, 28] and is an important mediator of platelet aggregation.

COX-2 on the other hand is a highly inducible enzyme under certain physiological conditions, although it is constitutively expressed in some tissues such as the brain, spinal cord, [29], and kidneys [30]. $PGH_2$ is catalytically converted to the various prostanoids *via* reduction, rearrangement or isomerisation by the terminal synthase enzymes (PGES, PGDS, PGFS, PGIS and TXS). These prostanoids include $PGD_2$, $PGE_2$, $PGF_{2\alpha}$, $PGI_2$ (prostacyclin) and $TXA_2$ (thromboxane $A_2$). They exert their biological effects in an autocrine or paracrine manner by binding to cell-surface receptors belonging to the family of seven transmembrane G-protein coupled rhodopsin receptors. These are designated DP, EP, FP, IP and TP for $PGD_2$, $PGE_2$, $PGF_{2\alpha}$, $PGI_2$, and $TXA_2$ respectively. Some prostanoids also bind to nuclear receptors, such as the peroxisome proliferator-activated receptors (PPARs). The $PGD_2$ dehydration product 15-deoxy-delta(12,14)-prostaglandin $J_2$ (15d-$PGJ_2$) is a natural PPARγ receptor ligand [31, 32], whereas $PGI_2$ is a natural ligand for PPARδ [31, 33]. Furthermore, indirect trans-activation of the PPARδ receptor has also been demonstrated by $PGE_2$ [34].

The action of different prostanoids in a particular tissue type is dependent on the cellular expression of their corresponding receptors and well as prostanoid production itself. These processes are also regulated by prostaglandin transporter (an influx transporter), multidrug resistance-associated protein 4 (an efflux transporter) and 15-prostaglandin dehydrogenase (a prostaglandin degradation enzyme) [3]. The prostanoid receptors activate a variety of intracellular signalling pathways to mediate their cellular effects. These pathways are detailed in a recent review by Riciotti and FitzGerald [35].

The LOX enzymes metabolize AA to the biologically active metabolites hydroperoxy–eicosatetraenoic acids (HPETEs), which upon reduction result in the formation of corresponding HETEs. Therefore, 5-, 8-, 12- and 15-HETE are the major AA metabolites formed by mammalian LOXs [36]. Conversely, the metabolism of linoleic acid preferentially results in the formation of hydroxy–octadecadienoic acids (HODEs), with 9- and 13-HODE the principle reaction products of linoleic acid oxygenation. In the case of the 5-LOX enzyme, HPETE is further metabolized to form the unstable epoxide leukotriene A4 (LTA4) in the presence of 5-lipoxygenase-activating protein. LTA4 is subsequently converted to 5(S)-hydroxy-6-trans8, 11,14-cis-eicosatetranoic acid (5-HETE), or hydrolyzed into LTB4 by leukotriene A4 hydrolase, or the cysteinyl leukotrienes, LTC4, LTD4 and LTE4, following enzymatic conjugation with gluthathione [37].

Cytochrome *P*-450 (CYP) epoxygenases convert arachidonic acid to four regioisomeric epoxyeicosatrienoic acids (5,6-EET, 8,9-EET, 11,12-EET, and 14,15-EET), which exert diverse biological activities in a variety of systems. Cytochrome *P*-450 2J2 (CYP2J2), a predominant human *P*-450 arachidonic acid epoxygenase that generates all four EETs, has been detected at the mRNA and/or protein level in heart, lung, liver, kidney, ileum, jejunum, and colon [38]. The pathway consists of two main branches, epoxygenases converting arachidonic acid to epoxyeicosatrienoic acids (EETs) and ω-hydroxylases converting arachidonic acid to hydroxyeicosatetraenoic acids (HETEs) [18]. Details of synthesis and degradation of EETs and HETEs are outlined in a recent review by Panigrahy *et al.* [18].

## 2. Altered Expression of Arachidonic Acid Signalling in NSCLC

A number of studies have demonstrated the prostanoid biosynthesis profile of malignant cells (in NSCLC) to be different to from that of normal lung tissue [39, 40]. Overexpression of cyclooxygenase-2 is a common occurance in NSCLC. A recent study of expression patterns in NSCLC found that COX-2 and mPGES-1 (microsomal PGES-1) levels were commonly increased, whereas levels of 15-PGDH (a prostaglandin degradation enzyme) were frequently decreased in human NSCLC samples relative to adjacent normal lung. This down-regulation in 15-PGDH expression led to the accumulation of multiple bioactive lipids in a mouse model of the disease [41] and supports earlier studies showing a similar loss in 15-PGDH levels in NSCLC [42]. Levels of the $PGE_2$ metabolite, PGE-M, were dramatically increased in humans with unresectable NSCLC and were significantly reduced by administration of the selective COX-2 inhibitor, celecoxib, suggesting that COX-2 contributes significantly to this over-production of $PGE_2$ [43].

A dramatic loss in PGIS mRNA levels was observed in primary human lung tumour samples, relative to matched normal controls [44]. These findings are in agreement with those of a previous report of decreased PGIS mRNA and immunohistochemical protein expression as well as very low levels of $PGF_{1\alpha}$ (the stable metabolite of $PGI_2$) in lung tumours compared to normal surrounding tissue [45]. Gene expression analysis of NSCLC showed a loss of PGIS content in human lung adenocarcinoma samples. However, a small subset of adenocarcinoma patients whose lung tumours retained PGIS expression demonstrated significantly enhanced survival. A statistically correlation was also observed between positive PGIS staining of lung tumour tissue and patient survival. It was therefore suggested that the detection of PGIS in tissue samples had strong prognostic value in predicting patient survival [46]. While the PGIS product, $PGI_2$, is one of the most abundant prostanoids in normal lung, it is only produced in very small amounts by human NSCLCs [39]. Comparative immunohistochemical analyses of NSCLC and normal human lung tissue have demonstrated that, while tumours were typically positive for TXS (thromboxane synthase) expression, PGIS expression was undetectable. In contrast, a moderate PGIS expression was observed in endothelial cells from pulmonary vessels of corresponding normal tissue [47]. Recent studies carried out by our group showed that PGIS protein expression was significantly reduced or lost in NSCLC protein samples, relative to matched normal controls, further supporting the notion that expression of this enzyme may be important for chemoprevention [48]. The precise mechanisms responsible for the down-regulation of PGIS in cancer are unclear, although several potential mechanisms have been investigated. Using transcription reporter assays, it was observed that single nucleotide polymorphisms in the PGIS promoter can affect transcriptional activity in human lung cancer [49]. PGIS expression was silenced in several lung cancer cell lines by CpG methylation (sites were mapped across the variable number of tandem repeats in the promoter and CpGs within intron and exon 1). FISH analysis demonstrated that lung cancer cell lines and tissues do not exhibit a loss of the PGIS genomic region, but have multiple copies. These observations suggest that an individuals' PGIS promoter haplotype may have a significant impact on a patients' predisposition for lung cancer. They also suggest an epigenetic mechanism, namely CpG methylation, which may be responsible for the down-regulation in PGIS expression. In support of these observations, the IP gene was not expressed at detectable levels in NSCLC cells, suggesting that expression of this receptor is not essential for tumour development and progression [44].

TXS is moderately expressed in bronchial epithelial cells and weakly expressed in vascular smooth muscle cells of normal lung tissue [47]. Recent observations in our laboratory have found TXS expression to be increased in NSCLC protein samples, relative to matched normal controls [50], suggesting that this enzyme may be a therapeutic target in the disease. The observed overexpression of TXS in these NSCLC samples, in the face of a loss of PGIS expression may also be of clinical significance in the disease. While the PGIS/TXS balance has been implicated in a range of disease states, it may also be of significant importance in cancer. Of particular interest, $TXB_2$ concentration was higher in samples from patients that smoked, when compared to those that did not smoke, suggesting that cigarette smoking influences the generation of this metabolite in lung cancer [51]. In support of these observations, smoking was previously shown to significantly increase $TXB_2$ production in both gastric and lung tissues [52].

The role of lipoxygenases in NSCLC carcinogenesis is complicated by the variety of LOX genes that have been identified in humans as well as varying profiles of LOX expression observed between studies on human tumour biopsies and experimentally-induced *in-vivo* models. The findings of studies carried out to examine LOX expression between matched normal and cancer tissues revealed that human 15-LOX-1 and -2 expression is usually lost in NSCLC, relative to matched cancer-free controls [53-55]. More recently, expression levels of 15-LOX metabolites, 15(S)-HETE and 13(S)-HODE were shown to be significantly reduced in human lung cancer tissue, relative to non-tumour controls. Reduced levels of these 15-LOX metabolites were also significantly correlated with reduced tumour development in a tobacco-induced mouse model of NSCLC [56]. Moussalli *et al.*, subsequently demonstrated that 15-LOX-1 downregulation in cancer cells is important for terminal cell differentiation dysregulation. As loss of terminal cell differentiation is one of the features which promotes tumourigenesis, this study suggests that 15-LOX-1 re-expression may be used therapeutically to inhibit tumourigenesis [53]. Conversely, both 5-LOX and platelet type 12-LOX are usually absent in normal lung epithelium, but are constitutively expressed in NSCLC. Data from the literature suggests that for the most part, LOX isoforms whose expression are lost during the progression of NSCLC cancer exhibit anti-tumour activity, while isoforms which are preferentially expressed in NSCLC, exhibit pro-tumourigenic effects. For example 15-LOX-1 expression was enhanced in tumours that were better differentiated and was inversely correlated with tumour grade [54].

## 3. Effect of the Arachidonic Acid Pathway on Tumour Cell Signalling and Proliferation

One of the main hallmarks of cancer states is the acquisition of limitless cellular replicative potential, or increased (and unopposed) proliferation of tumour cells [57]. Many cellular pathways are involved in the process by which cells choose between growth arrest, apoptosis or survival. The balance of COX and LOX signalling pathways with different growth factor receptor-induced signalling cascades has been implicated in the modulation of NSCLC tumour cell growth. This balance has also been implicated in a number of other identified hallmarks of cancer and is illustrated in Figure 2.

It has been hypothesized that changes in prostanoid profile affect cancer growth. It is well known that COX-2 derived $PGE_2$ stimulates tumour cell growth and progression. Studies carried out in the last number of years have been interested in the mechanisms underlying these effects. A role for EP2 in mediating the proliferative effects of $PGE_2$ on lung carcinoma cells has been demonstrated. PPAR$\gamma$ ligands inhibited lung cancer cell growth by inhibiting EP2 expression, an effect mediated through Erk signalling [58]. A more recent study has shown that $PGE_2$ stimulates the expression of integrin-linked kinase (ILK). The authors found that this effect was mediated through EP4 signalling, with subsequent induction of Sp1 protein and DNA-binding activity in the ILK promoter [59]. A number of NSAIDs have been shown to inhibit both $PGE_2$ levels and NSCLC cell growth. These NSAIDs also altered expression of markers of epithelial mesenchymal transition, suggesting that they may be beneficial in NSCLC prevention and/or treatment [60]. Overexpression of 15-PDGH significantly reduced tumour growth *in-vivo* further supporting a pro-tumour role for $PGE_2$ [42].

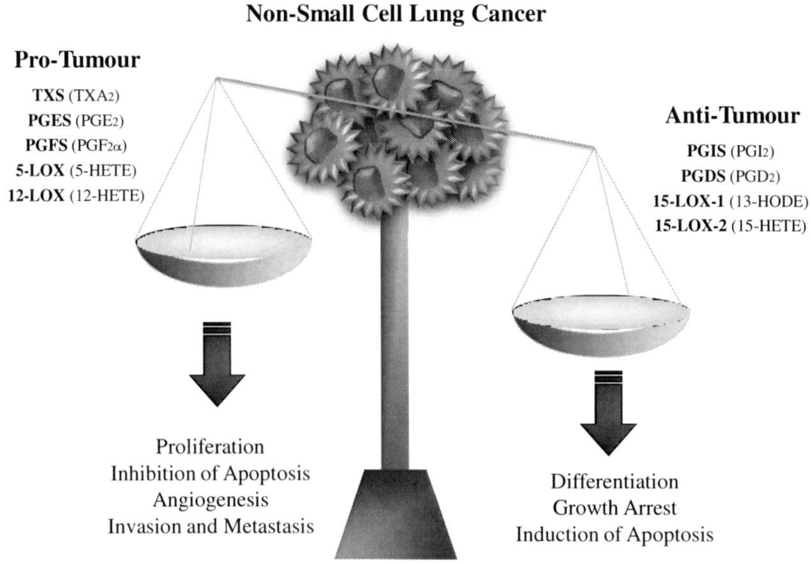


Figure 2. Tumour development is modulated by both pro- and anti-tumour eicosanoid pathways. The expression pattern of tissue-specific synthases (downstream of COX-signalling) and LOX isozymes, and the biological activity of their corresponding products, indicates a critical balance of pro- versus anti-tumour enzymes that may influence the course of tumour development and progression in NSCLC. Adapted from Cathcart *et al.*, 2011. *Cancer and Metastasis Reviews* [111].

In addition to $PGE_2$, the hydration product of $PGD_2$, 15d-$PGJ_2$, significantly reduced lung tumour growth *in-vitro* [61, 62], while growth inhibition was also observed *in-vivo*. This was associated with increased apoptosis, but was not influenced by PPARγ inhibition, suggesting that these effects are at least partly mediated by PPARγ independent mechanisms [61].

PGIS over-expression protected against lung cancer development in a variety of murine tumourigenesis models, including tobacco smoke exposure. In the carcinogenesis models used for PGIS overexpressing animals, an increase in $PGI_2$ production was consistently required for chemoprevention to occur [63, 64]. Expression of PPAR is increased in lung cancer and is thought to play a key role in malignant transformation [65]. Eicosanoids such as $PGI_2$ have been shown to modulate PPAR activity. $PGI_2$ analogues can activate the PPARδ receptor and significantly reduce the growth of the A-549 (adenocarcinoma) NSCLC cell line [66]. Both PGIS and $PGI_2$ may also modulate PPARγ activity with an almost two-fold induction in PPARγ expression observed following lung-specific PGIS overexpression [63, 64]. Ligand-activated PPARγ expression also results in growth arrest of human NSCLC cell lines [67]. Transgenic mice with PPARγ overexpression developed fewer lung tumours, suggesting that PPARγ may be a critical target for $PGI_2$-mediated lung cancer chemoprevention [68].

The role of thromboxane synthase expression in tumour growth has been investigated in a variety of tumour states [69-72]. Recent studies carried out in our laboratory demonstrated a significant reduction in tumour cell growth of two NSCLC cell lines following selective TXS inhibition with ozagrel, suggesting that this enzyme may be a survival factor in the disease [50]. The thromboxane $A_2$ receptor (TP) also induced cell proliferation in several cell lines. A recent report has shown that TP activation by its agonist I-BOP, induced expression of Nurr1, stimulating human lung cancer cell proliferation [73]. Nurr1 is an orphan nuclear receptor, which has been implicated in cell proliferation, differentiation, and apoptosis. These observations provide strong evidence that this receptor may mediate TP-agonist induced proliferation in lung cancer cells.

The cross-talk of LOX-derived products with different growth factor receptor-induced signalling pathways is involved in the regulation of tumour cell growth. The products of lipoxygenase metabolism may exert their biological effects in an intracrine manner through PPAR activation, or they may interact with specific transmembrane G-protein coupled receptors in an autocrine or paracrine manner [17]. Extensive research carried out within the last number of years has shown that targeted inhibition of LOX isoforms can suppress the proliferation of a wide variety of tumour cells. NSCLC cell growth was significantly inhibited *in-vitro* following treatment with either a non-selective LOX inhibitor or selective 5-LOX inhibitors, while non-selective LOX inhibition also inhibited tumour growth *in-vivo* [74]. A combined approach of 5-LOX inhibition and PPARγ antagonism inhibited the growth of NSCLC cells in a super-additive fashion, suggesting that combined arachidonic acid and PPARγ targeting is a promising approach for tumour growth inhibition [75]. Our lab have recently demonstrated a similar significant inhibition in tumour growth following selective 12-LOX inhibition with Baicalein, an effect which was observed both *in-vitro* (cell lines) and *in-vivo* (xenograft mouse model) (unpublished data).

# 4. Arachidonic Acid Mediated Regulation of Tumour Cell Death

Early tumour growth is modulated by the balance between increased tumour cell proliferation and decreased cell death. A second hallmark of cancer required for sustained tumour growth involves the evasion of apoptosis or programmed cell death. Programmed cell death is defined as an active, energy-dependant, well-defined process whereby cells commit suicide [57]. It is a physiological process by which unwanted or damaged cells are eliminated during tissue development and haemostasis [76]. Impaired apoptosis is thought to be crucial for tumour growth, conferring multiple selective advantages on tumour cells, allowing them to persist in a hostile environment, escape death, and evolve into more aggressive clones. Many anti-cancer agents, including radiation, induce apoptosis as an underlying tumour cell death mechanism [77, 78]. A functional link between the induction of apoptosis and interference with the eicosanoid biosynthesis pathway is well known. Indeed, one of the most widely investigated and supported potential mechanisms for the anti-cancer effects of COX-2 inhibition is the induction of tumour cell apoptosis [79]. However, COX-independent functions of the effects of COX-inhibitors on apoptosis in NSCLC have also been identified such as cytochrome c and AIF (apoptotic inducing factor) release, leading to subsequent caspase activation [80].

While $PGD_2$ was orginially thought to be involved in processes of inflammation, it has been recently demonstrated that $PGD_2$ has anti-proliferative and pro-apoptotic ability against tumourigenesis. $PGD_2$ promotes tumour cell death through the intrinsic apoptotic pathway, although the process does not seem to involve the DP receptors. While $PGD_2$ metabolites were effective inducers of apoptosis, 15d-$PGJ_2$ is most likely the main inducer of apoptosis in A-549 cells [81]. The 15d-$PGJ_2$ induction in apoptosis has been associated with ROS production and a decrease in glutathione (GSH) levels. While 15d-$PGJ_2$-induced apoptosis is induced by PPARγ agonists, apoptosis is not dependant on PPARγ activation [82]. The pro-apoptotic effect of 15d-$PGJ_2$ is further enhanced when combined with traditional chemotherapeutic agents, an effect which was associated with inhibition of Bcl2 and cyclin D1 expression as well as overexpression of caspase and p53 pathway genes [61]. PPAR ligands such as 15d-$PGJ_2$ can induce apoptosis in lung cancer cells by inducing the cyclin-dependant kinase inhibitor P21 and reducing cyclin D1 gene expression [62, 83]. Treatment of lung cancer cells with either $PGE_2$ or $PGF_{2\alpha}$ failed to induce apoptosis [62]. However 15-PGDH over-expression induced apoptosis in NSCLC cells, with evidence of DNA fragmentation, caspase activation, and reduced expression of Bcl-2 [42]. Very few studies have been carried out to examine the role of PGIS in apoptosis, particularly tumour cell apoptosis. While TXS inhibitors have been shown to induce apoptosis in cancer cells, the mechanism underlying this apoptotic effect is unclear [50]. TXS inhibition has recently been associated with over-production of reactive oxygen species and a reduction in NF-kB, while anti-oxidants can block the effects of TXS inhibition [84].

Induction of apoptosis was observed in NSCLC cells following selective 5-LOX inhibition [75]. 12-LOX inhibition has also been shown to induce apoptosis in NSCLC cells. Cell cycle arrest in the S-phase was also reported, with decreased levels of CDK-1 and cyclin B1, proteins shown to regulate S-phase transition to G2/M phase [85]. The effect of 12-LOX inhibition with baicalein on apoptosis has also been assessed in both adenocarcinoma and squamous cell carcinoma cell lines, with over 30% apoptosis observed following 72 h treatment. The authors also demonstrated a synergistic effect on tumour growth and apoptosis following combined treatment with baicalein and conventional chemotherapeutic agents [17]. Further studies will need to be carried out to assess the individual role of the LOX-isoforms and their respective metabolites in NSCLC development and progression.

## 5. The Role of Arachidonic Acid Signalling in NSCLC Tumour Angiogenesis

Angiogenesis may be defined as the process of generating new capillaries from a pre-existing blood supply [57]. Although indispensable in development, angiogenesis is highly regulated, and its persistence in adults in usually linked with disease, including cancer, chronic inflammatory disease and diabetic retinopathy [86, 87]. The induction of angiogenesis is necessary for the supply of oxygen and nutrients to tumours >2 mm in diameter, and is therefore essential for successful tumour growth [88]. In order to grow and spread, solid tumours secrete a variety of angiogenesis-promoting factors, which tip the delicate balance in favour of angiogenesis [89]. It has been demonstrated that the greater the number of vessels in tumour areas of highest vessel density, the lower the overall survival rate of the patients [90].

The prostanoids and their corresponding synthases can contribute, at least in part, to NSCLC development/progression *via* their role in the regulation of angiogenesis. Expression of the potent angiogenic factor, VEGF, is up-regulated through a COX-2-dependant mechanism in NSCLC. This effect is thought to be mediated *via* PKC signalling and downstream prostaglandin activation [91]. The lymphangiogenic factor, VEGF-C, but not

VEGF-D was significantly elevated in lung cancer cells overexpressing COX-2. EP1 is involved in COX-2 mediated VEGF-C upregulation and mediates its effects through transactivation of the HER-2/Neu tyrosine kinase receptor pathway [92]. COX-2 overexpression in NSCLC cells enhanced the expression of angiogenic chemokines CXCL5 and CXCL8. In a mouse model, the increased growth of COX-2 overexpressing tumours was inhibited by neutralization of these chemokines, suggesting a link between COX-2 and angiogenesis in NSCLC [93]. Reactivation of 15-PGDH in lung cancer cells significantly reduces tumour angiogenesis and growth *in-vivo*. PGD synthase deficiency enhances lung cancer progression *in-vivo*, an effect mediated *via* increased vascular leakage, angiogenesis, and monocyte/mast cell infiltration [94]. Evidence for the role of $TXA_2$ in angiogenesis is some-what contradictory, with both inhibition and induction of angiogenesis being documented. The thromboxane $A_2$ mimetic, U-46619 has been shown to stimulate endothelial cell migration. Inhibition of $TXA_2$ synthesis, which was stimulated by basic fibroblast growth factor or VEGF, reduced endothelial cell migration, implicating $TXA_2$ in angiogenesis [95].

$TXA_2$ has been shown to act as a potent stimulator of angiogenesis, both directly, and by inducing VEGF (vascular endothelial growth factor) and PDGF (platelet-derived growth factor) secretion from platelets following aggregation [96, 97]. The angiogenic effects of the TXS-pathway have also been demonstrated *in-vivo*, using a transgenic line of zebrafish Tg (fli 1: EGFP), which specifically expressed green flourescent protein in vessels. In this model, selective TXS inhibition had clear effects on intersegmental vessel morphology following 48 h incubation, suggesting an anti-angiogenic mechanism for this drug [98]. However, the role of this pathway in tumour angiogenesis in NSCLC has not yet been examined. While the role of LOX signalling in tumour angiogenesis in NSCLC has not been well investigated, Harats *et al.*, demonstrated the anti-angiogenic effects of 15-LOX in a mouse model of lewis lung carcinoma. They reported that 15-LOX inhibited tumour growth and metastasis growth in transgenic mice, an effect which was associated with a complicated network of small blood vessels [91].

## 6. Regulation of Adhesion, Migration and Invasion of NSCLC by Arachidonic Acid Pathways

The first phase in tumour invasion involves receptor-mediated adhesion of tumour cells to matrix proteins, followed by a second phase of matrix-breakdown by tumour-secreted proteases. This process creates an intra-cellular space into which invading cells can migrate [99]. Tumour spread to distant organs is the most clinically important property of malignant tumours and is known as metastasis. Metastasis allows the cancer to survive surgical excision of the primary tumour, and is responsible for increased tumour burden and difficulty in clinical management [100]. Tumour cell invasion is essential for the dissemination of metastatic cells across extracellular matrices and spread to distant organ sites, with tumour cell metastasis implicated in most cancer deaths [89].

While the role of LOX and EPOX pathways in the adhesion, migration and invasion of NSCLC has not been investigated, a number of studies have examined the contribution of the COX pathway to these pro-tumour mechanisms.

Tumour COX-2 expression is well known to be associated with enhanced tumour invasion. Downstream of COX-2 signalling, $PGE_2$ has been implicated in tumour invasion in NSCLC *via* EP4 signalling. This effect was also mediated through enhanced expression of invasion factors CD44 and MMP-2 [101]. $PGE_2$ has been associated with tumour progression in lung cancer [102]. $PGE_2$ expression in the lung tumour microenvironment is thought to initiate a mitogenic signalling cascade involving EP4, betaArrestin-1 and c-Src to mediate tumour cell migration [103]. Expression of EP2 in squamous cell carcinomas was significantly associated with lymph node metastasis, while overexpression was also correlated with both p16INK4A methylation and a poor prognosis [104]. EP4 also plays an important role in lung cancer metastasis. In a mouse model, tumour metastasis to the lungs was significantly reduced when mice were treated with a specific EP4 anagonist or when EP4 expression was knocked-down by RNA interference. *In-vitro* tumour cell adhesion, motility, invasion, colony formation and Akt phosphorylation were also significantly inhibited following EP4 antagonism [102]. In support of these observations, levels of the prostaglandin catabolic enzyme 15-PGDH, were negatively correlated with those of the pro-adhesive and invasive CD44 [42]. Prostacyclin has been shown to significantly reduce metastasis formation in a lewis lung carcinoma injected murine model. Treatment with $PGI_2$ significantly reduced initial lewis lung carcinoma cell density. In addition, lung weight was reduced by over 50% and the number of visible metastatic nodes by over 90% [105]. $PGI_2$ treatment also reduced the growth of lung micrometastases [106]. TXS expression was associated with increased micro-vessel density (a prognostic factor, predictive of metastasis and poor survival) and metastasis in patients presenting with NSCLC [107]. Early *in-vivo* studies with TXS inhibitors have failed to report any beneficial effects on metastasis or spread to the lymph nodes [108]. However, when used in combination with a TP antagonist, TXS inhibitors inhibited metastasis formation from tail vein injected B16a cells, as well as spontaneous metastasis formation from subcutaneous B16a and Lewis lung carcinoma tumours [109]. A potential role for the thromboxane receptor in tumour cell invasion and metastasis has also recently been examined. TP was shown to mediate tumour cell invasion *via* induction of matrix metalloproteinase (MMP) expression. Both MMP-1 and MMP-9 were implicated in this TP-mediated effect although other MMPs may also be induced [110].

## 7. Modulation of the Immune System in NSCLC by Arachidonic Acid

Tumours often possess the characteristics of inflamed tissue, including immune cell infiltration into the tumour and surrounding stroma. Chronic inflammation is thought to be largely responsible for the recruitment of these cells. One of the hallmarks of the inflammatory process is the production of inflammatory cytokines, including prostaglandins, leukotrienes and HETEs. While chronic inflammation is strongly implicated as a risk factor for cancer, the mechanisms by which the inflammatory process promotes tumour development have not yet been fully uncovered. Of all the mediators of arachidonic acid signalling, COX-2 and $PGE_2$ are by far the most studied with regard to their roles in inflammation and immune modulation in cancer. Studies to date suggest that the immunomodulatory role of $PGE_2$ on the immune system allows cancer cells to avoid attack, thereby promoting tumour progression [3]. The role of the arachidonic acid pathway in immunomodulation in cancer is discussed in depth in a number of recent reviews [3, 17, 111]. An immunosuppressive environment is of particular importance in the pathogenesis of NSCLC. The selective COX-2 inhibitor, celecoxib, inhibits NF-kappaB activation, an effect mediated through inhibition of IKK (I kappa B alpha kinase) and Akt inactivation [112, 113]. This effect was also correlated with suppression of NF-kappaB regulated proteins, COX-2, cyclin D1 and MMP-9 (matrix metalloproteinase-9) [113].

CD4+CD25+ Treg cell activities have been shown to increase in lung cancer and are thought to play a role in suppression of anti-tumour immune responses. Tumour-infiltrating Foxp3+ (the most specific Treg cell marker) Tregs are positively associated with COX-2 expression and negatively associated with recurrence-free survival in NSCLC [114]. Sharma *et al.*, have demonstrated that inhibition of the COX-2/$PGE_2$ pathway suppresses Treg cell activity, thereby enhancing anti-tumour responses [115]. $PGE_2$ is a potent suppressor of natural killer (NK) cell activity *in-vivo*, while its release can promote lung tumour metastasis through this immunomodulatory mechanism [116]. While COX and LOX pathways are both powerful mediators of inflammation, there is nothing reported in the literature regarding the role of the remaining prostanoids and leukotrienes in immune-modulation in NSCLC. This is an area that warrants further investigation.

# 8. Targeting Arachidonic Acid Pathways Using Pharmacological and Natural Agents

Is is well known that the arachidonic acid pathway plays a major role in NSCLC carcinogenesis. An association between regular aspirin use and decreased rates of a number of cancers has been demonstrated, although the evidence regarding lung cancer and aspirin use is unclear. Recent analysis of randomised controlled trials of daily aspirin to reduce the risk of vascular disease demonstrated a 30% reduction in deaths due to lung cancer in people taking aspirin for five or more years [117].

This report of targeting of the arachidonic acid pathway was published just prior to three subsequent trials demonstrating that targeting the same pathway with different agents effectively reverses proliferation or histologic changes in the lungs of former smokers [118-120].

A number of studies have been carried out in previous years to determine a potential role for targeting of the arachidonic acid pathway in NSCLC prevention and/or treatment. These studies have assessed a role for both pharmacological inhibitors and natural agents and have also investigated dual targeting approaches with traditional chemotherapeutics and other novel agents. These therapeutic approaches will be discussed in the subsequent sections.

## Pharmacological Agents

There has been a significant interest in COX-2 and its role in the development and progression of cancer over the past number of years, with a number of clinical trials examining selective COX-2 inhibition as a potential therapeutic strategy. A number of studies have shown a correlation between COX-2 expression and poor prognosis in NSCLC [121-123]. In addition, COX-2 inhibitors have been shown to modulate existing cancer therapies in NSCLC [124]. However, chronic use of high concentrations of selective COX-2 inhibitors have recently been associated with a significantly increased of cardiovascular events in susceptible individuals [125]. In addition, data from murine studies evaluating the role of non-selective or selective COX-2 inhibition have failed to yield overwhelmingly positive results. Surprisingly, COX-2 inhibition with celecoxib results in no change in tumour multiplicity and an increase in tumour size in an initiator-promoter model of lung tumourigenesis [126]. Increased COX-2 expression is associated with increased levels of downstream enzymes required for prostanoid synthesis [47]. The tumour-promoting effects of COX-2 overexpression may therefore be attributable to specific downstream products of arachidonic acid metabolism. The selective targeting of downstream effectors of the cyclooxygenase signalling pathway may therefore be a promising approach for the prevention and/or treatment of NSCLC, with the potential of avoiding the cardiovascular effects associated with selective COX-2 inhibition, while maintaining anti-tumour reactivity.

COX-inhibition reduces levels of a number of downstream arachidonic acid metabolites, including prostacyclin, which has demonstrated anti-metastatic and anti-proliferative properties [106, 127]. $PGI_2$ overexpression also prevents lung cancer development in a range of murine models, including cigarette smoke exposure [64, 68, 118-120]. While $PGE_2$ has been strongly implicated in carcinogenesis, overexpression of $PGE_2$ synthase demonstrated no increase in lung carcinogenesis *in-vivo* [128, 129]. Based on preclinical studies, a multicenter double-blind phase II study has been carried out to investigate the use of Iloprost (an oral prostacyclin analogue) for chemoprevention of non-small cell lung cancer. Iloprost is a stable analogue of epoprostanol, which is the synthetic analogue to $PGI_2$ and can be delivered through intravenous, inhaled, or oral routes [130]. Patients on the trial were assessed for the histologic progression of endobronchial dysplasia. Former smokers who received iloprost demonstrated a statistically significant improvement in histologic lung tissue measurements following just six months of treatment. The authors concluded that iloprost is a promising agent for cancer chemoprevention, and warrants testing in a larger phase III trial [131]. Iloprost activated PPAR$\gamma$ in both non-transformed bronchial epithelial cell lines and NSCLC cell lines, with activation in NSCLC associated with a reduction in tumour growth, invasion and metastasis [132]. Mice with PPAR$\gamma$ expression developed fewer lung tumours following urethane exposure and treatment with iloprost than wild-type mice. In this case, the tumour protective effect of iloprost treatment was independent of IP expression, suggesting an alternative membrane receptor may be responsible for the iloprost-mediated PPAR$\gamma$ activation [68]. PPAR$\gamma$ activation is therefore a second alternative mechanism which, in addition to $PGI_2$, may be ready for future chemoprevention trials [68]. While Iloprost is the first agent to show improvement of endobronchial dysplasia in lung cancer chemoprevention trials, the $PGE_2$ receptor (EP2) may also be a potential target for chemoprevention studies. Keith *et al.*, demonstrated that $PGE_2$ promotes lung tumourigenesis *via* EP2 activation [133]. Further studies are therefore warranted to assess EP2 as a chemopreventative agent in NSCLC.

## Natural Arachidonic Acid Modulators

The natural product, curcumin (derived from the spice tumeric), which exhibits anti-inflammatory and anti-carcinogenic properties, has also been shown to inhibit COX-2, PGES, $PGE_2$ and 5-LOX [134, 135]. The chemopreventative action of curcumin is proposed to be *via* modulation of arachidonic acid metabolism. A recent phase II colorectal chemoprevention trial demonstrated that this chemical was well tolerated and suggested that it can decrease aberrant crypt foci formation [136]. This was associated with significantly increased curcumin conjugate levels, but did not affect $PGE_2$ or 5-HETE levels, suggesting that other mechanisms may also mediate these short-term chemopreventative effects. Curcumin inhibited interferon-alpha induced expression of COX-2 and NF-kappaB in NSCLC cells and also increased the apoptotic effects of cisplatin [137, 138]. More recently, curcumin was shown to induce NSCLC apoptosis in a dose-dependent manner, an effect which coincided with up-regulation of pro-apoptotic gene expression (*Bax*, *Bad*) and down-regulation of anti-apoptotic gene expression (*Bcl-2*, *Bcl-XL*, *XIAP*) [139]. In addition to the array of pharmacological agents under investigation for their effect on LOX metabolism, a number of naturally occurring agents that may interact with lipoxygenase activity are constantly being discovered, such as dietary carotenoids including lycophyll (present in tomatoes) that may modify the enzymatic function of 5-LOX through binding to the catalytic site with high affinity [140]. There are also numerous plant phenols including baicalein, kaempferol, quercetin, nordihydroguaretic acid and resveratrol which are known for their chemopreventative as well as LOX-inhibitory activity in different tumour models [141]. The 12-LOX inhibitor, baicalein, a flavonoid isolated from an important medicinal plant Scutellariae Radix (the root of Scutellaria baicalensis Georgi) has been shown to induce apoptosis in a range of human cancer cell types [142-144]. A potential role for baicalein in NSCLC prevention has also been investigated. Treatment with baicalein counteracted the histological and molecular changes associated with pulmonary carcinoegenesis in a Swiss albino mouse model. The authors proposed that the chemotherapeutic effect observed in this study is a result of the anti-inflammatory and antioxidant effects on baicalein *in-vivo* [145]. Resveratrol, trans-3,5,4'-trihydroxystilbene, was first isolated in 1940 as a constituent of the roots of white hellebore (Veratrum grandiflorum O. Loes), but has since been found in various plants, including grapes, berries and peanuts. Resveratrol has been shown to suppress the expression of 5-LOX and to inhibit the proliferation of a wide variety of tumour cells, including lymphoid and myeloid cancers; multiple myeloma; cancers of the breast, prostate, stomach, colon, pancreas, and thyroid; melanoma; head and neck squamous cell carcinoma; ovarian carcinoma; and cervical carcinoma [146]. The growth-inhibitory effects of resveratrol are mediated through cell-cycle arrest; up-regulation of p21Cip1/WAF1, p53 and Bax; down-regulation of survivin, cyclin D1, cyclin E, Bcl-2, Bcl-xL and clAPs; and activation of caspases. It has been shown to suppress the activation of several transcription factors, including NF-kappaB, AP-1 and Egr-1; to inhibit protein kinases including IkappaBalpha kinase, JNK, MAPK, Akt, PKC, PKD and casein kinase II; and to down-regulate products of genes other than 5-LOX including COX-2, VEGF, IL-1, IL-6, IL-8, AR and PSA. Resveratrol inhibited NSCLC cell growth by 50% and also induced apoptosis. Furthermore, it significantly enhanced the anti-proliferative and apoptotic effects of the traditional chemotherapeutic, paclitaxel and enhanced radiosensitivity of NSCLC cells [147, 148]. The migratory and invasive abilities of NSCLC cells were significantly reduced following resveratrol treatment, further suggesting that it may be a promising therapeutic agent for NSCLC treatment [149]. Tea has been proposed to have a protective role in carcinogenesis. This was recently investigated by Mao *et al.*, who demonstrated that white tea extract (WTE) induced apoptosis *in-vitro*. This effect was at least partly mediated through activation of PPARγ and 15-LOX signalling pathways, with enhanced caspase 3 activation [150].

## Dual Targeting Approaches: Traditional Therapies and Novel Molecular Agents

An early study of COX-2 inhibition in combination with conventional chemotherapy in early stage NSCLC patients demonstrated that celecoxib treatment enhanced the response to pre-operative paclitaxil and carboplatin [151]. However, two subsequent phase III trials of celecoxib in combination with chemotherapy in late stage NSCLC patients demonstrated no survival benefit for the addition of celecoxib to conventional chemotherapy [152, 153]. A number of important differences were noted between these trials and that of Edelman *et al.*, which may explain the discrepancies observed, such as different chemotherapy regimens. Retrospective analysis carried out on a number of phase II trials have shown that celecoxib in combination with other anti-tumour agents improves outcomes in patients with high COX-2 expression [154-156]. Preliminary results of a phase II trial combining the selective COX-2 inhibitor apricoxib with chemotherapy in NSCLC patients (who were selected on the basis of urinary prostaglandin $E_2$ metabolite suppression following 5 days of apricoxib treatment) demonstrated markedly improved progression-free survival. Edelman *et al.*, recently commented that the only way to conclusively demonstrate a role for COX-2 inhibition in NSCLC treatment is through a prospective randomised trial, which selects patients for therapy on the basis of COX-2 expression [157]. Such a trial (CALGB30811) is currently underway. A randomised phase II trial failed to demonstrate the value of the combined approach of COX-2 (celecoxib) and 5-LOX (zileuton) inhibition for the treatment of patients with advanced lung cancer. In addition, a benefit for either agent alone alone in addition to chemotherapy was not observed. However, patients with increased COX-2 expression demonstrated improved survival following treatment with the selective COX-2 inhibitor than COX-2 expressing patients not receiving the drug, suggesting an advantage for this approach in patients with increased COX-2 expression [158]. The PPARγ ligand 15d-$PGJ_2$ has also been examined in combination with conventional chemotherapy for the treatment of NSCLC. 15d-$PGJ_2$ and docetaxel significantly reduced tumour volume in a mouse model, relative to untreated controls or either agent alone, suggesting that this combined approach has therapeutic potential in NSCLC treatment [61]. A number of studies have also been carried out to assess a dual targeting approach for NSCLC chemoprevention. Combined inhibition of both COX-2 and 5-LOX pathways enhanced growth arrest and death of both premalignant and malignant human lung cell lines [159]. A more recent study examined the effect of licofelone, a dual inhibitor of COX-2 and 5-LOX on pulmonary carcinogenesis *in-vivo*. Licofelone treatment dose-dependantly inhibited tumour incidence and multiplicity and also dose-dependantly inhibited COX-2, 5-LOX, proliferating cell nuclear antigen and increased apoptosis [160]. This suggests that licofelcone may be chemopreventative in NSCLC and warrants further investigation. Keith *et al.*, examined the effects of PGIS overexpression in combination with endothelial growth factor receptor (EGFR) inhibition with gefitinib in a murine model of pulmonary carcinogenesis. While gefitinib had no chemopreventative effect in this model, it enhanced the effect of PGIS overexpression, suggesting the potential for this combined approach [161].

**Table 1. The effects of arachidonic acid derived eicosanoids on the hallmarks of NSCLC**

| Eicoasanoid | Cancer Hallmark | Study Type | Result | Author |
|---|---|---|---|---|
| $PGD_2$ | Apoptosis | Cell line | - | Tsubouchi *et al.*, 2000[62] |
| | Proliferation | Cell line/xenograft | + | Tsubouchi *et al.*, 2000[62] |
| | Proliferation | Cell line | + | Han *et al.*, 2004[83] |
| | Apoptosis | Cell line | - | Han *et al.*, 2004[83] |
| | Proliferation | Cell line | + | Fulzele *et al.*, 2007[61] |
| | Apoptosis | Cell line | - | Fulzele *et al.*, 2007[61] |
| | Apoptosis | Cell line | - | Wang *et al.*, 2011[81] |
| | Apoptosis | Cell line | - | Wang *et al.*, 2011[82] |
| $PGE_2$ | Apoptosis | Cell line | NE | Tsubouchi *et al.*, 2000[61] |
| | Invasion | Cell line | + | Dohadwala *et al.*, 2002[101] |
| | Immune Response | Murine Model | - | Yaker *et al.*, 2003[116] |
| | Proliferation | Cell line | + | Han *et al.*, 2004[58] |
| | Immune Response | Murine Model | - | Sharma et al., 2005[115] |
| | Invasion/Metastasis | Cell line/xenograft | + | Yang *et al.*, 2006[102] |
| | Proliferation | Cell line | + | Zheng *et al.*, 2009[59] |
| | Proliferation | Cell line | + | Moody *et al.*, 2010[60] |
| | Migration | Cell line | + | Kim *et al.*, 2010[103] |
| $PGF_{2\alpha}$ | Apoptosis | Cell line | NE | Tsubouchi *et al.*, 2000[62] |
| $PGI_2$ | Metastasis | Murine model | - | Honn *et al.*, 1983[109] |
| | Metastasis | Murine model | NE | Stamford *et al.*, 1986[108] |
| | Metastasis | Murine model | - | Schirner *et al.*, 1997[106] |
| | Proliferation | Cell line | - | Fukumoto *et al.*, 2005[65] |
| | Metastasis | Murine model | - | Cuneo *et al.*, 2007[105] |
| $TXA_2$ | Metastasis | Murine Model | + | Honn *et al.*, 1983[109] |
| | Metastasis | Murine model | NE | Stamford *et al.*, 1986[108] |
| | Proliferation | Cell line | + | Li *et al.*, 2009[73] |
| | Proliferation | Cell line | + | Cathcart *et al.*, 2011[50] |
| | Apoptosis | Cell line | - | Cathcart *et al.*, 2011[50] |
| | Invasion | Cell line | + | Li *et al.*, 2012[110] |
| 5-LOX | Proliferation | Cell line | + | Moody *et al.*, 1998[74] |
| | Proliferation | Cell line | + | Avis *et al.*, 2005[75] |
| | Apoptosis | Cell line | - | Avis *et al.*, 2005[75] |
| 12-LOX | Apoptosis | Cell line | - | Leung *et al.*, 2007[84] |
| | Apoptosis | Cell line | - | Pidgeon et al., 2007[17] |
| 15-LOX | Proliferation | Murine model | + | Harats *et al.*, 2005[91] |
| | Angiogenesis | Murine model | + | Harats *et al.*, 2005[91] |
| | Metastasis | Murine model | + | Harats *et al.*, 2005[91] |

This table references studies which have examined the role of COX and LOX-derived eicosanoids on the hallmarks of NSCLC (+, cancer hallmark increased; - cancer hallmark reduced; NE, no effect).

# Conclusion

While a number of mechanisms have been identified in NSCLC carcinogenesis, a role for arachidonic acid derived eicosanoids in the disease is also evident. The COX signalling pathway is the most widely investigated of the three arachidonic acid signalling pathways. The most recent research efforts have focussed on examining down-stream effectors of COX-metabolism in NSCLC development and progression. The involvement of both COX ($PGE_2$, $TXA_2$) and LOX (5-LOX, 12-LOX and 15-LOX) signalling pathways in NSCLC is supported by a growing body of literature. The co-localization of these enzymes, their downstream metabolites, and their effects on carcinogenesis suggests that targeting these pathways may represent novel and promising therapeutic approaches for NSCLC prevention/treatment.

While smoking cessation will clearly have the greatest effect on lung cancer development, effective chemoprevention may also play a major role. Manipulation of prostaglandin production is an attractive chemoprevention strategy. Phase III chemoprevention trials will determine if iloprost is a novel approach for lung cancer chemoprevention. In terms of NSCLC treatment; further clinical trials of selective COX-2 inhibition are warranted, in which patients with advanced disease are selected on the basis of COX-2 expression. There is an urgent need for additional studies examining selective COX-2 inhibition in NSCLC, so that clinicians can conclusively determine whether inhibition of this pathway can significantly improve survival in patients with NSCLC. The identification of specific arachidonic acid-derived eicosanoids involved in NSCLC development and progression will also allow further development of targeted and personalised therapies for prevention and/or treatment.

These agents may have anti-tumour efficacy alone or in combination with other targeted therapies and/or traditional chemotherapeutic approaches. At present, analogues of $PGE_2$, $PGF_{2\alpha}$ and $PGI_2$ as well as TP and leukotriene antagonists are approved for clinical use, while inhibitors of mPGES-1, 5-LOX and its activating factor, and antagonists of DP1, DP2 and EP2 are undergoing clinical evaluation [35]. While targeting of both COX and LOX pathways remains promising as potential therapeutics for NSCLC carcinogenesis, further pre-clinical and clinical studies will be required to identify the signalling mechanisms associated with these pathways and to support preliminary findings.

# References


[1] Cuendet M, Pezzuto JM. The role of cyclooxygenase and lipoxygenase in cancer chemoprevention. *Drug Metabol. Drug Interact*. 2000;17(1-4):109-57.

[2] Klurfeld DM, Bull AW. Fatty acids and colon cancer in experimental models. *The American journal of clinical nutrition*. 1997;66(6 Suppl):1530S-8S. Epub 1997/12/12.

[3] Wang D, Dubois RN. Eicosanoids and cancer. *Nat. Rev. Cancer*. 2010;10(3):181-93. Epub 2010/02/20.

[4] Greene ER, Huang S, Serhan CN, *et al.* Regulation of inflammation in cancer by eicosanoids. *Prostaglandins Other Lipid Mediat* 2011:Epub. Epub 2011/08/26.

[5] Smith WL. The eicosanoids and their biochemical mechanisms of action. *Biochem. J.* 1989;259(2):315-24.

[6] Dannenberg AJ, Subbaramaiah K. Targeting cyclooxygenase-2 in human neoplasia: rationale and promise. *Cancer Cell.* 2003;4(6):431-6.
[7] Antonarakis ES, Heath EI, Walczak JR, *et al.* Phase II, randomized, placebo-controlled trial of neoadjuvant celecoxib in men with clinically localized prostate cancer: evaluation of drug-specific biomarkers. *J. Clin. Oncol.* 2009;27(30):4986-93. Epub 2009/09/02.
[8] Dragovich T, Burris H, 3rd, Loehrer P, *et al.* Gemcitabine plus celecoxib in patients with advanced or metastatic pancreatic adenocarcinoma: results of a phase II trial. *Am. J. Clin. Oncol.* 2008;31(2):157-62. Epub 2008/04/09.
[9] Jakobsen A, Mortensen JP, Bisgaard C, *et al.* A COX-2 inhibitor combined with chemoradiation of locally advanced rectal cancer: a phase II trial. *Int. J. Colorectal Dis.* 2008;23(3):251-5. Epub 2007/12/08.
[10] Papadimitrakopoulou VA, William WN, Jr., Dannenberg AJ, *et al.* Pilot randomized phase II study of celecoxib in oral premalignant lesions. *Clin. Cancer Res.* 2008;14(7):2095-101. Epub 2008/04/03.
[11] Bombardier C, Laine L, Reicin A, *et al.* Comparison of upper gastrointestinal toxicity of rofecoxib and naproxen in patients with rheumatoid arthritis. VIGOR Study Group. *N. Engl. J. Med.* 2000;343(21):1520-8, 2 p following 8.
[12] Bresalier RS, Sandler RS, Quan H, *et al.* Cardiovascular events associated with rofecoxib in a colorectal adenoma chemoprevention trial. *N. Engl. J. Med.* 2005;352(11):1092-102.
[13] Helin-Salmivaara A, Virtanen A, Vesalainen R, *et al.* NSAID use and the risk of hospitalization for first myocardial infarction in the general population: a nationwide case-control study from Finland. *Eur. Heart J.* 2006;27(14):1657-63. Epub 2006/05/30.
[14] Kearney PM, Baigent C, Godwin J, *et al.* Do selective cyclo-oxygenase-2 inhibitors and traditional non-steroidal anti-inflammatory drugs increase the risk of atherothrombosis? Meta-analysis of randomised trials. *BMJ.* 2006;332(7553):1302-8. Epub 2006/06/03.
[15] Solomon SD, McMurray JJ, Pfeffer MA, *et al.* Cardiovascular risk associated with celecoxib in a clinical trial for colorectal adenoma prevention. *N. Engl. J. Med.* 2005;352(11):1071-80.
[16] Yang VW, Shields JM, Hamilton SR, *et al.* Size-dependent increase in prostanoid levels in adenomas of patients with familial adenomatous polyposis. *Cancer Res.* 1998;58(8):1750-3.
[17] Pidgeon GP, Lysaght J, Krishnamoorthy S, *et al.* Lipoxygenase metabolism: roles in tumor progression and survival. *Cancer Metastasis Rev.* 2007;26(3-4):503-24. Epub 2007/10/19.
[18] Panigrahy D, Kaipainen A, Greene ER, *et al.* Cytochrome P450-derived eicosanoids: the neglected pathway in cancer. *Cancer Metastasis Rev.* 2010;29(4):723-35. Epub 2010/10/14.
[19] Hanahan D, Weinberg RA. The hallmarks of cancer. *Cell.* 2000;100(1):57-70.
[20] Hanahan D, Weinberg RA. Hallmarks of cancer: the next generation. *Cell.* 2011;144(5):646-74. Epub 2011/03/08.
[21] de Leval X, Dassesse T, Dogne JM, *et al.* Evaluation of original dual thromboxane A2 modulators as antiangiogenic agents. *J. Pharmacol. Exp. Ther.* 2006;318(3):1057-67.
[22] Zeldin DC. Epoxygenase pathways of arachidonic acid metabolism. *J. Biol. Chem.* 2001;276(39):36059-62. Epub 2001/07/14.

[23] Serhan CN. Systems approach to inflammation resolution: identification of novel anti-inflammatory and pro-resolving mediators. *J. Thromb. Haemost.* 2009;7 Suppl 1:44-8. Epub 2009/07/28.
[24] Gao H, Welch WJ, DiBona GF, *et al.* Sympathetic nervous system and hypertension during prolonged TxA2/PGH2 receptor activation in rats. *Am. J. Physiol.* 1997;273(2 Pt 2):H734-9.
[25] Needleman P, Moncada S, Bunting S, *et al.* Identification of an enzyme in platelet microsomes which generates thromboxane A2 from prostaglandin endoperoxides. *Nature.* 1976;261(5561):558-60. Epub 1976/06/17.
[26] Fu JY, Masferrer JL, Seibert K, *et al.* The induction and suppression of prostaglandin H2 synthase (cyclooxygenase) in human monocytes. *J. Biol. Chem.* 1990;265(28):16737-40.
[27] Funk CD. Prostaglandins and leukotrienes: advances in eicosanoid biology. *Science.* 2001;294(5548):1871-5.
[28] Patrignani P, Panara MR, Greco A, *et al.* Biochemical and pharmacological characterization of the cyclooxygenase activity of human blood prostaglandin endoperoxide synthases. *J. Pharmacol. Exp. Ther.* 1994;271(3):1705-12.
[29] Hoffmann C. COX-2 in brain and spinal cord implications for therapeutic use. *Curr. Med. Chem.* 2000;7(11):1113-20.
[30] Harris RC, McKanna JA, Akai Y, *et al.* Cyclooxygenase-2 is associated with the macula densa of rat kidney and increases with salt restriction. *J. Clin. Invest.* 1994;94(6):2504-10.
[31] Forman BM, Chen J, Evans RM. Hypolipidemic drugs, polyunsaturated fatty acids, and eicosanoids are ligands for peroxisome proliferator-activated receptors alpha and delta. *Proc. Natl. Acad. Sci. USA.* 1997;94(9):4312-7. Epub 1997/04/29.
[32] Kliewer SA, Sundseth SS, Jones SA, *et al.* Fatty acids and eicosanoids regulate gene expression through direct interactions with peroxisome proliferator-activated receptors alpha and gamma. *Proc. Natl. Acad. Sci. USA.* 1997;94(9):4318-23.
[33] Gupta RA, J. T, Krause WF, *et al.* Prostacyclin mediated activation of peroxisome proliferator-activated receptor delta in colorectal cancer. *Proceedings of the National Academy of Sciences of the United States of America.* 2000;97:13275-80.
[34] Wang D, Wang H, Shi Q, *et al.* Prostaglandin E(2) promotes colorectal adenoma growth via transactivation of the nuclear peroxisome proliferator-activated receptor delta. *Cancer Cell.* 2004;6(3):285-95. Epub 2004/09/24.
[35] Ricciotti E, FitzGerald GA. Prostaglandins and inflammation. *Arterioscler Thromb Vasc Biol.* 2011;31(5):986-1000. Epub 2011/04/22.
[36] Funk CD. Molecular biology in the eicosanoid field. *Progress in nucleic acid research and molecular biology.* 1993;45:67-98. Epub 1993/01/01.
[37] Fabre JE, Goulet JL, Riche E, *et al.* Transcellular biosynthesis contributes to the production of leukotrienes during inflammatory responses in vivo. *J. Clin. Invest.* 2002;109(10):1373-80. Epub 2002/05/22.
[38] Wu S, Moomaw CR, Tomer KB, *et al.* Molecular cloning and expression of CYP2J2, a human cytochrome P450 arachidonic acid epoxygenase highly expressed in heart. *J. Biol. Chem.* 1996;271(7):3460-8. Epub 1996/02/16.
[39] Hubbard WC, Alley MC, Gray GN, *et al.* Evidence for prostanoid biosynthesis as a biochemical feature of certain subclasses of non-small cell carcinomas of the lung as

determined in established cell lines derived from human lung tumors. *Cancer Res.* 1989;49(4):826-32.

[40] McLemore TL, Hubbard WC, Litterst CL, *et al.* Profiles of prostaglandin biosynthesis in normal lung and tumor tissue from lung cancer patients. *Cancer Res.* 1988;48(11):3140-7.

[41] Hughes D, Otani T, Yang P, *et al.* NAD+-dependent 15-hydroxyprostaglandin dehydrogenase regulates levels of bioactive lipids in non-small cell lung cancer. *Cancer Prev Res* (Phila). 2008;1(4):241-9. Epub 2009/01/14.

[42] Ding Y, Tong M, Liu S, *et al.* NAD+-linked 15-hydroxyprostaglandin dehydrogenase (15-PGDH) behaves as a tumor suppressor in lung cancer. *Carcinogenesis.* 2005;26(1):65-72. Epub 2004/09/11.

[43] Murphey LJ, Williams MK, Sanchez SC, *et al.* Quantification of the major urinary metabolite of PGE2 by a liquid chromatographic/mass spectrometric assay: determination of cyclooxygenase-specific PGE2 synthesis in healthy humans and those with lung cancer. *Analytical biochemistry.* 2004;334(2):266-75. Epub 2004/10/21.

[44] Kreutzer M, Fauti T, Kaddatz K, *et al.* Specific components of prostanoid-signaling pathways are present in non-small cell lung cancer cells. *Oncol Rep.* 2007;18(2):497-501. Epub 2007/07/06.

[45] Nana-Sinkam P, Golpon H, Keith RL, *et al.* Prostacyclin in human non-small cell lung cancers. *Chest.* 2004;125(5 Suppl):141S. Epub 2004/05/12.

[46] Stearman RS, Dwyer-Nield L, Zerbe L, *et al.* Analysis of orthologous gene expression between human pulmonary adenocarcinoma and a carcinogen-induced murine model. *Am. J. Pathol.* 2005;167(6):1763-75. Epub 2005/11/30.

[47] Ermert L, Dierkes C, Ermert M. Immunohistochemical expression of cyclooxygenase isoenzymes and downstream enzymes in human lung tumors. *Clin. Cancer Res.* 2003;9(5):1604-10.

[48] Cathcart MC, Gray SG, Baird AM, *et al.* Prostacyclin synthase expression and epigenetic regulation in nonsmall cell lung cancer. *Cancer.* 2011. Epub 2011/04/28.

[49] Stearman RS, Grady MC, Nana-Sinkam P, *et al.* Genetic and epigenetic regulation of the human prostacyclin synthase promoter in lung cancer cell lines. *Mol. Cancer Res.* 2007;5(3):295-308. Epub 2007/03/22.

[50] Cathcart MC, Gately K, Cummins R, *et al.* Examination of thromboxane synthase as a prognostic factor and therapeutic target in non-small cell lung cancer. *Mol. Cancer.* 2011;10(1):25. Epub 2011/03/11.

[51] Chen GG, Lee TW, Yip JH, *et al.* Increased thromboxane B(2) levels are associated with lipid peroxidation and Bcl-2 expression in human lung carcinoma. *Cancer Lett.* 2006;234(2):193-8. Epub 2005/05/07.

[52] Fahn HJ, Wang LS, Kao SH, *et al.* Smoking-associated mitochondrial DNA mutations and lipid peroxidation in human lung tissues. *Am. J. Respir Cell Mol. Biol.* 1998;19(6):901-9. Epub 1998/12/09.

[53] Moussalli MJ, Wu Y, Zuo X, *et al.* Mechanistic contribution of ubiquitous 15-lipoxygenase-1 expression loss in cancer cells to terminal cell differentiation evasion. *Cancer Prev. Res.* (Phila). 2011;4(12):1961-72. Epub 2011/09/02.

[54] Gonzalez AL, Roberts RL, Massion PP, *et al.* 15-Lipoxygenase-2 expression in benign and neoplastic lung: an immunohistochemical study and correlation with tumor grade and proliferation. *Hum. Pathol.* 2004;35(7):840-9. Epub 2004/07/17.

[55] Subbarayan V, Xu XC, Kim J, *et al.* Inverse relationship between 15-lipoxygenase-2 and PPAR-gamma gene expression in normal epithelia compared with tumor epithelia. *Neoplasia*. 2005;7(3):280-93. Epub 2005/04/01.

[56] Yuan H, Li MY, Ma LT, *et al.* 15-Lipoxygenases and its metabolites 15(S)-HETE and 13(S)-HODE in the development of non-small cell lung cancer. *Thorax*. 2010;65(4):321-6. Epub 2010/04/15.

[57] Cathcart MC, Reynolds JV, O'Byrne KJ, *et al.* The role of prostacyclin synthase and thromboxane synthase signaling in the development and progression of cancer. *Biochim. Biophys. Acta*. 2010;1805(2):153-66. Epub 2010/02/04.

[58] Han S, Roman J. Suppression of prostaglandin E2 receptor subtype EP2 by PPARgamma ligands inhibits human lung carcinoma cell growth. *Biochem. Biophys. Res. Commun*. 2004;314(4):1093-9. Epub 2004/01/31.

[59] Zheng Y, Ritzenthaler JD, Sun X, *et al.* Prostaglandin E2 stimulates human lung carcinoma cell growth through induction of integrin-linked kinase: the involvement of EP4 and Sp1. *Cancer Res*. 2009;69(3):896-904. Epub 2009/01/30.

[60] Moody TW, Switzer C, Santana-Flores W, *et al.* Dithiolethione modified valproate and diclofenac increase E-cadherin expression and decrease proliferation of non-small cell lung cancer cells. *Lung Cancer*. 2010;68(2):154-60. Epub 2009/07/25.

[61] Fulzele SV, Chatterjee A, Shaik MS, *et al.* 15-Deoxy-Delta12,14-prostaglandin J2 enhances docetaxel anti-tumor activity against A549 and H460 non-small-cell lung cancer cell lines and xenograft tumors. *Anticancer Drugs*. 2007;18(1):65-78. Epub 2006/12/13.

[62] Tsubouchi Y, Sano H, Kawahito Y, *et al.* Inhibition of human lung cancer cell growth by the peroxisome proliferator-activated receptor-gamma agonists through induction of apoptosis. *Biochem. Biophys. Res. Commun*. 2000;270(2):400-5. Epub 2001/02/07.

[63] Keith RL, Miller YE, Hoshikawa Y, *et al.* Manipulation of pulmonary prostacyclin synthase expression prevents murine lung cancer. *Cancer Res*. 2002;62(3):734-40.

[64] Keith RL, Miller YE, Hudish TM, *et al.* Pulmonary prostacyclin synthase overexpression chemoprevents tobacco smoke lung carcinogenesis in mice. *Cancer Res*. 2004;64(16):5897-904.

[65] Michalik L, Desvergne B, Wahli W. Peroxisome-proliferator-activated receptors and cancers: complex stories. *Nat. Rev. Cancer*. 2004;4(1):61-70. Epub 2004/01/07.

[66] Fukumoto K, Yano Y, Virgona N, *et al.* Peroxisome proliferator-activated receptor delta as a molecular target to regulate lung cancer cell growth. *FEBS Lett*. 2005;579(17):3829-36.

[67] Keshamouni VG, Reddy RC, Arenberg DA, *et al.* Peroxisome proliferator-activated receptor-gamma activation inhibits tumor progression in non-small-cell lung cancer. *Oncogene*. 2004;23(1):100-8. Epub 2004/01/09.

[68] Nemenoff R, Meyer AM, Hudish TM, *et al.* Prostacyclin prevents murine lung cancer independent of the membrane receptor by activation of peroxisomal proliferator--activated receptor gamma. *Cancer Prev. Res*. (Phila Pa). 2008;1(5):349-56. Epub 2009/01/14.

[69] Moussa O, Riker JM, Klein J, *et al.* Inhibition of thromboxane synthase activity modulates bladder cancer cell responses to chemotherapeutic agents. *Oncogene*. 2007.

[70] Moussa O, Yordy JS, Abol-Enein H, *et al.* Prognostic and functional significance of thromboxane synthase gene overexpression in invasive bladder cancer. *Cancer Res.* 2005;65(24):11581-7.
[71] Pradono P, Tazawa R, Maemondo M, *et al.* Gene transfer of thromboxane A(2) synthase and prostaglandin I(2) synthase antithetically altered tumor angiogenesis and tumor growth. *Cancer Res.* 2002;62(1):63-6.
[72] Sakai H, Suzuki T, Takahashi Y, *et al.* Upregulation of thromboxane synthase in human colorectal carcinoma and the cancer cell proliferation by thromboxane A2. *FEBS Lett.* 2006;580(14):3368-74.
[73] Li X, Tai HH. Activation of Thromboxane A2 Receptors Induces Orphan Nuclear Receptor Nurr1 Expression and Stimulates Cell Proliferation in Human Lung Cancer Cells. *Carcinogenesis.* 2009. Epub 2009/07/03.
[74] Moody TW, Leyton J, Martinez A, *et al.* Lipoxygenase inhibitors prevent lung carcinogenesis and inhibit non-small cell lung cancer growth. *Experimental lung research.* 1998;24(4):617-28. Epub 1998/07/11.
[75] Avis I, Martinez A, Tauler J, *et al.* Inhibitors of the arachidonic acid pathway and peroxisome proliferator-activated receptor ligands have superadditive effects on lung cancer growth inhibition. *Cancer Res.* 2005;65(10):4181-90. Epub 2005/05/19.
[76] Perl M, Chung CS, Ayala A. Apoptosis. *Crit. Care Med.* 2005;33(12 Suppl):S526-9. Epub 2005/12/13.
[77] Kaufmann SH, Earnshaw WC. Induction of apoptosis by cancer chemotherapy. *Exp. Cell Res.* 2000;256(1):42-9. Epub 2000/03/31.
[78] Milas L, Gregoire V, Hunter N, *et al.* Radiation-induced apoptosis in tumors: effect of radiation modulating agents. *Adv. Exp. Med. Biol.* 1997;400B:559-64. Epub 1997/01/01.
[79] Castelao JE, Bart RD, 3rd, DiPerna CA, *et al.* Lung cancer and cyclooxygenase-2. *Ann. Thorac. Surg.* 2003;76(4):1327-35.
[80] Sanchez-Alcazar JA, Bradbury DA, Pang L, *et al.* Cyclooxygenase (COX) inhibitors induce apoptosis in non-small cell lung cancer through cyclooxygenase independent pathways. *Lung Cancer.* 2003;40(1):33-44. Epub 2003/03/28.
[81] Wang JJ, Mak OT. Induction of apoptosis in non-small cell lung carcinoma A549 cells by PGD(2) metabolite, 15d-PGJ(2). *Cell biology international.* 2011;35(11):1089-96. Epub 2011/10/18.
[82] Wang JJ, Mak OT. Induction of apoptosis by 15d-PGJ2 via ROS formation: an alternative pathway without PPARgamma activation in non-small cell lung carcinoma A549 cells. *Prostaglandins Other Lipid Mediat.* 2011;94(3-4):104-11. Epub 2011/03/15.
[83] Han S, Sidell N, Fisher PB, *et al.* Ligands of peroxisome proliferator-activated receptor gamma inhibit lung cancer cell growth and induce apoptosis by stimulation of P21 expression. *Chest.* 2004;125(5 Suppl):134S. Epub 2004/05/12.
[84] Leung KC, Li MY, Leung BC, *et al.* Thromboxane synthase suppression induces lung cancer cell apoptosis via inhibiting NF-kappaB. *Exp. Cell Res.* 2010;316(20):3468-77. Epub 2010/07/22.
[85] Leung HW, Yang WH, Lai MY, *et al.* Inhibition of 12-lipoxygenase during baicalein-induced human lung nonsmall carcinoma H460 cell apoptosis. *Food Chem. Toxicol.* 2007;45(3):403-11. Epub 2006/10/20.

[86] Folkman J. Angiogenesis in cancer, vascular, rheumatoid and other disease. *Nat. Med.* 1995;1(1):27-31.

[87] Carmeliet P, Jain RK. Angiogenesis in cancer and other diseases. *Nature.* 2000;407(6801):249-57. Epub 2000/09/23.

[88] Hanahan D, Folkman J. Patterns and emerging mechanisms of the angiogenic switch during tumorigenesis. *Cell.* 1996;86(3):353-64. Epub 1996/08/09.

[89] Herbst RS, Onn A, Sandler A. Angiogenesis and lung cancer: prognostic and therapeutic implications. *J. Clin. Oncol.* 2005;23(14):3243-56. Epub 2005/05/12.

[90] Weidner N, Semple JP, Welch WR, *et al.* Tumor angiogenesis and metastasis--correlation in invasive breast carcinoma. *N. Engl. J. Med.* 1991;324(1):1-8. Epub 1991/01/03.

[91] Harats D, Ben-Shushan D, Cohen H, *et al.* Inhibition of carcinogenesis in transgenic mouse models over-expressing 15-lipoxygenase in the vascular wall under the control of murine preproendothelin-1 promoter. *Cancer Lett.* 2005;229(1):127-34. Epub 2005/09/15.

[92] Su JL, Shih JY, Yen ML, *et al.* Cyclooxygenase-2 induces EP1- and HER-2/Neu-dependent vascular endothelial growth factor-C up-regulation: a novel mechanism of lymphangiogenesis in lung adenocarcinoma. *Cancer Res.* 2004;64(2):554-64. Epub 2004/01/28.

[93] Pold M, Zhu LX, Sharma S, *et al.* Cyclooxygenase-2-dependent expression of angiogenic CXC chemokines ENA-78/CXC Ligand (CXCL) 5 and interleukin-8/CXCL8 in human non-small cell lung cancer. *Cancer Res.* 2004;64(5):1853-60. Epub 2004/03/05.

[94] Murata T, Aritake K, Matsumoto S, *et al.* Prostagladin D2 is a mast cell-derived antiangiogenic factor in lung carcinoma. *Proc. Natl. Acad. Sci. USA.* 2011;108(49):19802-7. Epub 2011/11/23.

[95] Nie D, Lamberti M, Zacharek A, *et al.* Thromboxane A(2) regulation of endothelial cell migration, angiogenesis, and tumor metastasis. *Biochem. Biophys. Res. Commun.* 2000;267(1):245-51.

[96] Rhee JS, Black M, Schubert U, *et al.* The functional role of blood platelet components in angiogenesis. *Thromb Haemost.* 2004;92(2):394-402. Epub 2004/07/23.

[97] Arisato T, Hashiguchi T, Sarker KP, *et al.* Highly accumulated platelet vascular endothelial growth factor in coagulant thrombotic region. *J. Thromb. Haemost.* 2003;1(12):2589-93. Epub 2003/12/17.

[98] Cathcart MC, O'Byrne KJ, Reynolds JV, *et al.* COX-derived prostanoid pathways in gastrointestinal cancer development and progression: novel targets for prevention and intervention. *Biochim. Biophys. Acta.* 2012;1825(1):49-63. Epub 2011/10/22.

[99] Giese A, Loo MA, Rief MD, *et al.* Substrates for astrocytoma invasion. *Neurosurgery.* 1995;37(2):294-301; discussion -2. Epub 1995/08/01.

[100] Fidler IJ, Ellis LM. The implications of angiogenesis for the biology and therapy of cancer metastasis. *Cell.* 1994;79(2):185-8. Epub 1994/10/21.

[101] Dohadwala M, Batra RK, Luo J, *et al.* Autocrine/paracrine prostaglandin E2 production by non-small cell lung cancer cells regulates matrix metalloproteinase-2 and CD44 in cyclooxygenase-2-dependent invasion. *J. Biol. Chem.* 2002;277(52):50828-33. Epub 2002/10/24.

[102] Yang L, Huang Y, Porta R, *et al.* Host and direct antitumor effects and profound reduction in tumor metastasis with selective EP4 receptor antagonism. *Cancer Res.* 2006;66(19):9665-72. Epub 2006/10/05.
[103] Kim JI, Lakshmikanthan V, Frilot N, *et al.* Prostaglandin E2 promotes lung cancer cell migration via EP4-betaArrestin1-c-Src signalsome. Mol *Cancer Res.* 2010;8(4):569-77. Epub 2010/04/01.
[104] Alaa M, Suzuki M, Yoshino M, *et al.* Prostaglandin E2 receptor 2 overexpression in squamous cell carcinoma of the lung correlates with p16INK4A methylation and an unfavorable prognosis. *Int. J. Oncol.* 2009;34(3):805-12. Epub 2009/02/13.
[105] Cuneo KC, Fu A, Osusky KL, *et al.* Effects of vascular endothelial growth factor receptor inhibitor SU5416 and prostacyclin on murine lung metastasis. *Anticancer Drugs.* 2007;18(3):349-55. Epub 2007/02/01.
[106] Schirner M, Schneider MR. Inhibition of metastasis by cicaprost in rats with established SMT2A mammary carcinoma growth. *Cancer Detect Prev.* 1997;21(1):44-50. Epub 1997/01/01.
[107] Yoshimoto A, Kasahara K, Kawashima A, *et al.* Characterization of the prostaglandin biosynthetic pathway in non-small cell lung cancer: a comparison with small cell lung cancer and correlation with angiogenesis, angiogenic factors and metastases. *Oncol. Rep.* 2005;13(6):1049-57. Epub 2005/05/05.
[108] Stamford IF, Melhuish PB, Carroll MA, *et al.* Survival of mice with NC carcinoma is unchanged by drugs that are thought to inhibit thromboxane synthesis or increase prostacyclin formation. *Br. J. Cancer.* 1986;54(2):257-63. Epub 1986/08/01.
[109] Honn KV. Inhibition of tumor cell metastasis by modulation of the vascular prostacyclin/thromboxane A2 system. *Clin. Exp. Metastasis.* 1983;1(2):103-14. Epub 1983/04/01.
[110] Li X, Tai HH. Increased expression of matrix metalloproteinases mediates thromboxane A2-induced invasion in lung cancer cells. *Curr. Cancer Drug Targets.* 2012;12(6):703-15. Epub 2012/04/21.
[111] Cathcart MC, Lysaght J, Pidgeon GP. Eicosanoid signalling pathways in the development and progression of colorectal cancer: novel approaches for prevention/intervention. *Cancer Metastasis Rev.* 2011;30(3-4):363-85. Epub 2011/12/03.
[112] Shishodia S, Koul D, Aggarwal BB. Cyclooxygenase (COX)-2 inhibitor celecoxib abrogates TNF-induced NF-kappa B activation through inhibition of activation of I kappa B alpha kinase and Akt in human non-small cell lung carcinoma: correlation with suppression of COX-2 synthesis. *J. Immunol.* 2004;173(3):2011-22. Epub 2004/07/22.
[113] Shishodia S, Aggarwal BB. Cyclooxygenase (COX)-2 inhibitor celecoxib abrogates activation of cigarette smoke-induced nuclear factor (NF)-kappaB by suppressing activation of IkappaBalpha kinase in human non-small cell lung carcinoma: correlation with suppression of cyclin D1, COX-2, and matrix metalloproteinase-9. *Cancer Res.* 2004;64(14):5004-12. Epub 2004/07/17.
[114] Shimizu K, Nakata M, Hirami Y, *et al.* Tumor-infiltrating Foxp3+ regulatory T cells are correlated with cyclooxygenase-2 expression and are associated with recurrence in resected non-small cell lung cancer. Journal of thoracic oncology : *official publication of the International Association for the Study of Lung Cancer.* 2010;5(5):585-90. Epub 2010/03/18.

[115] Sharma S, Yang SC, Zhu L, *et al.* Tumor cyclooxygenase-2/prostaglandin E2-dependent promotion of FOXP3 expression and CD4+ CD25+ T regulatory cell activities in lung cancer. *Cancer Res.* 2005;65(12):5211-20. Epub 2005/06/17.

[116] Yakar I, Melamed R, Shakhar G, *et al.* Prostaglandin e(2) suppresses NK activity in vivo and promotes postoperative tumor metastasis in rats. *Ann. Surg. Oncol.* 2003;10(4):469-79. Epub 2003/05/08.

[117] Rothwell PM, Fowkes FG, Belch JF, *et al.* Effect of daily aspirin on long-term risk of death due to cancer: analysis of individual patient data from randomised trials. *Lancet.* 2011;377(9759):31-41. Epub 2010/12/15.

[118] Keith RL, Blatchford PJ, Kittelson J, *et al.* Oral iloprost improves endobronchial dysplasia in former smokers. *Cancer Prev. Res.* (Phila). 2011;4(6):793-802. Epub 2011/06/04.

[119] Kim ES, Hong WK, Lee JJ, *et al.* Biological activity of celecoxib in the bronchial epithelium of current and former smokers. *Cancer Prev. Res.* (Phila). 2010;3(2):148-59. Epub 2010/01/28.

[120] Mao JT, Roth MD, Fishbein MC, *et al.* Lung cancer chemoprevention with celecoxib in former smokers. *Cancer Prev. Res.* (Phila). 2011;4(7):984-93. Epub 2011/07/08.

[121] Achiwa H, Yatabe Y, Hida T, *et al.* Prognostic significance of elevated cyclooxygenase 2 expression in primary, resected lung adenocarcinomas. *Clin. Cancer Res.* 1999;5(5):1001-5.

[122] Khuri FR, Wu H, Lee JJ, *et al.* Cyclooxygenase-2 overexpression is a marker of poor prognosis in stage I non-small cell lung cancer. *Clin. Cancer Res.* 2001;7(4):861-7.

[123] Brabender J, Park J, Metzger R, *et al.* Prognostic significance of cyclooxygenase 2 mRNA expression in non-small cell lung cancer. *Ann. Surg.* 2002;235(3):440-3.

[124] Hida T, Kozaki K, Muramatsu H, *et al.* Cyclooxygenase-2 inhibitor induces apoptosis and enhances cytotoxicity of various anticancer agents in non-small cell lung cancer cell lines. *Clin. Cancer Res.* 2000;6(5):2006-11. Epub 2000/05/18.

[125] Topol EJ. Failing the public health--rofecoxib, Merck, and the FDA. *N. Engl. J. Med.* 2004;351(17):1707-9.

[126] Kisley LR, Barrett BS, Dwyer-Nield LD, *et al.* Celecoxib reduces pulmonary inflammation but not lung tumorigenesis in mice. *Carcinogenesis.* 2002;23(10):1653-60. Epub 2002/10/12.

[127] Honn KV, Cicone B, Skoff A. Prostacyclin: a potent antimetastatic agent. *Science.* 1981;212(4500):1270-2. Epub 1981/06/12.

[128] Blaine SA, Meyer AM, Hurteau G, *et al.* Targeted over-expression of mPGES-1 and elevated PGE2 production is not sufficient for lung tumorigenesis in mice. *Carcinogenesis.* 2005;26(1):209-17. Epub 2004/10/09.

[129] Pai R, Soreghan B, Szabo IL, *et al.* Prostaglandin E2 transactivates EGF receptor: a novel mechanism for promoting colon cancer growth and gastrointestinal hypertrophy. *Nat. Med.* 2002;8(3):289-93.

[130] Gomberg-Maitland M, Olschewski H. Prostacyclin therapies for the treatment of pulmonary arterial hypertension. *Eur. Respir. J.* 2008;31(4):891-901. Epub 2008/04/02.

[131] Keith RL. Oral iloprost for the chemoprevention of lung cancer. 13th *World Conference on Lung Cancer* 2009;Abstracts.

[132] Bren-Mattison Y, Van Putten V, Chan D, *et al.* Peroxisome proliferator-activated receptor-gamma (PPAR(gamma)) inhibits tumorigenesis by reversing the

undifferentiated phenotype of metastatic non-small-cell lung cancer cells (NSCLC). *Oncogene.* 2005;24(8):1412-22. Epub 2004/12/21.
[133] Keith RL, Geraci MW, Nana-Sinkam SP, *et al.* Prostaglandin E2 receptor subtype 2 (EP2) null mice are protected against murine lung tumorigenesis. *Anticancer Res.* 2006;26(4B):2857-61. Epub 2006/08/05.
[134] Koeberle A, Northoff H, Werz O. Curcumin blocks prostaglandin E2 biosynthesis through direct inhibition of the microsomal prostaglandin E2 synthase-1. *Mol. Cancer Ther.* 2009;8(8):2348-55. Epub 2009/08/13.
[135] Hong J, Bose M, Ju J, *et al.* Modulation of arachidonic acid metabolism by curcumin and related beta-diketone derivatives: effects on cytosolic phospholipase A(2), cyclooxygenases and 5-lipoxygenase. *Carcinogenesis.* 2004;25(9):1671-9. Epub 2004/04/10.
[136] Carroll RE, Benya RV, Turgeon DK, *et al.* Phase IIa clinical trial of curcumin for the prevention of colorectal neoplasia. *Cancer Prev. Res.* (Phila). 2011;4(3):354-64. Epub 2011/03/05.
[137] Chanvorachote P, Pongrakhananon V, Wannachaiyasit S, *et al.* Curcumin sensitizes lung cancer cells to cisplatin-induced apoptosis through superoxide anion-mediated Bcl-2 degradation. *Cancer Invest.* 2009;27(6):624-35. Epub 2009/03/14.
[138] Lee J, Im YH, Jung HH, *et al.* Curcumin inhibits interferon-alpha induced NF-kappaB and COX-2 in human A549 non-small cell lung cancer cells. *Biochem. Biophys. Res. Commun.* 2005;334(2):313-8. Epub 2005/07/12.
[139] Wu SH, Hang LW, Yang JS, *et al.* Curcumin induces apoptosis in human non-small cell lung cancer NCI-H460 cells through ER stress and caspase cascade- and mitochondria-dependent pathways. *Anticancer Res.* 2010;30(6):2125-33. Epub 2010/07/24.
[140] Hazai E, Bikadi Z, Zsila F, *et al.* Molecular modeling of the non-covalent binding of the dietary tomato carotenoids lycopene and lycophyll, and selected oxidative metabolites with 5-lipoxygenase. *Bioorg. Med. Chem.* 2006;14(20):6859-67. Epub 2006/07/14.
[141] Bednar W, Holzmann K, Marian B. Assessing 12(S)-lipoxygenase inhibitory activity using colorectal cancer cells overexpressing the enzyme. *Food Chem. Toxicol.* 2007;45(3):508-14. Epub 2006/10/10.
[142] Kuntz S, Wenzel U, Daniel H. Comparative analysis of the effects of flavonoids on proliferation, cytotoxicity, and apoptosis in human colon cancer cell lines. *Eur. J. Nutr.* 1999;38(3):133-42. Epub 1999/08/12.
[143] Pidgeon GP, Kandouz M, Meram A, *et al.* Mechanisms controlling cell cycle arrest and induction of apoptosis after 12-lipoxygenase inhibition in prostate cancer cells. *Cancer Res.* 2002;62(9):2721-7. Epub 2002/05/01.
[144] Tong WG, Ding XZ, Adrian TE. The mechanisms of lipoxygenase inhibitor-induced apoptosis in human breast cancer cells. *Biochem. Biophys. Res. Commun.* 2002;296(4):942-8. Epub 2002/08/30.
[145] Chandrashekar N, Selvamani A, Subramanian R, *et al.* Baicalein inhibits pulmonary carcinogenesis-associated inflammation and interferes with COX-2, MMP-2 and MMP-9 expressions in-vivo. *Toxicol. Appl. Pharmacol.* 2012;261(1):10-21. Epub 2012/03/01.
[146] Aggarwal BB, Bhardwaj A, Aggarwal RS, *et al.* Role of resveratrol in prevention and therapy of cancer: preclinical and clinical studies. *Anticancer Res.* 2004;24(5A):2783-840. Epub 2004/11/03.

[147] Kubota T, Uemura Y, Kobayashi M, *et al.* Combined effects of resveratrol and paclitaxel on lung cancer cells. *Anticancer Res.* 2003;23(5A):4039-46. Epub 2003/12/12.
[148] Liao HF, Kuo CD, Yang YC, *et al.* Resveratrol enhances radiosensitivity of human non-small cell lung cancer NCI-H838 cells accompanied by inhibition of nuclear factor-kappa B activation. *Journal of radiation research.* 2005;46(4):387-93. Epub 2006/01/06.
[149] Liu PL, Tsai JR, Charles AL, *et al.* Resveratrol inhibits human lung adenocarcinoma cell metastasis by suppressing heme oxygenase 1-mediated nuclear factor-kappaB pathway and subsequently downregulating expression of matrix metalloproteinases. *Molecular nutrition and food research.* 2010;54 Suppl 2:S196-204. Epub 2010/05/13.
[150] Mao JT, Nie WX, Tsu IH, *et al.* White tea extract induces apoptosis in non-small cell lung cancer cells: the role of peroxisome proliferator-activated receptor-{gamma} and 15-lipoxygenases. *Cancer Prev. Res.* (Phila). 2010;3(9):1132-40. Epub 2010/07/30.
[151] Altorki NK, Keresztes RS, Port JL, *et al.* Celecoxib, a selective cyclo-oxygenase-2 inhibitor, enhances the response to preoperative paclitaxel and carboplatin in early-stage non-small-cell lung cancer. *J. Clin. Oncol.* 2003;21(14):2645-50. Epub 2003/07/16.
[152] Koch A, Bergman B, Holmberg E, *et al.* Effect of celecoxib on survival in patients with advanced non-small cell lung cancer: a double blind randomised clinical phase III trial (CYCLUS study) by the Swedish Lung Cancer Study Group. *Eur. J. Cancer.* 2011;47(10):1546-55. Epub 2011/05/14.
[153] Groen HJ, Sietsma H, Vincent A, *et al.* Randomized, placebo-controlled phase III study of docetaxel plus carboplatin with celecoxib and cyclooxygenase-2 expression as a biomarker for patients with advanced non-small-cell lung cancer: the NVALT-4 study. *J. Clin. Oncol.* 2011;29(32):4320-6. Epub 2011/10/13.
[154] Fabi A, Metro G, Papaldo P, *et al.* Impact of celecoxib on capecitabine tolerability and activity in pretreated metastatic breast cancer: results of a phase II study with biomarker evaluation. *Cancer Chemother Pharmacol.* 2008;62(4):717-25. Epub 2007/12/12.
[155] Fidler MJ, Argiris A, Patel JD, *et al.* The potential predictive value of cyclooxygenase-2 expression and increased risk of gastrointestinal hemorrhage in advanced non-small cell lung cancer patients treated with erlotinib and celecoxib. *Clin. Cancer Res.* 2008;14(7):2088-94. Epub 2008/04/03.
[156] Rini BI, Weinberg V, Dunlap S, *et al.* Maximal COX-2 immunostaining and clinical response to celecoxib and interferon alpha therapy in metastatic renal cell carcinoma. *Cancer.* 2006;106(3):566-75. Epub 2005/12/22.
[157] Edelman MJ, Hodgson L, Wang X, *et al.* Cyclooxygenase-2 (COX-2) As a Predictive Marker for the Use of COX-2 Inhibitors in Advanced Non-Small-Cell Lung Cancer. *J. Clin. Oncol.* 2012;30(16):2019-20. Epub 2012/04/05.
[158] Edelman MJ, Watson D, Wang X, *et al.* Eicosanoid modulation in advanced lung cancer: cyclooxygenase-2 expression is a positive predictive factor for celecoxib + chemotherapy--Cancer and Leukemia Group B Trial 30203. *J. Clin. Oncol.* 2008;26(6):848-55. Epub 2008/02/19.
[159] Schroeder CP, Yang P, Newman RA, *et al.* Simultaneous inhibition of COX-2 and 5-LOX activities augments growth arrest and death of premalignant and malignant human lung cell lines. *J. Exp. Ther. Oncol.* 2007;6(3):183-92. Epub 2007/06/08.

[160] Sharma S, Lee J, Zhou J, *et al.* Chemopreventive efficacy and mechanism of licofelone in a mouse lung tumor model via aspiration. *Cancer Prev. Res.* (Phila). 2011;4(8):1233-42. Epub 2011/05/13.
[161] Keith RL, Karoor V, Mozer AB, *et al.* Chemoprevention of murine lung cancer by gefitinib in combination with prostacyclin synthase overexpression. *Lung Cancer.* 2010;70(1):37-42. Epub 2010/02/02.

# Index

## D



## E



## F

## G



## H



## I



## J



## K



## L



## M

## N



## O



## P

## R



## S



## T



## U



## V



## X



## Z